Essentials of
Community-based Rehabilitation

Essentials of Community-based Rehabilitation

Satya Bhushan Nagar
Coordinator
DCBR Program, Department of Physiotherapy
Head
Department of Community-based rehabilitation
Ex-Coordinator
Department of Physiotherapy
Coordinator, Community Activities of Medical Field
Janardan Rai Nagar Rajasthan Vidyapeeth Deemed University
Udaipur, Rajasthan, India
Member, Rajasthan Paramedical Council
Government of Rajasthan, India

Forewords
Umasankar Mohanty
Indumathi Rao

JAYPEE

JAYPEE BROTHERS MEDICAL PUBLISHERS
The Health Sciences Publisher
New Delhi | London

Jaypee Brothers Medical Publishers (P) Ltd

Headquarters

EMCA House
23/23-B, Ansari Road, Daryaganj
New Delhi 110 002, India
Landline: +91-11-23272143,
+91-11-23272703
+91-11-23282021, +91-11-23245672
E-mail: jaypee@jaypeebrothers.com

Corporate Office

Jaypee Brothers Medical Publishers (P) Ltd.
4838/24, Ansari Road, Daryaganj
New Delhi 110 002, India
Phone: +91-11-43574357
Fax: +91-11-43574314
E-mail: jaypee@jaypeebrothers.com

Overseas Off ces

J.P. Medical Ltd
83, Victoria Street, London
SW1H 0HW (UK)
Phone: +44-20 3170 8910
Email: info@jpmedpub.com

EU GPSR Authorised Representative
Logos Europe, 9 rue Nicolas Poussin
17000, La Rochelle, France
Phone: +33 (0) 6 67 93 73 78
E-mail: Contact@logoseurope.eu

Website: www.jaypeebrothers.com Website:
www.jaypeedigital.com

Essentials of Community-based Rehabilitation

First Edition: 2017, Reprint: **2025**

ISBN 978-93-86261-22-9

Printed in India

Dedicated to
My Grand Parents

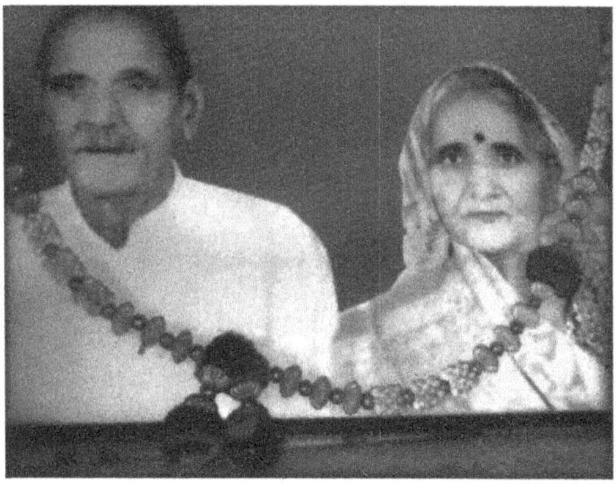

Late Pandit Sh Damodar Prasad Nagar
and
Late Smt Sona Devi Nagar

Foreword

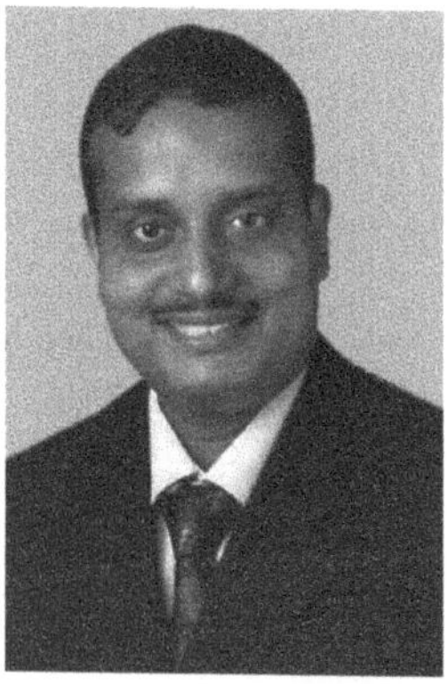

I have immense pleasure in forewording this book titled *Essentials of Community-based Rehabilitation* brought out by my close professional associate Dr Satya Bhushan Nagar, a renowned physiotherapy academician and rehabilitation professional.

Community-based rehabilitation (CBR) was initiated by WHO following the Declaration of Alma-Ata in 1978 in an effort to enhance the quality of life for people with disabilities and their families, meet their basic needs, and ensure their inclusion and participation. While initially a strategy to increase access to rehabilitation services in resource-constrained settings, CBR is now a multisectoral approach working for the equalization of opportunities and social inclusion of people with disabilities while combating the perpetual cycle of poverty and disability. CBR is implemented through the combined efforts of people with disabilities, their families and communities, and relevant government and non-government health, education, vocational, social and other services. CBR is changing, and it has to change. Even today, CBR focuses on taking rehabilitation services to the population in many parts of the world where it has not yet reached!

Dr Nagar has given an overview to concepts, principles, components, and other aspect of CBR. This book also includes disability evaluation or assessment criteria, professional ethics regarding physiotherapy, ergonomics at workplace. This book aims at the students of physiotherapy, occupational therapy, and rehabilitation studying in various colleges or universities all over the country. Since it conforms to the syllabus of undergraduate physiotherapy and rehabilitation program laid down by several universities, I am sure that this book would definitely benefit physiotherapy students and rehabilitation professionals. In my opinion, essential of CBR lives up to the promise of its title. I am delighted that the author has found the time and dedication needed to write this semper excelsius masterly book which will enable him to share his experience as an author and teacher to wider audience.

I am sure the content of the book will cater to the needs of students and physiotherapy professionals in community-based rehabilitation. I congratulate Dr Nagar for his intense effort to provide a textbook of CBR with essential contents and I wish him great success.

Umasankar Mohanty
BPT (Hons), MPT (Manual Therapy) PhD MISEP MIAP FAGE
PhD Guide, Department of Physiotherapy
Lovely Professional University
President
Manual Therapy Foundation of India
President
The Indian Association of Physiotherapists
Member
International Society of Educators in Physiotherapy

Foreword

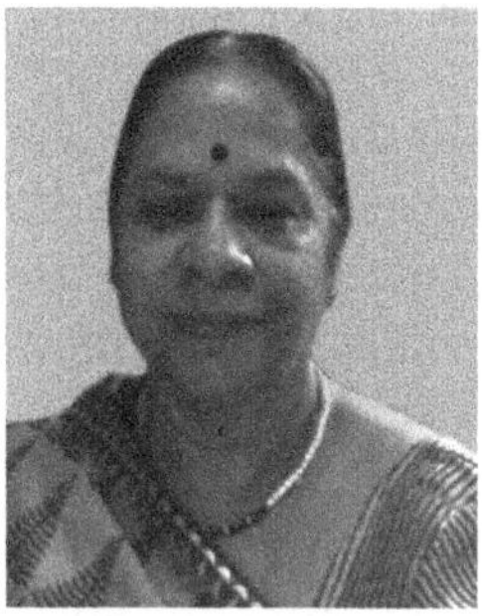

The Constitution of India has included disability and aging in its state list. Disability is also a Panchayat Raj subject as per PRI Act. Further, India has signed and ratified UN convention on persons with disabilities in 2006. Indian Parliament passed a legislation titled Equal Opportunities Act in 1995 in the winter session of Parliament.

The goal of a national or state level policy is to promote an inclusive, community-based, barrier-free opportunities for fullest actualization of potential in every individual with a rights-based vision for persons with disabilities with a clearly defined goals/objectives and strategies relevant to diverse socioeconomic-geographic diversities in India.

Persons with disabilities have potential and right to the enjoyment of the full range of civil and political, educational, health and socio-economic and cultural rights embodied in the Indian constitution.

India straddles two worlds simultaneously: It is both a developed and developing nation. It is the fourth largest economy in terms of purchasing-power parity, in the top ten most industrialized countries, and a global leader in information technology. It is the world's largest democracy and a rising power.

The Constitution of India ensures equality, freedom, justice and dignity of all individuals and mandates an inclusive society, including persons with disabilities. India is a signatory to the declaration on the full participation and equality of people with disabilities in the Asia Pacific Region and Biwako Millennium Framework for Action towards an inclusive, barrier-free and rights-based society. Further, the Eleventh Five Year Plan of India (GOI, 2008) and now Twelfth Plan (2012–2017) have marked "Inclusive Growth" as its focus and have earmarked substantial financial provisions to make this inclusion a reality. Strategy also puts us all on similar grounds.

India has signed and ratified the UN Convention for Persons with Disabilities in 2006. In India, the Persons with Disabilities (Equal Opportunities, Protection of Rights and Full Participation) Act 1995 defines disability as one or more of the following: blindness, low vision, leprosy cured, hearing impairment, locomotor disability, mental retardation and mental illness. A new draft comprehensive bill on disability, which is based on UN convention on the right of persons with disabilities (UNCRPD) principles, is waiting for the Parliament approval in India.

There is no universally agreed definition of disability. Historically, disability is understood to be a medical condition—a problem located within the individual. Since then, disability activists who have conceptualized disability as primarily a social phenomenon have challenged this medical or individual model. This social model draws a clear distinction between "impairments" and "disability". It argues that it is the society that disables people with impairments, by failing to recognize and accommodate difference, and through the attitudinal, environmental and institutional barriers that it erects against people with impairments. Disability thus arises from a complex interaction between social, economic and health conditions.

Social inclusion is a multidimensional and cross-sectional concept, which needs to be, mainstreamed into various areas at national, regional and local levels. It does not lie, not only within one tier or section of society, nor does it rely on only one area of policy to exact changes. There is a larger and infinitely more comprehensive aim to social inclusion that encompasses many areas of society and humanity.

Understanding how the dimensions of inclusion are structured and realizing its diverse nature in diverse cultures and socioeconomic threshold is necessary for this. As inequality and exclusion are produced systematically, and they can be tackled. It is necessary to distinguish inequality from being different. While we can be different, we all need to be provided with equal opportunities and access. Accommodating people with diverse needs to build a common future is a core value of an inclusive society. Developing a concept of inclusion in which people get together are interconnected, and sharing a sense of belongingness as well as sense of responsibility is necessary.

If this concept of social inclusion is promoted, cycles of exclusion and traditional blockades, structural and perceived, will begin to dismantle. This would constitute an important step towards an inclusive society. Equally, while the actual fiscal responsibilities involved in creating inclusive societies may initially present a challenge, the viewpoint should be promoted that the investment in motivating participation in all sectors of society is an investment in a successful and sustainable future and a more balanced society, meeting the needs of all its members, where investment in inclusion and the resulting change in society are actually beneficial to all.

A majority of persons with disabilities live in rural areas

The country's disabled population has increased by 22.4% between 2001 and 2011. The number of disabled, which was 2.19 crore in 2001, rose in 2011 to 2.68 crore—1.5 crore males and 1.18 crore females. Rural areas have more disabled people than urban areas. In Maharashtra, Andhra Pradesh, Odisha, Jammu and Kashmir and Sikkim, the disabled account for 2.5% of the total population, while Tamil Nadu and Assam are among those where the disabled population is less than 1.75% of the total population.

According to World Bank Report 2009 titled "From Commitment to Outcomes" which states that while official estimates of disability are low (around 2%), alternative estimates using better methods and more inclusive definitions suggest a higher incidence of disability (of at least 5-8%). Many systematic studies of NGOs in Karnataka shows the prevalence of disability in 0-14 age group children is around 4-6%.

Poverty and disability link

Persons with disabilities are most disadvantaged group of people in a community. Though they have immense talent like any other person unless there is a positive attitude to include them in the mainstream development they would remain poor, illiterate, unemployed and dependent in their life. But if we include them in the development program with a positive attitude they can contribute to the community-nation building.

A society for all

Disability centered/friendly policy initiatives taken by NDA government to enable persons with disabilities in India in 2014-2016. CBR helps include persons effectively in the national development program.

1. Accessible India Campaign—2015
2. HRD Ministry's National Education Policy—2014
3. National Health Policy—2016
4. National Bill on Allied and Health Professionals—2015
5. National Youth Policy which includes Sports—2015
6. National Skill Development Framework—2014

7. Disability Rights Drafts Bill pending the approval of the parliament.
8. Rural Development and Panchayat Raj (RDPR) on mandatory inclusion of person with disability in all the development program.

CBR is a proven strategy to achieve the goals of inclusion of All—leaving none behind.

"Sabka Saath Sab Ka Vikas" is the vision of India. Hon'ble Prime Minister of India, Sri Narendra Bhai Modi Ji urges to use the word "Divyang". The community has a major role to play in the rehabilitation process. In order to get the Vision to Action, we need CBR and trained human resources for CBR, resource manuals on CBR.

One of the major barriers to rehabilitation is the attitude of the community. The participation of the community will ensure that all attitudinal and social barriers to the rehabilitation process are minimized.

The role and inherent potential of the family to overcome problems of disability must be recognized as a basic building block of the rehabilitation process.

The ultimate goal in rehabilitation is empowerment of persons with disabilities. Empowerment comes from enjoying the equity in the community. Empowerment of a person with disabilities has several dimensions. Equal opportunities and active participation in the family, community and development program continues to be a major focus for the community based-rehabilitation program. Economic independence is one of the key factors that lead a person to achieve the goal of empowerment.

The conventional approaches in rehabilitation, such as special schools, social and vocational rehabilitation centers, special employment schemes, residential schools, hostels, etc. are expensive models. It would be impossible to find the financial and human resources required to reach all disabled people in India through this approach.

There are several accepted political goals, such as the universalization of elementary education, mass literacy programs, poverty eradication programs, health for needy people and other developmental programs. These are aimed at improving the quality of life of underprivileged groups, such as people with disabilities. Yet, it is a common experience that disabled people seldom participate in such mainstream programs. Hence, it is important to develop a plan for people with disabilities aiming at a large coverage with good quality services in a sustainable manner, by optimal utilization of resources available at the state level. For these reasons, it is imperative to adopt an efficient and cost-effective approach such as community-based rehabilitation (CBR).

CBR strategy is an effort to design a system for change—for improving service delivery in order to reach all in need, for providing more equal opportunities and for promoting and protecting the human rights of disabled people".

Inclusion is accepted globally and locally as the underlying principle on which rehabilitation programs should be built on. However, there is a need for some exclusive measure to achieve the goal of inclusion. The exclusive measures are required because people with disability not only belong to poorer of the poorest sections in the society, but they are also fighting the social images about them. Self-image elevating activities are necessary in addition to image boosting activities in the community. A sense of belonging is intrinsically vital, as most feel isolated and neglected.

Democratization at grassroots has picked up tremendous momentum in the last decade. Panchayath Raj System is one example of decentralization of policy decision-making and implementation of all development programs.

In India, Mahatma Gandhi emphasized the need for self-reliance and self-sustainable villages as early as the beginning of last century. The concept of Self-help and Gram Swaraj are not foreign concepts to us. The ancient village management system was also based on the principle of "sharing and caring".

Somewhere along the line, after independence, people started playing the role of "recipient of services and benefits" and became beneficiaries. This passive role of the community did not help in the long run.

Neither government nor the community can afford to start separate services for separate sets of people. The District CBR Society is to help meet different needs of the community without disintegrating families from their communities.

There has been an increasing realization that the chances of sustaining programs without the community's participation at all levels of implementation are close to nil. The decentralization of power structures/increased number of grassroots NGO projects has strengthened the learning that community should be involved right from project conceptualization to implementation/evaluation stage. Various project-planning skills, such as rural appraisals/logical framework analysis, etc. have been developed to ensure community participation in planning of projects.

The second resource book on CBR by Dr Nagar fills a major deficit in our society. The book is comprehensive with 28 Chapters, with illustrations which makes reading easy.

I recommend this book *Essentials of Community-based Rehabilitation,* to all professionals working in the field of disability, inclusive development and health sectors.

I hope to see more books from Dr Nagar in future.

Indumathi Rao
Regional Advisor
CBR Network
South Asia, Bengaluru
Karnataka, India

Preface

Community-based Rehabilitation (CBR) brings rehabilitation know-how to villages and urban slums, and CBR personnel facilitate people to take responsibility for their own lives. CBR is a systematized approach within general community development whereby persons with disabilities are enabled to live a fulfilling life within their own community, making maximum use of local resources, and helping the community become aware of its responsibility in ensuring the inclusion and equal participation of PWDs. In the process, PWDs are also made aware of their own role and responsibility, as they are part of the community. People with disabilities are estimated to form 7-10% of the population in any country, and around 2% would need some form of rehabilitation services. Yet, only 0.01-0.02% of the population in developing countries actually get such services. There are presently about 200 million moderately and severely disabled people in developing countries, where disabilities are mostly poverty related. The incidence of disability has always been on the increasing trend and about 60% of disabilities. In order to further promote the development of CBR in coordination with the social and economic development of this region, there is a need to develop a set of comprehensive guidelines for CBR evaluation. Such guidelines should be scientific, practical, easy to use, and should cover various aspects and stages of the practice. CBR is strategy within community development for rehabilitation, equalization of opportunities and social inclusion of all children and adults with disabilities. A disability is an umbrella term, covering impairments, activity limitations, and participation restrictions. An impairment is a problem in body function or structure; an activity limitation is a difficulty encountered by an individual in executing a task or action; while a participation restriction is a problem experienced by an individual in involvement in life situations. Thus, disability is a complex phenomenon, reflecting an interaction between features of a person's body and those of the society in which he/she lives. Where rehabilitation is community-based, then the decision making and responsibility for the habilitation of those disabled individuals are in the community, and do not originate outside the community.

"The community-based rehabilitation strategy is an effort to design a system for change for improving service delivery in order to reach all in need, for providing more equal opportunities and for promoting and protecting the human rights of disabled people" (Helander, 1993, page 5). WHO has developed community-based rehabilitation program designed to integrate with programs for primary health care. Since then CBR as a tool for government and non-government intervention has been expanding very rapidly all over the world. People with disabilities, their families, and their communities have benefited from CBR.

CBR practices in countries with vast differences in race, culture, language, socioeconomic-political development, and religious belief have provided a collection of diversified and rich experiences. This book has been launched to meet a specific need of undergraduate student of physiotherapy and rehabilitation it will give overview of concept, principle, criteria, components and aspects of community-based rehabilitation.

CBR evaluation and its practical significance. It will help Rehabilitation professional to assess disability and to implement CBR program. The first edition of the book will bring about to design a system for change for improving service delivery in order to reach all in need, for providing more equal opportunities and for promoting and protecting the human rights of disabled persons.

I am extremely thankful to supreme power, who by his immeasurable infinite grace enabled me to write this book, No venture of this kind is possible without the blessing of my Parents Smt Daya Devi and Shri Krishna Chandra Nagar. To whom I shall remain ever indebted.

I also wish to express my thanks to my brother Dr Satish Nagar and his wife Smt Sadhna Nagar and their wards Ayush and Aryan, who has helped me in each and every step of preparation of this book. I will be failing in my duty if I do not mention the name of my wife Mrs Sonal and my Dear son Aman and daughter Anushree and my in-laws Smt Girish and Suryakant Nagar for their understanding and unstinted support during the long months of collecting the material and writing of the book. I would like to be grateful to my teachers who made me able to do such kind of work. It is a pleasure to acknowledge the valuable suggestions and kind support received from professor SS Sarangdevot, Hon'ble Vice Chancellor Janardan Rai

Nagar Rajasthan Vidhyapeeth Deemed University, Udaipur, Rajasthan, India, Dr Indumathi Rao, Regional Advisor CBR Network, Professor Umasankar Mohanty President IAP, Professor Sanjeev Jha, Advisor IAP, and Professor Jagmohan Singh, Professor NS Rao, and my colleagues and my dear friends and Students. May this book give an effective stimulus to physiotherapy students and rehabilitation professionals to gain knowledge of CBR and disability.

Satya Bhushan Nagar

Contents

Abbreviations

AA	:	Alcoholics anonymous
ADHD	:	Attention deficit hyperactivity disorder
ADL	:	Activities of daily living
AHRTAG	:	Appropriate health resources and technologies action group
CBR	:	Community-based rehabilitation
CHA	:	Community health aide
CP	:	Cerebral palsy
CW	:	Community worker
DPI	:	Disabled People's International
EEC	:	European Economic Community
GDP	:	Gross domestic product
IAP	:	Indian Association of Physiotherapists
IBR	:	Institution-based rehabilitation
IDA	:	International Development Association
ILEP	:	International Federation of Anti-Leprosy Associations
ILO	:	International labour organization
ILS	:	Intermediate Level Supervisor
IYDP	:	International Year of Disabled People
LS	:	Local supervisor
MR	:	Mental retardation
MRT	:	Mapnet Resource Teacher
NDLRP	:	National district level rehabilitation program
NGO	:	Non-governmental organization
OAS	:	Organization of American States
OAU	:	Organization of African Unity
PHC	:	Primary health care
PHW	:	Public health worker
RDP	:	Declaration on the Rights of Disabled Persons
RI	:	Rehabilitation International
RMR	:	Declaration on the Rights of Mentally Retarded Persons
TCPD	:	Training in the Community for People with Disabilities (a Manual published by WHO, 1989)
TP	:	Training package
UDHR	:	Universal Declaration of Human Rights
UK	:	United Kingdom
UN	:	United Nations
UNCSDHA	:	United Nations Centre for Social Development and Humanitarian Affairs

UNDESD	:	United Nations Department of Economic and Social Development
UNDP	:	United Nations Development Programme
UNESCO	:	United Nations Educational, Scientific and Cultural Organization
UNHCR	:	United Nations High Commissioner for Refugees
UNICEF	:	United Nations Children's Fund
UNOV	:	United Nations Office at Vienna
USA	:	United States of America
US$	:	United States of America, dollars
WCPT	:	World Confederation for Physical Therapy
WHO	:	World Health Organization
WPA	:	World Programme of Action Concerning Disabled Persons

PLATE 1

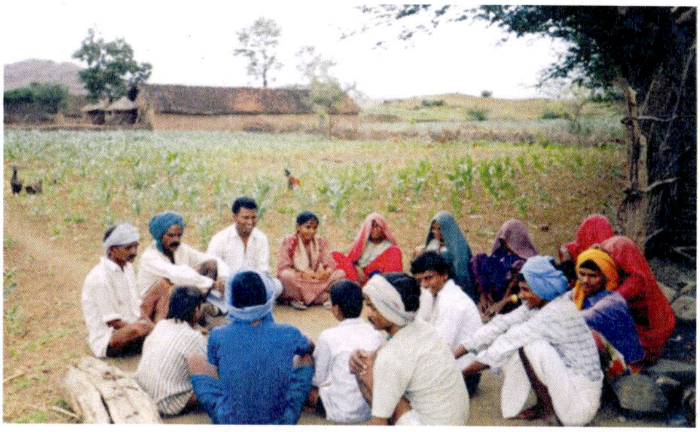

Fig. 2.1: Community meeting

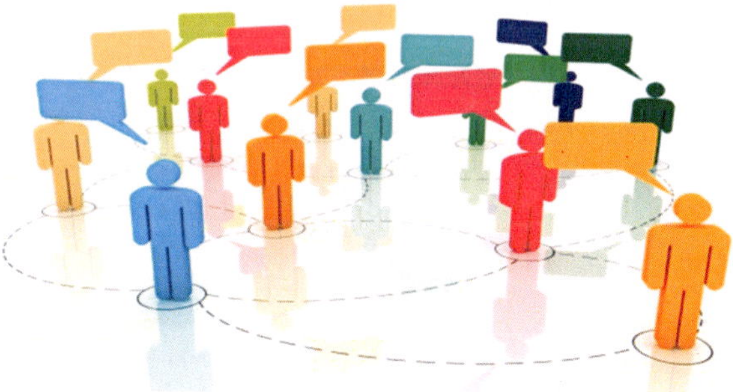

Fig. 5.1: Community network

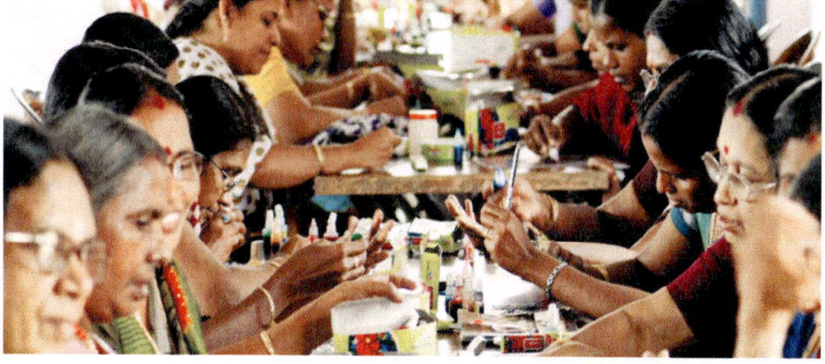

Fig. 6.1: Self-help group of women

PLATE 2

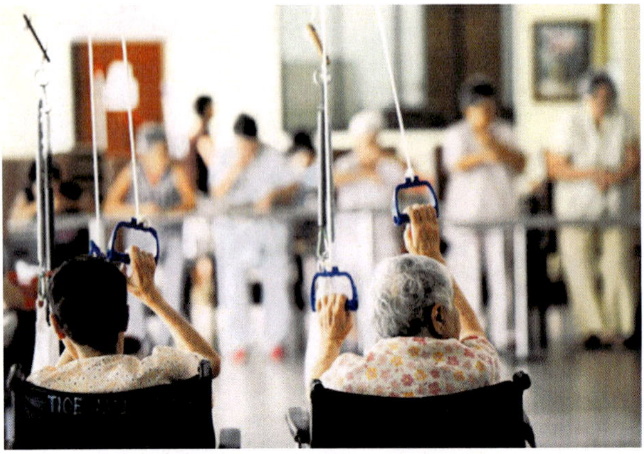

Fig. 11.1: Geriatric rehabilitation

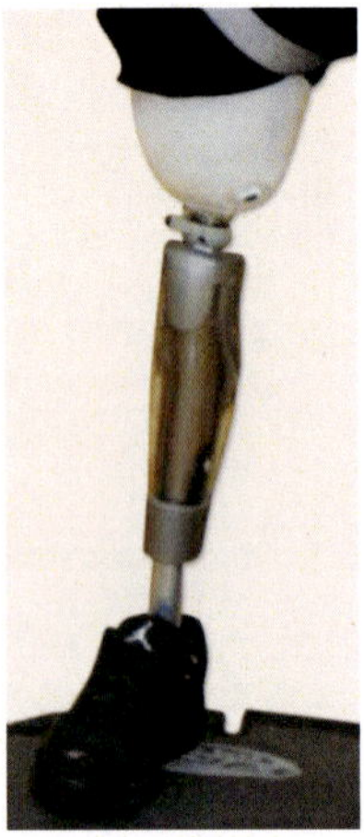

Fig. 22.1: Below knee prosthesis

PLATE 3

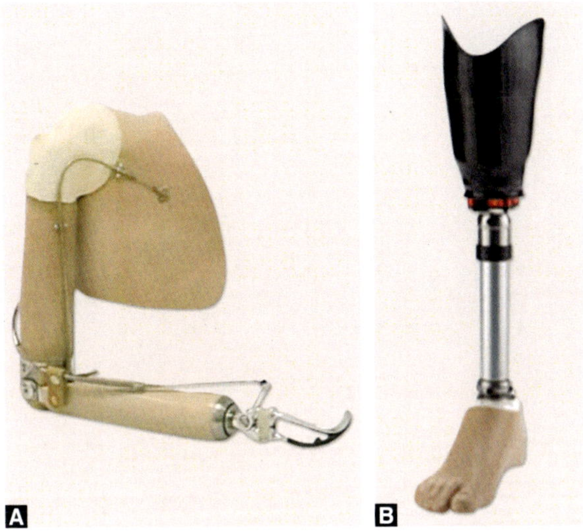

Figs 22.2A and B: Exoskeletal prostheses

CHAPTER

1

Introduction to Rehabilitation Medicine

INTRODUCTION: REHABILITATION MEDICINE AND PHYSIATRY

Medicine evolves to reflect the needs of society. This evolution is commonly viewed to be driven by scientific research advances. However, factors on a macroscopic, population level can be equally influential.

Three such factors in the 20th century led to the creation of a new specialty, physical medicine and rehabilitation. For much of the last century, medicine revolved around the concept of saving lives. The result has been prolonged quantity of life with an increase in the prevalence of chronic disease. During the same decades, armed conflicts not only redefined geographic maps but also enhanced the public's awareness of people with disabilities; in some instances, this group came to represent a new segment of society. In addition, the polio epidemic of the 1950s left many people with friends and family members with disabilities, and the presidency of Franklin Roosevelt in the United States led to an awareness that a disability does not have to be a social handicap. The recognition of the inherent value of people with disabilities and of their needs resulted in the development of the specialty of physical medicine and rehabilitation. At its most basic, this specialty focuses on maximizing a person's independence through medical, psychological or physical treatments or through modifications to their environment.

Common causes of disability requiring complex rehabilitation include cardiovascular diseases, respiratory ailments and arthritis. Less common but potentially devastating conditions such as spinal cord injury, acquired brain injury, amputation and congenital neurologic or musculoskeletal conditions often require lifelong medical follow-up. Each of these conditions presents its own subset of medical complications and rehabilitation needs. Fortunately for the physician, some of the complications and needs overlap between conditions. For example, understanding the principles of spasticity management can help the clinician to treat the child with cerebral palsy, the adult with a spinal cord injury and the elderly patient with a stroke.

It is very difficult to define the physiatry in a single word. While the fields of neurology or orthopedic deal with nerve and brain or bones and joints, like as physiatry focuses on assisting the general improvement of functional recovery in disabled patients. Historically physiatry originated from two different fields, physical medicine and rehabilitation. According to Dorland dictionary, the word" *physio*" which means nature and" *iatrke*" which means operation or medicine. Therefore, the physiatry involves treating and diagnosing diseases using light, heat, cold, and electricity. Between the late 1930s and early 1940s doctor who treated arthritis using ultrasound or microwaves were called physical therapy physicians which is the origin of the term physiatrist.

DEFINITION: REHABILITATION MEDICINE

Physical medicine and rehabilitation (PM and R), also known as physiatry or rehabilitation medicine, is a branch of medicine that aims to enhance and restore functional ability and quality of life to those with physical impairments or disabilities.

Scope of Rehabilitation Medicine

Common conditions that are treated by rehabilitation physicians include

- Amputation
- Spinal cord injury

- Sports injury
- Stroke
- Musculoskeletal pain syndromes such as low back pain
- Fibromyalgia, and
- Traumatic brain injury.

Cardiopulmonary rehabilitation involves optimizing function in those afflicted with heart or lung disease. Chronic pain management is achieved through a multidisciplinary approach involving psychologists, physical therapists, exercise therapists, anesthesiologists, and interventional procedures when indicated.

Stroke, in addition to the previous methodology, is often treated with the help of a speech therapist and recreational therapist when possible. Physical medicine and rehabilitation physicians utilized electrodiagnostic medicine studies to help diagnose patients with symptoms of numbness, cramps or tingling.

Amputation

Amputation is the removal of a limb by trauma, medical illness, or surgery. As a surgical measure, it is used to control pain or a disease process in the affected limb, such as malignancy or gangrene. In some cases, it is carried out on individuals as a preventative surgery for such problems. A special case is that of congenital amputation, a congenital disorder, where fetal limbs have been cut off by constrictive bands. In some countries, amputation of the hands, feet or other body parts is or was used as a form of punishment for people who committed crimes. Amputation has also been used as a tactic in war and acts of terrorism; it may also occur as a war injury. In some cultures and religions, minor amputations or mutilations are considered a ritual accomplishment. Unlike some non-mammalian animals (such as lizards that shed their tails, salamanders that can regrow many missing body parts, and hydras, flatworms and starfish that can regrow entire bodies from small fragments), once removed, human extremities do not grow back, unlike portions of some organs, such as the liver. A transplant or prosthesis is the only options for recovering the loss.

Spinal Cord Injury

A spinal cord injury (SCI) is damage to the spinal cord that causes changes in its function, either temporary or permanent (Fig. 1.1). These changes translate into loss of muscle function, sensation or

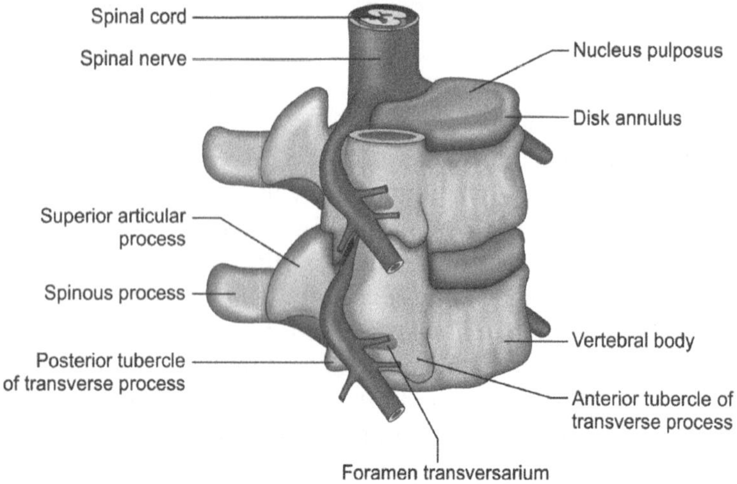

Fig. 1.1: Spinal cord with associated structure

autonomic function in parts of the body served by the spinal cord below the level of the lesion. Injuries can occur at any level of the spinal cord and can be classified as complete injury, a total loss of sensation and muscle function, or incomplete, meaning some nervous signals are able to travel past the injured area of the cord. Depending on the location and severity of damage along the spinal cord, the symptoms can vary widely, from pain or numbness to paralysis to incontinence. The prognosis also ranges widely, from full recovery in rare cases to permanent tetraplegia (also called quadriplegia) in injuries at the level of the neck, and paraplegia in lower injuries. Complications that can occur in the short- and long-term after injury include muscle atrophy, pressure sores, infections, and respiratory problems.

In the majority of cases, the damage results from physical trauma such as car accidents, gunshots, falls, or sports injuries, but it can also result from no traumatic causes such as infection, insufficient blood flow, and tumors. Efforts to prevent SCI include individual measures such as using safety equipment, societal measures such as safety regulations in sports and traffic, and improvements to equipment. Known since ancient times to be a catastrophic injury and long believed to be untreatable, SCI has seen great improvements in its care since the middle of the 20th century. Treatment of spinal cord injuries starts with stabilizing the spine and controlling inflammation to prevent further damage. Other interventions needed can vary widely depending on the location and extent of the injury, from bed rest to surgery. In many cases, spinal cord injuries require substantial, long-term physical and occupational therapy in rehabilitation, especially if they interfere with activities of daily living. Research into new treatments for spinal cord injuries includes stem cell implantation, engineered materials for tissue support, and wearable robotic exoskeletons.

Stroke

Stroke, also known as cerebrovascular accident (CVA), cerebrovascular insult (CVI), or brain attack, is when poor blood flow to the brain results in cell death. There are two main types of stroke: ischemic, due to lack of blood flow, and hemorrhagic, due to bleeding. They result in part of the brain not functioning properly. Signs and symptoms of a stroke may include an inability to move or feel on one side of the body, problems understanding or speaking, feeling like the world is spinning, or loss of vision to one side among others. Signs and symptoms often appear soon after the stroke has occurred. If symptoms last less than one or two hours it is known as a transient ischemic attack (TIA). Hemorrhagic strokes may also be associated with a severe headache. The symptoms of a stroke can be permanent. Long-term complications may include pneumonia or loss of bladder control (Fig. 1.2).

The main risk factor for stroke is high blood pressure. Other risk factors include tobacco smoking, obesity, high blood cholesterol, diabetes mellitus, previous TIA, and atrial fibrillation among others. An ischemic stroke is typically caused by blockage of a blood vessel. A hemorrhagic stroke is caused by bleeding either directly into the brain or into the space surrounding the brain. Bleeding may occur due to a brain aneurysm. Diagnosis is typically with medical imaging such as a CT scan or MRI scan along with a physical exam. Other tests such as an electrocardiogram (ECG) and blood tests are done to determine risk factors and rule out other possible causes. Low blood sugar may cause similar symptoms.

Prevention includes decreasing risk factors as well as possibly aspirin, statins, surgery to open up the arteries to the brain in those with problematic narrowing, and warfarin in those with atrial fibrillation. A stroke often requires emergency care. An ischemic stroke, if detected within three to four and half hours, may be treatable with a medication that can break down the clot. Aspirin should be used. Some hemorrhagic strokes benefit from surgery. Treatment

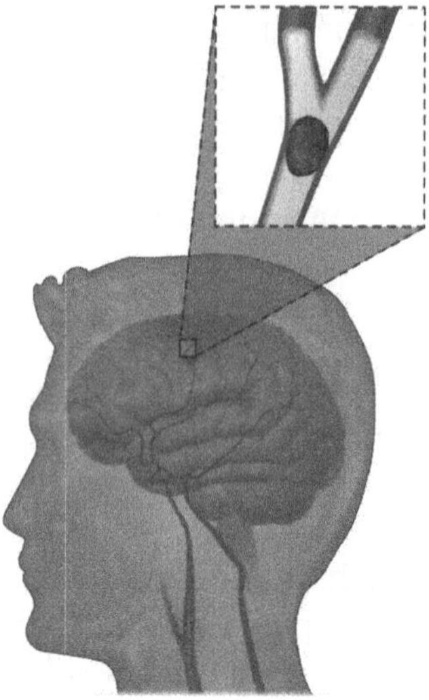

Fig. 1.2: Illustration of an embolic stroke showing a blockage lodged in a blood vessel

to try recover lost function is called stroke rehabilitation and ideally takes place in a stroke unit; however, these are not available in much of the world.

In 2013, approximately 6.9 million people had an ischemic stroke and 3.4 million people had a hemorrhagic stroke. In 2010, there were about 33 million people who had previously had a stroke and were still alive. Between 1990 and 2010 the number of strokes which occurred each year decreased by approximately 10% in the developed world and increased by 10% in the developing world. In 2013, stroke was the second most frequent cause of death after coronary artery disease, accounting for 6.4 million deaths (12% of the total). About 3.3 million deaths resulted from ischemic stroke while 3.2 million deaths resulted from hemorrhagic stroke. About half of people who have had a stroke live less than one year. Overall, two-thirds of strokes occurred in those over 65 years old.

Low Back Pain

Low back pain is a common disorder involving the muscles, nerves, and bones of the back. Pain can vary from a dull constant ache to a sudden sharp feeling. Low back pain may be classified by duration as acute (pain lasting <6 weeks), sub-chronic (6–12 weeks), or chronic (>12 weeks). The condition may be further classified by the underlying cause as mechanical, non-mechanical, or referred pain. The symptoms of low back pain usually improve within a few weeks from the time they start, with 40–90% of people completely better by 6 weeks (Fig. 1.3).

In most episodes of low back pain, a specific underlying cause is not identified or even looked for, with the pain believed to be due to mechanical problems such as muscle or joint strain. If the pain does not go away with conservative treatment or if it is accompanied by "red flags" such as unexplained weight loss, fever, or significant problems with feeling or movement, further testing may be needed to look for a serious underlying problem. In most cases, imaging tools such as X-ray computed tomography are not useful and carry their own risks. Despite this, the use of imaging in low back pain has increased. Some low back pain is caused by damaged intervertebral Disks, and the straight leg raise test is useful to identify this cause. In those with chronic pain, the pain processing system may malfunction, causing large amounts of pain in response to non-serious events.

The treatment of acute nonspecific low back pain of rapid onset is typically with simple pain medication and the continuation of as much normal activity as the pain allows. Medications are recommended for the duration that they are helpful, with paracetamol (also known as acetaminophen) as the preferred first medication. A number of other options are available for those who do not improve with usual treatment. Opioids may be useful if simple pain medications are not enough, but they are not generally recommended due to side effects.

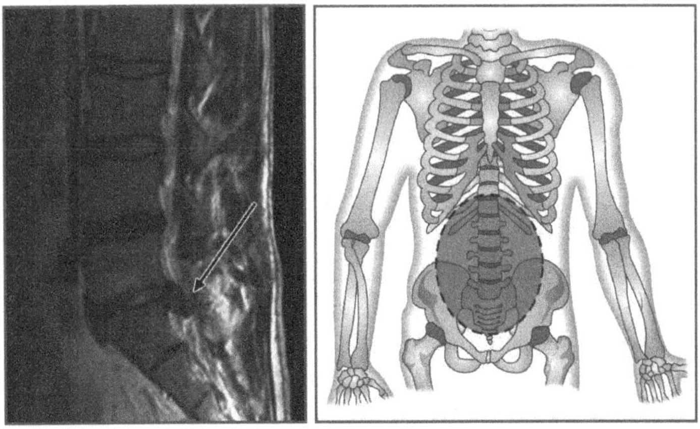

Fig. 1.3: A herniated disk as seen an MRI, one possible cause of low back pain

Surgery may be beneficial for those with Disk-related chronic pain and disability or spinal stenosis. No clear benefit has been found for other cases of non-specific low back pain. Low back pain often affects mood, which may be improved by counseling or antidepressants. Additionally, there are many alternative medicine therapies, including the Alexander technique and herbal remedies, but there is not enough evidence to recommend them confidently. The evidence for chiropractic care and spinal manipulation is mixed. Approximately 9 to 12% of people (632 million) have LBP at any given point in time, and nearly 25% report having it at some point over any one-month period. About 40% of people have LBP at some point in their lives, with estimates as high as 80% among people in the developed world. Difficulty most often begins between 20 and 40 years of age. Men and women are equally affected. Low back pain is more common among people aged 40–80 years, with the overall number of individuals affected expected to increase as the population ages.

FIBROMYALGIA

Fibromyalgia (FM) is a medical condition characterized by chronic widespread pain and a heightened pain response to pressure. Other symptoms include feeling tired to a degree that normal activities are affected, sleep problems, and troubles with memory. Some people also report restless leg syndrome, bowel or bladder problems, numbness and tingling, and sensitivity to noise, lights or temperature. Fibromyalgia is frequently associated with depression, anxiety, and posttraumatic stress disorder other types of chronic pain are also frequently present.

The cause of fibromyalgia is unknown but believed to involve a combination of genetic and environmental factors with half the risk attributed to each. The condition runs in families and many genes are believed to be involved. Environmental factors may include psychological stress, trauma, and certain infections. The pain appears to result from processes in the central nervous system and the condition is referred to as a "central sensitization syndrome". Fibromyalgia is recognized as a disorder by the US National Institutes of Health and the American College of Rheumatology. There is no specific diagnostic test. Diagnosis involves first ruling out other potential causes and verifying that a set number of symptoms are present.

The treatment of fibromyalgia can be difficult. Recommendations often include getting enough sleep, exercising regularly, and eating a healthy diet. Cognitive behavioral therapy may also be helpful. Dietary supplements also lack evidence to support their use. While fibromyalgia can last a long time, it does not result in death or tissue damage.

Fibromyalgia is estimated to affect 2–8% of the population. Females are affected about two times more often than males. Rates appear similar in different areas of the world and among different cultures. Fibromyalgia was first defined in 1990 with updated criteria in 2011. There is controversy about the classification, diagnosis, and treatment of fibromyalgia. While some feel the diagnosis of fibromyalgia may negatively affect a person, other research finds it to be beneficial. The term "fibromyalgia" is from New Latin, *fibro-*, meaning "fibrous tissues", Greek myo-, "muscle", and Greek algos, "pain"; thus the term literally means "muscle and connective tissue pain".

Traumatic Brain Injury

Traumatic brain injury (TBI), also known as intracranial injury, occurs when an external force traumatically injures the brain. TBI can be classified based on severity, mechanism (closed penetrating head injury), or other features (e.g. occurring in a specific location or over a widespread area). Head injury usually refers to TBI, but is a broader category because it can involve damage to structures other than the brain, such as the scalp and skull (Fig. 1.4).

TBI is a major cause of death and disability worldwide, especially in children and young adults. Males sustain traumatic brain injuries more frequently than do females. Causes include falls, vehicle accidents, and violence. Prevention measures include use of technology to protect those suffering from automobile accidents, such as seat belts and sports or motorcycle helmets, as well as efforts to reduce the number of automobile accidents, such as safety education programs and enforcement of traffic laws.

Brain trauma can occur as a consequence of a focal impact upon the head, by a sudden acceleration/deceleration within the cranium or by a complex combination of both movement and sudden impact. In addition to the damage caused at the moment of injury, brain trauma causes secondary injury, a variety of events that take place in the minutes and days following the injury. These processes, which

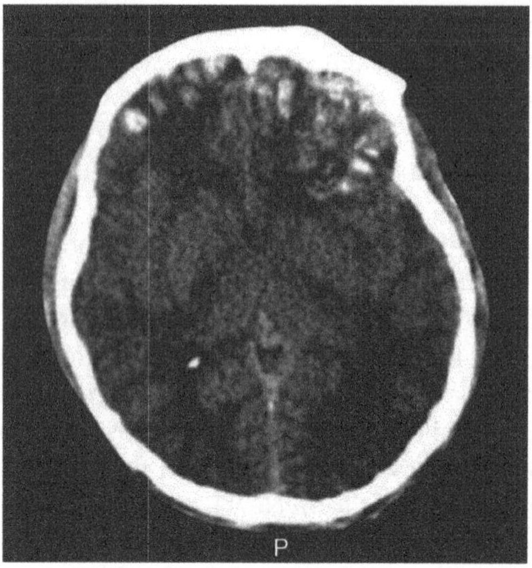

Fig. 1.4: CT scan of patient with brain trauma. Emergent CT imaging revealed a sagittally oriented skull fracture extending from the vertex to the foramen magnum as well as a transverse parietal and temporal bone fracture

include alterations in cerebral blood flow and the pressure within the skull, contribute substantially to the damage from the initial injury.

TBI can cause a host of physical, cognitive, social, emotional, and behavioral effects, and outcome can range from complete recovery to permanent disability or death. The 20th century saw critical developments in diagnosis and treatment that decreased death rates and improved outcome. Some of the current imaging techniques used for diagnosis and treatment include computed tomography and MRI (magnetic resonance imaging). Depending on the injury, treatment required may be minimal or may include interventions such as medications, emergency surgery or surgery years later. Physical therapy, speech therapy recreation therapy, occupational therapy and vision therapy may be employed for rehabilitation. Counseling, supported employment, and community support services may also be useful.

DEFINITION: REHABILITATION

Rehabilitation is the utilization of the existing capacities of the handicapped person by the combined and coordinated use of medical, social, educational and vocational measures to the optimum level of his or her functional ability.

Rehabilitation Process

1. The rehabilitation process is different for everyone. Rehabilitation programs should be individualized, catering to each person's unique needs. Just as no two people are exactly alike, no two-brain injuries are exactly alike. The person with a brain injury and his or her family should always be the most important members of the treatment team. Cultural, religious, social and economic backgrounds must always be taken into consideration when planning a person's rehabilitation program.
2. Rehabilitation channels the body's natural healing abilities and the brain's relearning process so than an individual recovers as quickly and efficiently as possible. Rehabilitation also involves learning new ways to compensate for abilities that have permanently changed due to brain injury. There is much that is still unknown about the brain and brain injury rehabilitation. Treatment methods and technology are rapidly advancing as knowledge of the brain and its functions increases.
3. The goal of rehabilitation is to help people regain the most independent level of functioning possible.

Models of Rehabilitation

In the past, rehabilitation services for people with brain injury were largely provided in a "medical model," located in a medical facility with a cadre of physicians, nurses, and trained professionals providing services. While this model still predominates, the trend today is toward more community-based rehabilitation models, and more options are available than ever before. Rehabilitation service delivery and funding are changing rapidly as managed care continues to replace the traditional fee-for-service and indemnity insurance plans.

Medical-based Rehabilitation

Early intervention is crucial. Rehabilitation should ideally start in the intensive care unit. At this point, rehabilitation is generally preventive in nature. Range of motion, bowel and bladder hygiene (i.e. initiation of regular bowel program and removing indwelling catheters), prevention of pressure sores, and orientation are all very important, right from the beginning. Frequently, rehabilitation activities initiated in the ICU can reduce complications and sometimes, the length of hospitalization.

Acute Rehabilitation: Once a person is medically stable, transfer to an acute rehabilitation facility often occurs. There, he/she will spend several hours a day in a structured rehabilitation program. This program usually includes a team of professionals with training and experience in brain injury rehabilitation such as Physical Therapists (PT), Occupational Therapists (OT), Speech-Language Pathologists (SLP), and Neuropsychologists. Additional staffs support the brain injury rehabilitation team's efforts, and often include case management, respiratory therapy, pharmacy, lab, nuclear medicine and radiology and dietary. A doctor with a specialty in Physical Medicine and Rehabilitation (PM&R), also known as a "physiatrist", may head up the team.

"Subacute" Rehabilitation: People who are minimally aroused for a prolonged period often have limited attention and stamina, and need a less intensive level of rehabilitation services, over a longer period of time. Subacute rehabilitation may be provided in a variety of settings, but is often in a skilled nursing facility or nursing home. It is important to note that the services provided by subacute programs vary widely, as there is no generally accepted definition of subacute services at this time.

It is important to recognize that "more therapy" does not make a person "better", but that "appropriate" therapy does. Subacute rehabilitation programs require the same appropriately trained professionals as acute rehabilitation programs do. The goals of subacute rehabilitation should include minimizing morbidity, maintaining functional positioning, hygiene, nutrition, and medication management, as well as providing support for the person with a brain injury and his/her family. Subacute rehabilitation programs may also be designed for persons who have made progress in the acute rehabilitation setting and are still progressing, but are not making rapid functional gains.

Day Treatment/Day Rehab: Day rehab (sometimes called "Day Hospital") provides intensive rehabilitation in a structured setting during the day and allows the person with a brain injury to return home to their family at night. The treatment team is often made up of a variety of the same sort rehabilitation professionals found in acute rehabilitation.

Community-based Rehabilitation

Outpatient Facilities: Following acute rehabilitation or subacute rehabilitation, a person with a brain injury may continue to receive outpatient treatment in specific areas (i.e. ongoing speech pathology to continue to work on cognition, or occupational therapy to work on driving, etc.). Often, this treatment can also be provided in the home by a home-health agency.

Home-based Rehabilitation

There are a few rehabilitation companies, which focus on providing acute rehabilitation within the home, or community setting. Once medically stable, some persons with a brain injury may be able to participate in such a program, if there is such a program in their community.

Community Re-entry: Community re-entry programs generally focus on developing higher-level motor and cognitive skills in order to prepare the person with a brain injury to return to independent living and potentially to work. Treatment may focus on safety in the community, interacting with others, initiation and goal setting and money management skills. Vocational evaluation and training may also be a component of this type of program. Community re-entry programs generally run for part or all of the day, with participants returning home to sleep and be with their families.

Transitional Living Programs: Transitional living programs provide housing for persons with brain injury, with the goal of regaining the ability to live as independently as possible. Sometimes, programs will have several different levels, depending on the level of need of the individual. In addition to physical, occupational, speech and recreation therapists, these programs usually have life skills technicians, who assist the person with a brain injury acquire skills and learn compensatory techniques, so they can live in the most independent setting.

REHABILITATION TEAM MEMBERS

A rehabilitation program is specifically designed for each individual depending on the injury, disorder, or illness. A multidisciplinary team approach for care and service is the basis of rehabilitation treatment. Multidisciplinary refers to the fact that many different disciplines work together toward a common goal. The team is usually directed by a physiatrist. Other specialists play important roles in the treatment and education process. Team members involved depend on many factors. These include patient need, facility resources, and insurance coverage for services.

The multidisciplinary rehabilitation team may include the following team members:

1. *Patient and family:* The patient and family are considered the most important members of the rehabilitation team.
2. *Physiatrist:* A healthcare provider who evaluates and treats rehabilitation patients. The physiatrist is usually the team leader. He/she is responsible for coordinating patient care services with other team members. A physiatrist focuses on restoring function to people with disabilities.
3. *Rehabilitation nurse:* A nurse who specializes in rehabilitative care and assists the patient in achieving maximum independence. The focus is on medical care, prevention of complications, and patient and family education.
4. *Clinical social worker:* A professional counselor who acts as a liaison for the patient, family, and rehabilitation treatment team. The social worker helps provide support and coordinate discharge planning and referrals. He/she may also help coordinate care with insurance companies.
5. *Physical therapist:* A therapist who helps restore function for patients with problems related to movement, muscle strength, exercise, and joint function.
6. *Occupational therapist:* A therapist who helps restore function for patients with problems related to activities of daily living (ADLs) including work, school, family, and community and leisure activities.
7. *Speech/language pathologist:* A therapist who helps restore function for patients with problems related to cognitive, communication, or swallowing issues.
8. *Psychiatrist, psychologist, or neuropsychologist:* A healthcare provider or counselor who conducts cognitive (thinking and learning) assessments of the patient. He/she also helps the patient and family adjust to the disability.
9. *Recreation therapist:* A therapist who coordinates therapeutic recreation programs to help promote social skills and leisure activities.

10. *Audiologist:* A healthcare professional who specializes in the evaluation and treatment of hearing and hearing loss.
11. *Registered Dietitian:* A nutritionist who evaluates and provides for the dietary needs of each patient. This is based on the patient's medical needs, eating abilities, and food preferences.
12. *Vocational therapist:* A counselor who assists people with disabilities to plan careers and find and keep satisfying jobs.
13. *Orthotist:* A healthcare professional who makes braces or splints used to strengthen or stabilize a part of the body.
14. *Prosthetist:* Healthcare professional who makes and fits artificial body parts, such as an artificial leg or arm.
15. *Case manager:* A rehabilitation case manager helps plan, organize, coordinate, and monitor services and resources for the patient.
16. *Respiratory therapist:* A therapist who helps treats and restores function for patients with airway and breathing problems.
17. *Chaplain:* A spiritual counselor who helps patients and families during crisis periods. He/she helps serve as a liaison between the hospital and the home church or place of worship.
18. *Biomedical engineer:* The field of rehabilitation is an interface between the medical and engineering profession. With the advance of technology, we have newer user friendly environment control units, communication aids, orthosis and limbs. All these have to designed by electronic and mechanical engineering professionals. The role of biomedical engineer is to inter act with the physiatrist, orthotist and speech pathologist to design a piece of equipment which will be of use to the person with disability.
19. *Vocational counselor:* The vocational counselor is an important professional in the sociovocational team who identifies the right vocation, skill or way of life of these patients. The skilled trainer trains the client in a particular vocation and the placement officer places him/her in suitable job.
20. *Music therapist:* The intervention of the music therapist involves instrumental or vocational performance by the person with disability or helping him/her appreciates music or attends musical events. This goes a way in:
    - Helping children or adults with cerebral palsy or other paralytic conditions to improve coordination and develop gross and fine motor skills through playing instruments

or exercising music. Some children with Down syndrome respond naturally to music.

- Relaxation, sedation, or control of pain or anxiety.
- Improving speech through articulation training or melodic intonation.
- Improving socialization skills, self-confidence, and esteem through group music activities.
- Improving quality of life for patients in palliative care.

CHAPTER

2

Community-based Rehabilitation

INTRODUCTION TO CBR

Community-based Rehabilitation (CBR) brings rehabilitation know-how to villages and urban slums, and CBR personnel facilitate people to take responsibility for their own lives. CBR is a systematized approach within general community development whereby persons with disabilities are enabled to live a fulfilling life within their own community, making maximum use of local resources and helping the community become aware of its responsibility in ensuring the inclusion and equal participation of PWDs. In the process, PWDs are also made aware of their own role and responsibility, as they are part of the community.

DEFINITION: COMMUNITY-BASED REHABILITATION

CBR is strategy within community development for rehabilitation, equalization of opportunities and social inclusion of all children and adults with disabilities.

—By UNESCO and WHO

CBR is a strategy for enhancing the quality of life of disabled people by improving service delivery, by providing more equitable opportunities and by promoting and protecting their human rights"

—By Einar Helander

"A strategy within community development for the rehabilitation, equalization of opportunities and social integration of all people with disabilities"

—By United Nations

Community-based rehabilitation, or CBR, is becoming increasingly recognized as an appropriate model of service delivery to provide effective rehabilitation and therapy services to rural and remote communities, with particular relevance for remote and rural indigenous communities.

In simple terms, CBR refers to the delivery of basic services to disabled people within their community, including all services necessary to improve the participation and functioning in daily activity. More broadly, CBR is implemented through the combined efforts of people with disabilities themselves, their families and communities, and appropriate health, education, vocation and social services.

CBR is an appropriate rehabilitation program for the rural people with disability, delivered at their door step with the use of local resources and with the involvement of local people (Fig. 2.1).

CBR is a need-based rehabilitation done in the community at the community level by utilizing the contribution of the community. The people with disability and their families are intensively involved in the decision making process as are the member of the community. CBR is self-help movement based on:

- Awareness concern of the community
- Initiative from the community

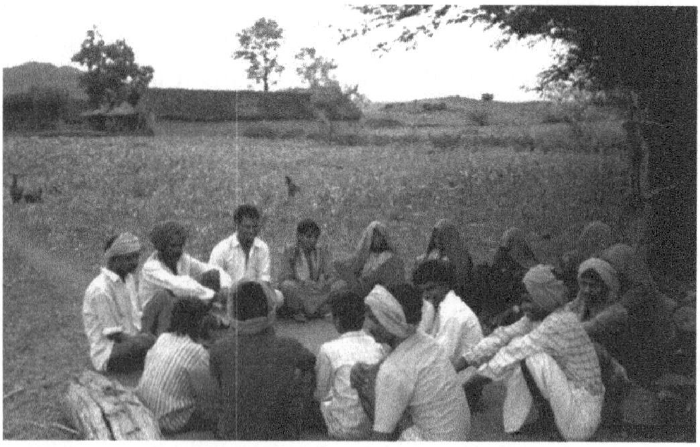

Fig. 2.1: Community meeting. *Source:* www.mhinnovation.net *(For color version see plate 1)*

- Planning from the community
- Implementation by the community
- Evaluation by the community
- Modification by the community
- Benefits to and from the community.

Principles of CBR

Community-based rehabilitation is founded on a set of principles described below.

To establish principles that are totally consistent and free from contradictions is not easy to do. There is nothing new or eccentric about the five ideas of highlighted here:

i. Equality
ii. Social justice
iii. Solidarity
iv. Integration
v. Dignity.

We should, however, note that these principles, for example, the one concerning equality, are not always part of the local or national culture. In others, nobody will object to them. However, they may not be applied.

Equality

All human beings are of inherently equal worth, are entitled to equal rights and share the same responsibilities. Human beings are born each a unique individual. Each develops along different lines. Each has different abilities. These differences do not make us unequal in worth. It is a fact that disabled people in most or all societies are denied equality in rights. This reflects the prevailing social attitudes of our societies, which are biased toward admiring and rewarding certain abilities while disregarding many other qualities. Disabled people face a situation similar to that of women in some societies, who, until recently, were denied the right to vote and earned lower salaries than men for the same work do. Some countries still will not let disabled people participate in political functions or give them a vote. Disabled people are responsible neither for their situation nor for such attitudes. They are the victims. Disability is caused primarily by environmental factors—such as disease, trauma and lack of prenatal care. Involuntarily affected by such factors, people with disabilities may see their hope for a better life deteriorate in the face of social insensitivity to their needs for equality. They may be denied the right to rehabilitation, education, employment and social integration. Insensitivity may lead to their rejection or even to the questioning of their right to life. One of the most fundamental questions relative to equality is "Who has the power over a disabled person?" Is it the authorities and experts, or is it the disabled individual himself/herself? If there is one characteristic that is common to the group of disabled people—standing out over and above such others as poverty, lack of services, and lack of access to education and employment—certainly that characteristic is powerlessness. One of the aims of a rehabilitation program should be to stress the abilities and competence of disabled people, to increase their responsibilities and rights, to apply more equal and more human standards to these fellow human beings, and to strengthen the process of empowerment. In order to achieve this, we have to overcome prejudice and reject arbitrary concepts of difference concerning disabled people, which have been reinforced over many centuries by tradition and dominant power structures, and which today represent formidable roadblocks on their way.

Social Justice

Social justice implies that services and opportunities provided for disabled people should be at the disposal of all and not be reserved for a numerically small group among them. It stands to reason that the ultimate goal is to make individualized care, training, schooling, and access to employment and income generation available to all disabled people. These are vital contributory factors to integration, self-actualization. Achievement of this objective is, however, many years away. In the meantime, guided by the principle of social justice, we should endeavor to build program that will eventually give all disabled people at least the essential services.

Basic ten rules for integrated living

1. *Family life:* As a person with a disability, you should have the freedom to find a partner, have children, and set up your own family. You should live with your family and be part of your community.
2. *Shelter:* You should have shelter and be able to move about freely at home and in your surroundings.

3. *Food:* As an infant, you should be breastfed. As a child and as an adult, you should have a fair share of your family's food.
4. *Schooling:* As a child with a disability, you should go to school with the non-disabled. Your teacher should have learned how to take care of your special needs and to include you in all school activities.
5. *Education and training:* You should get the opportunities for education and training that you need in order to prepare yourself to work and to live independently.
6. *Leisure time:* You should be free to join others on social, cultural and religious occasions.
7. *Public services:* You should have access to all public services and all public buildings. Roads and public transport should be designed in such a way as to let you move and mix freely and independently in society.
8. *Association:* You should not be denied membership of any associations or organizations open to all, and you should be free to form or join an association of disabled people, should you so wish.
9. *Economic opportunities:* You should have the same opportunities to work as other people; any loss of income caused by your disability should be compensated.
10. *Political participation:* You should be allowed to vote and to participate in government as other citizens do. Your voice should be heard in matters of concern to you and regarding services provided for you.

Social justice further implies that one should not seek to accord disabled people privileges that go beyond what they would have been entitled to had they been able-bodied. It is true, disabled people today rarely enjoy their legitimate human rights. Positive discrimination is widely believed to be a means to remedy this situation. Rather than attempting to formulate yet another and another bill of rights—all of which eventually will fail for the same reasons—one should look into the underlying causes of the non-application of legitimate existing rights and remedy that situation.

Solidarity

The responsibility for fostering human life is shared by all. Solidarity should be shown toward those among us who are dependent and need help—children, the elderly, and those who have a disability.

Solidarity of purpose and efforts toward this end should be seen as a privilege of all and not as charity for some.

In industrialized countries, it is common to have systems designed to transfer resources (cash, pensions, subventions, and services) from one group to another, for example, from the employed to the unemployed. Normally, disabled people should benefit from such transfers if they do not earn enough to enable them to live decent lives. In developing countries, the extended family, the tribe, or the clan plays a similar function. Dependency is not a characteristic limited to disabled people. On the contrary, all human beings are dependent on each other during many years of their lives. Solidarity is one of the main principles of our societies, without which none of us could survive.

Integration

All members of the society should join in the mainstream of community life. Disabled people are often Excluded from the activities of a particular society because they are looked upon as "special" or "strange."

There is a clear correlation between the policy of providing special, segregated services and the attitudes of most non-disabled people in favoring the segregation of disabled people.

Segregation of services, housing, jobs, and education transportation and so on, is mainly caused by social factors and cultural prejudice.

Segregation is a vicious circle. As long as disabled people are out of sight, nobody will get to know them, and fear and anxiety about meeting these hidden members of society will grow. Integration of disabled people in all aspects of life will, in the long-term perspective, help them to achieve friendship with and esteem by others, and finally, to attain the degree of human dignity now denied to most of them. Ten basic rules for integrated living are suggested, which exemplify this principle.

Dignity

The final guiding principle is dignity. All disabled people should live a life in dignity. The term "dignity" may be defined as follows: "the quality that earns or deserves respect." Dignity for a disabled person is possible when:

- It is recognized that all human beings have equal worth and equal rights;

- All are willing—in the spirit of solidarity—to share the opportunities and means needed for self-actualization;
- He/she is fully participating in the life of the community.

Objectives of CBR Program

Based on the above principles, the broad long-term objective or goal for rehabilitation is: "to promote a development that eventually will allow all disabled people to live a life in dignity.

To achieve this end requires actions aimed at, among others:

- Providing all the rehabilitation services needed;
- Reducing or eliminating environmental barriers;
- Compensating disabled people for any loss in their standard of living caused by disability;
- Promoting social integration and self-actualization;
- Protecting and ensuring the security of disabled people;
- Empower disabled people, so they can exercise their rights and have adequate representation and influence in the society where they live. The realization of these actions will depend on the willingness of society to provide the necessary resources and social means in a spirit of solidarity. This can only be brought about by a change of prevalent attitudes and behavior. Sensitization and education of the public at large are important mean for reaching the ultimate aim of gaining equality for disabled people. Another requirement is that governments take over the leading role and assume the responsibility for disabled people in the same way as they do for non-disabled citizens. Obviously, it will take many years to translate this broad objective into practice, so we need to devise realistic, long-term, step-by-step approaches along with a strategy for their application.

General Approaches to CBR

There are three approaches to CBR

- Learning from the people
- Building and upgrading the system from below
- Do not look for instant or easy solutions.

Learning from the people: The first element in the approach to CBR is to learn from the people. In the conventional rehabilitation model, efforts had been made to transfer the technology, types of professionals and service systems existing in the industrialized world. This has largely failed. The essence of the CBR approach is to find out what is locally initiated, in terms of successful technology, service and management systems, in each developing country and to build on this experience. Not until the applied local approach builds on this general principle will the development be sustainable. Such a review of existing technology, service and management systems should not be confined to the disability area. There is a host of development projects initiated by local communities, and analyzing their achievements as well as their failures will teach us a great deal. Such development projects may be concerned with, for example, community water supply, agriculture, primary health care and elementary schools. We should therefore set out by looking for the inventive parents who have successfully trained their blind child to walk around in the village, or their mentally retarded adolescent to work in the fields. We should seek the advice of the schoolteacher who has included disabled children in the local school, as well as that of the artisan who has made crutches and wooden legs.

We should learn management from local community leaders, and principles of community work from existing cooperatives and development committees, and we should learn to respect the abilities and experience of the local people and listen carefully to their views. Hence, the principle is to look for what there is already and to learn from the people—this should be the point of departure of any development effort.

Building and upgrading the system from below: The conventional system often started off by providing a "national center" or similar, in the belief that later on this center would develop ramifications and decentralized services. In reality this has rarely been the case. National center's stayed national center's, and more often than not they turned into ivory towers.

The CBR system endeavors to start development from below, by first encouraging the establishment of community services and, at a later stage, linking them to a referral system. The referral system should be created once the community needs are known, preferably after a certain period of implementation.

In a system built from below, the educational objectives for professional staff working at referral centers will be formulated in response to local requirements while taking into consideration how existing resources could be restructured and decentralized. At its inception, a CBR system will necessarily be simple. Over time it should be upgraded from below, by improving community workers' competence through in-service training program. Parents or other family members who act as trainers of disabled individuals will develop their abilities through experience.

Local school teachers could learn more about how to integrate disabled children in the class, possibly with the assistance of a mobile resource teacher. Community leaders could start projects for integrated, informal ability training and help disabled people to an income-generating activity. Human rights could be protected if the community provides mediation. And disabled people could obtain more say and better representation of their views. CBR program owe much of their success to the principle of building and upgrading the system from below.

Do not look for instant or easy solutions: There are no quick or easy solutions. It will take years to adapt the technology to suit individual requirements, to inspire community involvement and organization to train all the necessary personnel, to set up service systems to cover entire populations, to build-up management resources, and to locate the necessary funds.

There is no such thing as a standardized CBR system, nor can this system be copied from country to country. Certain patterns can be duplicated, and experience can be shared, but each country has to make its own adaptations. Other problems such as those related to prejudice and application of human rights will take even.

Longer to resolve, given our very limited experience in how to apply awareness-building, sensitization and public education program. All governments seeking to improve the quality of life for their disabled citizens should bear in mind that sustained, active efforts will be needed for a period of 15 to 25 years, if not more. The involvement of governments is necessary, for there is no other way to create a well-functioning network of services. But governments have limited funds and should not "promise to do everything". No nations have more resources than those, which can be mobilized through their own people; for rehabilitation services, a participatory approach is needed, involving people.

CRITERIA OF THE CBR PROGRAM

The development and implementation of CBR program should be based on the following criteria:

1. People with disabilities must be included in CBR program at all stages and levels, including initial program design and implementation. In order to give significance to their involvement, they must have distinct decision-making roles.
2. The primary objective of CBR program activities is the improvement of the quality of life of people with disabilities.
3. One focus of CBR program activities is working with the community to create positive attitudes towards people with disabilities and to motivate community members to support and participate in CBR activities.
4. The other focus of CBR program is providing assistance for people with all types of disabilities (physical, sensory, psychological and mental); for people of all ages, including older people; for people affected by leprosy; for people affected by epilepsy; and for other people who may be identified by the community as needing special assistance.
5. All activities in CBR program must be sensitive to the situation of girls and women. This is because in many communities throughout the Asian and Pacific region women are not treated equally. When they are disabled, the problems that they face in life are doubled. Furthermore, women are usually the primary family care-givers for all people with disabilities.
6. CBR programs must be flexible, so that they can operate at the local level and within the context of local conditions. There should not be only one model of CBR because different social and economic contexts and different needs of individual communities will require different solutions. Flexible, local programs will ensure community involvement and result in a variety of program models which are appropriate for different places.
7. CBR program must coordinate service delivery at the local level. Community members seldom understand the different roles and specializations that are part of providing assistance to people with disabilities. They tend only to see the problem of disability and only to want access to "one window" for help. They may focus only on where to go and who to see about a specific "problem", rather than understanding the totality of what constitutes a fulfilling life for a community member who has a disability.

COMPONENTS OF CBR PROGRAM

The components of a CBR program should include:

1. *Creating a positive attitude towards people with disabilities:* This component of CBR program is essential to ensure equalization of opportunities for people with disabilities within their own community. Positive attitudes among community members can be created by involving them in the process of program design and implementation, and by transferring knowledge about disability issues to community members.
2. *Provision of functional rehabilitation services:* Often people with disabilities require assistance to overcome or minimize the effects of their functional limitations (disabilities). In communities where professional services are not accessible or available, CBR workers should be trained to provide primary rehabilitation therapy in the following areas of rehabilitation:
   - Medical
   - Eye care service
   - Hearing services
   - Physiotherapy
   - Occupational therapy
   - Orientation and mobility training
   - Speech therapy
   - Psychological counseling
   - Orthotics and prosthetics
   - Other devices.
3. *Provision of education and training opportunities:* People with disabilities must have equal access to educational opportunities and to training that will enable them to make the best use of the opportunities that occur in their lives. In communities where professional services are not accessible or available, CBR workers should be trained to provide basic levels of service in the following areas:
   - Early childhood intervention and referral, especially to medical rehabilitation services
   - Education in regular schools
   - Non-formal education where regular schooling is not available
   - Special education in regular or special schools
   - Sign language training
   - Braille training
   - Training in daily living skills.

4. *Creation of micro- and macro-income-generation opportunities:* People with disabilities need access to micro- and macro-income-generation activities, including obtaining financial credit through existing systems, wherever possible. In slums and rural areas, income-generation activities should focus on locally appropriate vocational skills. Training in these skills is best conducted by community members who, with minimal assistance, can easily transfer their skills and knowledge to people with disabilities.
5. *Provision of care facilities:* Often, people with extensive disabilities are in need of assistance. When they have no families or their families are incapable of caring for them, in order for them to survive, long-term care facilities must be provided in the community where they can get the assistance that they need. Moreover, day-care facilities may be needed to provide respite for families who either work or need time off for other activities.
6. *Prevention of the causes of disabilities:* Many types of disability can be prevented by relatively simple measures. Proper nutrition is one of the more significant ways of preventing disabilities. Another important area of disability prevention is the detection of disability in young children and intervention early in their development, to minimize the effect of impairment. There are many other areas of disability prevention that are also important. These include activities to decrease the number of accidents in the home, on the road and at work, as well as other initiatives to encourage people to pursue healthy lifestyles over the course of their lives.
7. *Management, monitoring and evaluation:* The effectiveness and efficiency of all CBR program components, both in the community and in the area of service delivery outside the community, depend on effective management practices. The impact of program activities must be measured on a regular basis. People must be trained in effective management practices. Data must be collected, reviewed and evaluated to ensure that program objectives are met. In this way, the success or failure of a CBR program can be honestly measured.

BASIC CONCEPT OF CBR

Decentralization of Responsibility and Resources

This publication focuses on understanding community-based rehabilitation (CBR). It does not try to define CBR, as it has become apparent in recent years that CBR defies definition. This is because its simplicity and complexity have led to confusion about what CBR means. The simplicity of CBR has to do with its history of starting with the delivery of primary rehabilitation therapy to people with disabilities in their communities. The complexity of CBR is the result of the current concept that CBR program should be multisectoral (or multidisciplinary), so that they can provide assistance in all of the areas which are central to improvement of the quality of life of people with disabilities. This complexity recognizes the need for close coordination, collaboration and cooperation between governmental and non-governmental organizations of all types and at all levels.

The basic concept inherent in the multisectoral approach to CBR is in both human and financial, to community-level organizations. In this approach, governmental and non-governmental institutional and outreach rehabilitation services must support community initiatives and organizations.

For the multisectoral approach to CBR to be successfully translated into action, both governmental and non-governmental service capacities need to be improved in most countries of the Asian and Pacific region. Of special importance is improvement of the capacity and skills for facilitating community involvement. Such improvement and related activities must be closely coordinated to ensure the optimum use of scarce resources. In accordance with the multisectoral concept, systems are developed, at the community level and among governmental and non-governmental organizations that interact and reach out to each other.

Empowerment of the Community

Another factor for the success of the multisectoral approach is the empowerment of the community to assume responsibility for ensuring that all its members, including those with disabilities, achieve equal access to all of the resources that are available to that community, and that they are enabled to participate fully in the social, economic and political life of the community. This approach ensures that what is done in the name of CBR actually fits into the reality of the community and is owned by the community.

MULTISECTORAL APPROACH TO CBR

The starting point for understanding CBR is the following approach agreed to in 1994 by ILO, UNESCO and WHO community-based rehabilitation (CBR) is a strategy within community development for the rehabilitation, equalization of opportunities and social integration of all people with disabilities. CBR is implemented through the combined efforts of disabled people themselves, their families and communities, and the appropriate health, education, vocational and social services.

This approach to CBR is multisectoral and includes all governmental and non-governmental services that provide assistance to communities. Many of the services which can provide opportunities for and assistance to people with disabilities are not traditionally considered relevant to CBR program and people with disabilities. Examples include community development organizations, agricultural extension services, and water and sanitation program.

In the ILO-UNESCO-WHO approach to CBR, the phrase "within community development" is understood to be the following strategy recommended by the United Nations. The utilization, [in an integrated program] of approaches and techniques which rely on local communities as units of action and which attempt to combine outside assistance with organized local self-determination and effort, and which correspondingly seek to stimulate local initiative and leadership as the primary instrument of change.

In the CBR context, community means: (a) a group of people with common interests who interact with each other on a regular basis; and/or (b) a geographical, social or government administrative unit. Whilst the architects of community-based rehabilitation conceived of the approach as involving all sectors of the society the majority of early attempts to translate the philosophy into practice grew out of health-based program. However, the goal of CBR is to contribute towards the empowerment of persons with disabilities, facilitating an independent lifestyle in which they participate in all aspects of community life. Multisectoral collaboration is therefore imperative if such a goal is to be achieved, as no one sector alone, can achieve such a broad objective. The breadth of the challenge necessitates a partnership between all the various sectors, i.e. health, education, labor, vocational, housing, welfare, sports and agriculture, in collaboration with NGOs, Disabled Peoples Organizations (DPOs), and the traditional and religious leaders within the community.

RATIONALE FOR A MULTISECTORAL APPROACH

In many ways, the needs of persons with disabilities are the same as their able-bodied peers. Such Needs cut across all sectors. Moreover the community represents disabled persons of all ages, at different stages of life different sectors come into play. No one sector can begin to respond to the comprehensive needs involved in the rehabilitation process. CBR program should seek to meet the needs of disabled persons of various etiologies and of all ages. If the initiating group does not have the expertise to address the needs of a specific target group, they should seek out the relevant partners to develop a more comprehensive approach.

PROBLEMS IN ACHIEVING A MULTISECTORAL APPROACH TO REHABILITATION

The one factor that unites disabled people throughout the world is the low priority, they are given within their countries. Where a response has been forthcoming, it is often limited in effectiveness because of the lack of collaboration between government departments. A unified response has not been forthcoming for a variety of reasons including:

- Lack of political commitment which is reflected in the absence of a national policy on disability issues
- Rigid ministerial demarcations which prevent collaboration as different sectors vie for resources
- Ministries have often developed an inertia of their own characterized by a fixed way of doing things
- Poor communication between ministries
- Competition between sectors, each of which wants to be perceived as the `lead' body
- Lack of a tradition of collaboration where the emphasis has instead been on vertical training which emphasizes particular professional orientation.

SECTORS AND ROLES FOR THE DEVELOPMENT AND IMPLEMENTATION OF COMMUNITY-BASED REHABILITATION

The initiative to start CBR programs and to facilitate their development may come from any one of the following groups. However, the effectiveness of CBR and the long-term development and sustainability of any CBR initiative will require the coordination, involvement and collaboration of all seven groups. The seven groups and their suggested roles are as follows:

1. *People with disabilities:* People with disabilities can and should contribute to all levels of CBR programs in every position within a program. They know what the effects of local conditions are on themselves. They are likely to have a good understanding of those effects on their peers with disabilities. They also know what impairment really means in the context of their family, community and nation. This knowledge enables them to be very effective members of a CBR team. They can be more effective than non-disabled people as role models for and counselors of other people with disabilities. People with disabilities have an important role in community education. As community educators, they serve as living examples of people with disabilities who make a significant contribution, provided that they are given the opportunity and the right type of assistance. CBR programs should also facilitate the development of self-help organizations of people with disabilities at the community level.
2. *Families of people with disabilities:* Families have the primary responsibility for caring for all of their members. They are the first line of support and assistance for people with disabilities at the local level. As such, families must be included in CBR program activities. Where the individual with a disability is not able, for whatever reason, to speak for himself/herself, a family member should represent him/her and should be considered a legitimate member of disabled people's organizations. Members of families with experience in caring for people with disabilities are the people who most often initiate CBR programs and are, or prove to be, the most effective contributors at all levels.
3. *Communities:* Community members should be involved in CBR programs at all levels because they already know the local environmental conditions, the local economy, the local political situation and how to work with them. They also know about the accessibility, availability and effectiveness of locally available rehabilitation services; who in the community cares enough about other people to become a program leader or worker; and, which community members have the knowledge and skills for training others in microeconomic activities. They are the people most

likely to want to live, work and stay in the community. Community involvement usually requires the agreement and approval, both formal and informal, of the community leaders.

4. *Governments (local, regional, national):* Governments have the most important role in the development and sustainability of CBR programs. Their cooperation, support and involvement are essential if CBR is to cover the total population and be sustainable. They should implement and coordinate the development of the entire program structure, including the development of the referral system, as well as the activities within the community. They also should provide resources for non-governmental organizations (NGOs) and community activities. Finally, they should ensure that discriminatory legislation is changed and that the rights of people with disabilities are guaranteed and protected.
5. *Non-governmental organizations, local, regional, national and international organizations:* NGOs, including organizations of people with disabilities, are often able to provide resources and skills to facilitate the development of new programs, especially in areas where none exist. They can develop new approaches to CBR and provide training programs for government employees, CBR workers, people with disabilities, families, and community members. NGOs are effective in facilitating the development of community members as CBR program leaders. They are often best able to provide long-term care facilities for those people with extensive disabilities whose families cannot or will not look after them.
6. *Medical professionals, allied health science professionals, educators, social scientists and other professionals:* Professionals are often in a position where they can, as trainers and educators, facilitate the development of new programs by making their knowledge and skills accessible to community members and CBR program workers. They can also ensure that they support community efforts by making themselves available and accessible on a referral basis. When they are in government service, they can advocate and promote the development of CBR programs as an effective way to provide local-level services quickly.

The private sector (business and industry): The private sector has a social obligation to return some of the benefits of its operations to the communities that support it. In the past, this support has largely taken the form of charity. Charity occurs when donors "give" whatever they feel is a needed or appropriate to person with disabilities. This approach to assisting people with disabilities is no longer appropriate and needs to be changed. Supporting CBR program activities eliminates the need for charity. CBR support is a much more appropriate way of directing resources to communities and people with disabilities. By supporting CBR programs, the private sector receives credit for its social involvement while being guaranteed that its support is put to effective and efficient use. Who but trained, knowledgeable community members would know what is most.

7. Needed by the people of their own community?

ASPECT OF CBR PROGRAM

1. Medical
2. Educational
3. Economical
4. Social

Medical

Medical aspect usually start with evaluation of the disability by a group of professional a comprehensive program is chart out which is followed by diligent grassroots level trained personnel. Usually, the relatives of the patient are also trained.

Educational

Whenever required education is imparted to those who need basic knowledge and skills. This gains more significance in the children suffering from cerebral palsy.

Economical

The education, vocational and a vocational skills imparted will provide a spring board for the patient to register himself for a job or open up opportunities for self-employment of avenues for economic betterment.

Social

The success of any CBR program depends on factor like effectiveness, individual values as well as social acceptability of the Program.

MODELS OF CBR

- *WHO model:* Uses trainers, booklets on health conditions.
- *Neighborhood model:* A resource center in the community adopts another center, trains personnel and in due course this becomes another resource center.
- *DRC model:* The District Rehabilitation Scheme (DRC) was launched by the Government of India in January 1985 on a pilot basis in collaboration with The National Institute of Disability Rehabilitation and Research, The US Department of Education and UNICEF. The DRC scheme had a considerable impact, but it was community located, not community-based.

CBR TEAM

1. First and for most the patient
2. His/her relatives
3. CBR workers
4. Locally available skilled workers, e.g. carpenter who could be trained to make appliances and aids.
5. Local leader
6. The school teacher
7. Multipurpose rehabilitation worker (A trained person who can identify disability and give the basic physiotherapy and prescribe orthotics)
8. PHC staff including medical officer and other health worker (an orientation program towards rehabilitation has recently been introduced by the Rehabilitation Council of India for PHC Doctors)
9. District administrative officer
10. The following member may provide specialized training and disability identification services.
    - Psychiatrist
    - Physiotherapist
    - Occupational therapist
    - Orthotists and prosthetic engineers.

OPINION MAKERS

1. *People with disability:* They can be more effective than nondisabled people as role model and counselors of other people with disabilities.

2. *Families of people with disabilities*
3. *Community members:* Community member know the local environmental conditions, the economy, The political situation, and how to work within them. *Governments*: (Local, Regional, National)
4. *Nongovernmental organizations*
5. *Medical professionals:* Allied health science professionals, educators, social scientist and other professionals are often used in their capacity as educators.
6. *The private sector:* (Business and industry) has a social obligation to return some of the benefits of its operations to the communities that support it.

DIFFERENCE BETWEEN INSTITUTION-BASED AND COMMUNITY-BASED REHABILITATION

1. *Institution-based rehabilitation:* In Institution-based rehabilitation, the focus of control is based in the institution. This service meets a small number of needs of a small number of disabled people. This is at best a limited approach, and at worst it can abuse the rights of disabled persons.
2. *Outreach program:* With Outreach, the focus of control is still based in the institution. More people can be 'reached,' but there will be limits according to distance from the institution, and according to whether the needs of the disabled people are similar to what the institution offers.
3. *Community-based rehabilitation:* With CBR, the focus of control should be with the community. So the starting point is exactly the opposite. The disabled people, family and community members decide what their priorities are, and then work together with local organizations, government, institutions, in order to access the relevant and appropriate services. Institutions have an important role as referral agencies (Table 2.1).

THE VALUE OF PHYSIOTHERAPY AND OCCUPATIONAL THERAPY IN COMMUNITY-BASED REHABILITATION

Physiotherapy and occupational therapy are two health disciplines which specifically focus on providing functional rehabilitation for people with disabilities. Both professions complement each other in

TABLE 2.1: Difference between CBR and IBR

S. No.	*Community-based rehabilitation*	*Institution-based (Medical) rehabilitation*
1.	Based on social model and human rights model	Based on medical model
2.	Concept of capacity building and empowerment	Concept of treatment—prescription
3.	Person with disability will be the decision taker	Professional is the decision taker
4.	Utilization of available resources in their own community	Utilization of professional service delivery model
5.	Targeted for larger population	Target of smaller population
6.	Minimal medical service/Basic services	High tech medical services
7.	Economic status of people with disability is not a barrier	Economic status is big barrier for getting the services
8.	Team member include person with disability, parents, care givers, family, local community, NDGs, voluntary organizations, governments... (Change according to the cultural/context)	Team member include person with disability, physician, physiotherapist, speech therapist orthotics and prosthetic technician, music therapist... (Change according to the medical condition)

their knowledge and skills and in their approaches to management of disability. However, the key to successful provision of services by these professions is in the ability of the practitioners to use a good clinical reasoning or problem-solving approach to management of disability and to be client and family focused in the provision of therapy (Table 2.2).

In persons with chronic disabilities, it is highly desirable that the person with the disability has access to the knowledge and skills of a good occupational therapist and physiotherapist at some stage of their lifetime, preferably as early as possible after the detection of the disability. In this way, relevant therapy can be instituted as soon as possible.

In countries such as India, where 85% of the population live in rural and remote areas of the country, access to such specialist services is a luxury rather than a right. Consequently, there is significant value in training mid-level workers to provide basic home-based therapy

TABLE 2.2: Differences between CBR and other rehabilitation

Sl. No.	*What is CBR?*	*What is not CBR?*
1.	Flexible	Rigid or a blue-print
2.	Active involvement of families and communities	An approach which only focuses on the physical or medical needs of a person
3.	A partnership approach with disabled people and parents of disabled children	Long-term residential care
4.	Capacity building of disabled people and their families, in the context of their community and culture	Delivering a service to disabled people as passive recipients
5.	Holistic in its approach to disabled people; addressing social, employment, educational, and other needs not just physical multi-sectoral	Only outreach from a center
6.	An approach which uses centers/institutions to respond to the needs of disabled people and their families	Rehabilitation training in isolation
7.	A system which is based in the community, but which uses district level and national level services for referral	Surveys on disability with no action
8.	An approach which aims to enable around 80% of disabled people's rehabilitation needs to be addressed in the community	Limited to one sector
9.	Integrated into existing services and promoting the social inclusion of disabled people	An approach which is determined by the needs of an institution or group of professionals
10.	An approach with a broad concept of 'rehabilitation'	An approach which requires that disabled people have to travel to a remote center or institution to meet their needs
11.	A long-term strategy	Segregated and separate from services for other people An approach with a narrow concept of 'rehabilitation' A short-term fix

on a day-to-day basis. It is our contention that such training requires a basic understanding of the principles of anatomy, physiology and pathology of disabilities; more importantly the workers need significant training in using a functional approach to assessment and management of disabilities, with particular emphasis on problem solving, documentation, realistic goal setting and understanding simple progression of rehabilitation programs for common disabilities which they encounter. After training, these workers continue to need access to 'expert' therapists who act as consultants to the mid-level workers. These 'experts' can provide advice on a regular basis and review complex cases, meanwhile contributing to the continuing education of the mid-level worker.

Since 1995, faculty from the University of Sydney have collaborated with Action Aid India and other non-government agencies to provide final year physiotherapy and occupational therapy students, who act as an 'expert' technical resource for the teaching and training of community-based rehabilitation workers (CBRW's) and other village health workers in selected CBR projects throughout South India. In our experience, there are several distinct principles that must be adopted in providing training to mid-level health workers:

1. An adult learning approach to presentation of materials must be used rather than the traditional pedagogical approach.
2. Interactive or experiential learning is much more successful and promotes thinking and reasoning rather than passive learning.
3. A functional approach to assessment and intervention is essential, rather than the traditional 'medical model' approach to diagnosis and treatment. A functional approach is more meaningful to the client and care-givers and provides greater motivation to improve, as the clients can see that the interventions affect their ability to perform normal activities of daily living.
4. Theoretical sessions must be interspersed with practical sessions whereby participants can practice their skills and implementation of knowledge on each other, before exposure to clients with disabilities.
5. Fieldwork practice sessions are essential, from the very beginning of any training program, so that participants can put into practice what they have learned in the 'classroom.'
6. Regular review of knowledge and skills, with concurrent feedback is highly recommended.

7. The level and complexity of knowledge and skills presentation must be tailored to the needs and educational standards of the participants.
8. Documentation is essential. It provides an objective baseline assessment for the functional status of the client, from which realistic, measurable treatment goals can established. Therapists can therefore evaluate efficacy of interventions and progression of therapy. It is essential that measurable outcomes are introduced. Such documentation can also be of value to CBR co-coordinators, in that they can measure the effectiveness of their CBR programs; they can also discover deficits in CBRW's knowledge and abilities, thereby knowing where continuing education needs to be provided (Table 2.3).

Table 2.3: Differences between institutional and CBR-based training manual

Sl. No.	*Area of difference*	*Institution*	*CBR*
1.	Duration and location of training	4 years degree- Institutionally trained'	3 months to 1 year locally trained
2.	Type of training	Trained to manage acute, complex cases, and in the use of sophisticated technology	Trained to teach family and clients to cope with consequences of disability within the community settings, using the available resources
3.	Extent of training	Interventions limited to skills training for the clients	Interventions to fulfill the needs of clients regarding daily living activities in their home environment
4.	Goal of the training	Interventions to discharge the patient from the hospital	Interventions to prepare the re-entry of the client to his home
5.	Setting for the intervention	Interventions take place in the institutions	Interventions take place in the client's home

Contd...

Contd...

Sl. No.	*Area of difference*	*Institution*	*CBR*
6.	Resources needed for the intervention	Solutions are based on high technology equipment	Solutions are based on resources from the community
7.	Knowledge base of the trainees	Users of manuals are highly trained and know medical terminology describing the state of the art technology	Users of manuals are lay people, poorly trained and unfamiliar with medical terminology
8.	Language of the manuals	Universal language can be used to write the manuals	Manuals have to be written in the context of local culture, tradition and dialect
9.	Type of clients	Minority of disabled persons who require sophisticated technology for their rehabilitation	Majority of the disabled persons who require only simple techniques for their rehabilitation

General discussion followed the presentation by the authors. Much discussion was generated around the issue of whether CBRWs should be multi-skilled in all areas of CBR or whether there is value in training different types of mid-level workers; that is, therapy workers, community workers, etc. It is the contention of the authors that no one system is appropriate for all CBR programs. It may be appropriate, for example, to have 'therapy workers in projects that have a large number of clients or a large area of coverage and where there is significant community development work to be done. In another project, it may be more appropriate for the CBRW to incorporate all areas of community-based rehabilitation—therapy, community involvement, income generation, etc. If the former scenario is adopted, it is essential for the lines of communication to be firmly established, so that all workers are focusing on a common goal, i.e. that the person with a disability is given maximum opportunity to become an active and equal member of the community.

CHAPTER

3

Community-based Rehabilitation and Empowerment

INTRODUCTION

Empowerment is an ongoing process, which enables an individual to fulfil his duties, responsibilities and protect her/his rights in the society.

COMMUNITY-BASED REHABILITATION AND EMPOWERMENT

Empowerment of people with disabilities is the ultimate goal of any community-based rehabilitation (CBR) program. The road to empowerment compels the community to create and promote equal opportunities, so that people with disabilities get an access to: Health services, education, housing facilities, work placements, emotional security, family bonds, marriage, leisure/free personal time, recreation and other needs.

And above all, the right to choose-full participation in decision-making on, issues concerning self, family, community.

PROGRAM OF ACTION CONCERNING DISABLED PERSONS

1981 was declared the International Year of Disabled Persons by the United Nations. This year was not recognized by the South African government. It was, nevertheless, promoted by the NGO sector whose adopted theme was 'Full Participation and Equality'. It was this that gave rise to the development of a disability rights movement in this country. The most important outcome of the International Year of Disabled Persons was the adoption of the World Program of Action Concerning Disabled Persons during the UN Decade of Disabled Persons (1983–1993). The purpose of the World Program of Action was to promote effective measures for the prevention of disability, rehabilitation and the realization of equal opportunities for persons with disabilities.

NATIONAL YEAR OF DISABLED PERSONS

1986, the International Year of Peace, was also not recognized by the South African government, which, apparently in an attempt to divert attention from the violence raging in the country at the time, declared a National Year of the Disabled.

Investigations carried out on the circumstances of disabled people by NGOs [including the Disabled People South Africa (DPSA) and the Government] revealed the complete absence of any workable policy on disability. Gross discrepancies in the few existing services were also revealed, in terms of both racial and rural/urban distribution.

Following the 1986 investigation, an Interdepartmental Coordinating Committee for the Care of the Disabled (ICCD), involving state departments and the NGO sector, was established. Its role was to implement the various recommendations arising out of the 1986 investigation. Because by the end of 1991, it had not succeeded in implementing a single one of its tasks, it was disbanded and a restructured South African Federal Council on the Rehabilitation of Disabled Persons (SAFCD) was given responsibility for policy development. In doing so, it was to build on the experience and creative interaction between service providers and representatives of organizations of disabled people over the preceding seven years. It was also decided that the Federal Council should interface with the political negotiating process rather than the government of the day. However, this structure also struggled due to lack of capacity and other factors.

RULES ON THE EQUALIZATION OF OPPORTUNITIES FOR PERSONS WITH DISABILITIES

The UN facilitated the drafting of the Standard Rules for the Equalization of Opportunities for Disabled Persons to provide governments with clearer guidelines on actions to be taken. The Standard Rules were adopted by the UN General Assembly on 20 December 1993.

AIMS OF THE STANDARD RULES

The aims of the standard rules are as follows:

1. They imply a strong moral and political commitment by the State to take action for the equalization of opportunities for persons with disabilities.
2. They offer an instrument for policy-making and action. The purpose is to ensure that all persons with disabilities may exercise the same rights and obligations as other citizens.
3. They outline crucial aspects of social policies in the disability field, and provide models for the political decision-making process required for the attainment of equal opportunities.
4. They propose national mechanisms for close collaboration between the State, organs of the UN, NGOs and DPOs.

OBJECTIVES OF THE STANDARD RULES

The objectives of the standard rules are to:

1. Stress that all action in the field of disability presupposes adequate knowledge and experience of the conditions and special needs of persons with disabilities;
2. Emphasize that the process through which every aspect of the organization of society is made accessible to all is a basic objective of socioeconomic development;
3. Outline crucial aspects of social policies in the field of disability, including, as appropriate, the active encouragement of technical and economic cooperation;

4. Provide models for the political decision-making process required for the attainment of equal opportunities, bearing in mind widely differing technical and economic levels, and the fact that the process must reflect keen understanding of the cultural context within which it takes place and the crucial role of persons with disabilities in it, and
5. Propose national mechanisms for close collaboration among states, the organs of the UN system, other inter-governmental bodies and organizations of persons with disabilities.

POLITICAL AND MORAL FOUNDATION

The International Bill of Human Rights comprises the Universal Declaration of Human Rights, the International Covenant on Economic, Social and Cultural Rights and the International Covenant on Civil and Political Rights, the Convention on the Rights of the Child and the Convention on the Elimination of All Forms of Discrimination against Women, as well as the World Program of Action concerning Disabled Persons. It constitutes the political and moral foundation for the standard rules on the equalization of opportunities for persons with disabilities. We should learn management from the local community, and principles of community work from existing co-operatives and development committees; we should learn to respect the abilities and experience of the local people, and listen carefully to their views. Hence, the principle is to look for what there is already and to learn from the people. This should be the point of departure of any development effort.

CHAPTER

4

Community-based Rehabilitation and Types of Evaluation

EVALUATION OF COMMUNITY-BASED REHABILITATION (CBR)

Evaluation means assessment. A working definition of evaluation of CBR refers to a standard to make objective judgments on the activities and outcomes of CBR program and the rehabilitation efficacy of people with disabilities in line with the goals, strategy, action plan, implementation of CBR program and the rehabilitation training scheme of the consumer. Generally speaking, there are three types of evaluation: goal evaluation, process evaluation and outcome evaluation. Relevance, effectiveness, efficiency, sustainability and impact are the core factors that should be considered in the evaluation of CBR.

Relevance

Does the program meet the needs and offer comprehensive rehabilitation services for people with disabilities and their families, and does it relevant to the program goals?

Effectiveness

Does the program achieve its objectives both in terms of quality and quantity, and does it make satisfactory result in service coverage and the rehabilitation efficacy of people with disabilities?

Efficiency

Does the program make the maximum outcome with the minimum income, and does it use the resource in the most efficient way?

Sustainability

Can the program continue once the external assistance is withdrawn?

Impact

What effect has the program had on its social settings, economic development, rehabilitation technique and institution, etc?

WHY EVALUATE A CBR PROGRAM?

Assess the pertinence, implementation process, effectiveness and efficiency in accordance with the action plan of CBR program.

Find out the changes happening in community development, attitude and sense to disability and rehabilitation, etc.

Judge whether the CBR service provided is effective, feasible, economical and practical.

Assess the cooperation among sectors of community, the implementation of CBR program, the approval, acceptance and participation of the community leaders, professionals, disabled people and their family members.

Identify whether the disabled people have achieved the rehabilitation goals.

Examine and explore the contents, methods, and process of evaluation in CBR program.

Systematic collect, analyses and interpret information about the activities and outcomes of CBR program in order to provide scientific basis for community leaders and person concerned.

In other words, the evaluation is a process of learning experience, drawing a lesson, revising plan, and improving ongoing program, a course of changing the evaluation management from traditional and experimental way to modern and scientific way, as well as a good chance of re-mobilization and re-guidance.

HOW TO EVALUATE A CBR PROGRAM?

For achieving the evaluation purpose mentioned above, it is necessary to follow the principles of evaluation and take appropriate evaluation measures.

Self-evaluation: The evaluators are said to be those who are inside the program or know the program very well. For examples, program administrators, executors, target people, service consumers, etc. They are familiar with the program and can make contribution to the evaluation activities.

Mutual-evaluation: The evaluation is made between (or among) two (or more) CBR programs. The evaluators come from outside their own community. They can exchange experiences, draw on each other's advantages and avoid disadvantages.

Higher authorities-evaluation: The evaluation is made by superior level departments that are in charge of the program. Therefore the program can get the understanding, support and suggestion from their higher authorities directly.

External-evaluation: The evaluation is carried out by organizations and persons from outside the country or the community. Outsiders can take a fresh look at the program and will not be personally involved, so the evaluation may be more objective.

Each type of evaluation has its own strengths and limitations. However, they should all be guided by the following principles: (a) be based on facts, (b) be comprehensive, (c) to include both quantitative and qualitative aspects, and (d) to include archival data and first hand field findings.

WHEN SHOULD THE EVALUATION BE DONE?

The development of CBR is an on-going process. For reaching the goals of a CBR program, there is a need for implementation to be in phases. Therefore, each phase's evaluation not only has to identify CBR program for the particular phase, but also improve the program's work for the next phase, and draw on the experiences and lessons for achieving the final goals of the CBR program.

There are many factors relating to the realization of rehabilitation goals for disabled people. The key factors are not the types and degrees of disabilities but the attitude towards disabled people, when the rehabilitation activities start, what kind of rehabilitation measures are used, and social factors, etc. For example, a person with visual impairment can reach a higher-level rehabilitation goal, but a person with better eyesight may only reach a lower level rehabilitation goal. Similarly, there is a need for achieving the best rehabilitation goal in each phase. Both evaluations for CBR program and individual consumer of CBR service should be an ongoing activity. Generally, evaluation should be built into the CBR program at regular intervals. For instance:

Monthly Evaluation

Evaluate in stages: 3-month, half a year, one year according to the program development.

Mid-term evaluation: It is essential to evaluate CBR program during the mid-time period. This is necessary to identify the problems based on the experience thus far and to make a decision on the activities to be carried out.

Eventual evaluation: Evaluation should be made at the end of the program, it should be the most important, detailed and overall of all the evaluation activities.

Follow-up evaluation: Some outcome or findings such as disability rate, attitude change, impact and sustainability can only be shown after a longer time. So, it is necessary to conduct evaluation at a specified future date.

Evaluation Process

(a) Making a detailed evaluation plan. (b) Collecting materials and conducting investigation. (c) Analysis results. (d) Making evaluation report, giving suggestion. (e) Feedback of results and putting them into practice.

WHAT KIND OF INFORMATION SHOULD BE KEPT?

The following is a list of the kind of information needed for evaluation: Community profile. Survey on a community profile can provide an outline or a brief description, and get basic information of a community, such as general description, ethnic, culture, religious, situation on socioeconomical development, environment, quality of life of disabled people, health and social activities, etc. People may think that they are familiar with their own community, and know it very well, but they may lack information, which is essential for a CBR program. So while paying attention to the survey of disabilities, we should not neglect the survey on the community profile.

A community profile includes the following contents:

i. *Geographical features of a community:* This tells about the location, size, area, resources, climates, etc.
ii. *Population:* This tells about the population size, nation, ethnic, cultural, religious, prevalence of diseases and disabilities, attitudes to disabled people, etc.
iii. *Physical and social environment:* This tells about the situation of economic, traffic, communication, barrier-free facilities, the number (the location, scale, equipment of hospitals, rehabilitation centers, schools, shelter workshops, welfare units, vocational training stations and recreation places, etc.
iv. *Institution and network:* This tells what you will need for launching CBR project, such as, the administrative set up, government departments, non-governmental organizations and implementation networks, for instance, primary health care network, social welfare network, disabled person's federation, women's organization, etc.
v. *Attitude towards people with disabilities:* Along with the socioeconomical development and social progress, the attitudes to people with disabilities have changed greatly. The word "attitude" has two meanings. One meaning is understanding, respect, care, help disabled people; another meaning is prejudice, discrimination, neglect, ignorance, refuse disabled people. Wrong attitudes will impede reaching the rehabilitation goals of disabled people and the progress of CBR program.
vi. *Map of a community with the lists of households:* The map should show roads, paths, fields, water sources markets, important rehabilitation places and all households in the program area and number in each household.

Survey of Disabled People in the Community

The survey of disabled people should include: The following contents:

i. General information of disabled person: Name, sex, age, nation, address, the name of household head, his/her work unit.

ii. The history of disability: The type and degree of disability, the causes of disability, rehabilitation or medical measures accepted and the assessment of abilities for living, learning working and social activity of disabled person.
iii. Rehabilitation needs: It includes needs that the disabled people may have in medical care, rehabilitation service, education, employment, participate family's life and social activities of disabled person. It is necessary to judge the priority among all the rehabilitation needs.
iv. Social aspects: It includes marriage status, family composition, source of income, employment status, attitude from family members and disabled person himself or herself, etc.

According to the individual information from the survey, we can analyze the following aspects:

i. The percentage of the number of households with disabled people in the total number of households surveyed.
ii. The percentage of people with disability in all people surveyed.
iii. Age distribution and age distribution according to their disability.
iv. Sex distribution and sex distribution according to their disability.
v. Statistics of disability types.
vi. Statistics of disability degree.
vii. Status analysis of disabled children.
viii. Income and employment status of disabled persons.
ix. Education level of disabled persons.
x. Marriage and family status of disabled persons.
xi. Rehabilitation needs according to their disability.
xii. The causes of disability according to disability type.

CBR Action Plan

CBR action plan is made according to the laws and regulations of the state and adapted to local conditions. Being a comprehensive developmental plan for CBR program, it includes the background of a community, situation analysis, expecting goals, activities, action measures, process, organization of implementation, financial management, monitoring, evaluation, and experience spread, etc. As an important part of a community developmental plan, CBR action plan is helpful to the overall evaluation of CBR.

Implementation Situation

i. Measure and process: It includes the action time, (year, month, date), place, measures, contents, goals, etc. For example, when was the CBR leading group established? Where is the office? Who are the members of leading group? What are the duty and task? etc.
ii. Executive organization and personnel: Who participate in the program? Who are the persons in charge of the program?, etc.
iii. Financial management: The budget, the source of fund, funding distribution and expenditure, etc.
iv. Monitoring and evaluation

Rehabilitation Training Record of Disabled People

A training file for disabled people should include:

i. General information of disabled people
ii. Rehabilitation program and suggestion
iii. Implementation of rehabilitation program "to find out if person need training and to assess progress")
iv. Comprehensive assessment in phase: According to the results of assessment at the first time, mid-time and eventual time, to give the mark of rehabilitation effect (high level, middle level and low level).
v. The new rehabilitation program of suggestion: According to the eventual evaluation results, revise the rehabilitation program and give suggestion. It marks the rehabilitation training and activities step in a new phase.

Statistical forms: According to all the requirement for CBR action plan, report the statistics results to sectors concerned level by level, statistics should be carried out at least half a year or every year. Statistics results are expected to show:

What changes have happened in number and services of institutions or units concerned CBR program? For instance, health facilities (health post, primary health center, district hospital, province hospital, national hospital or center); schools (pre-schools, primary schools, secondary schools, vocational training center's, special education schools or classes); recreation facilities, etc.

What changes have happened in number, function, service, length, payment of personnel in CBR program, such as administrators, professionals, local supervisors CBR workers, family guides, etc.

- Situation on making and implementation of laws (including regulations and local statutes)
- Situation on training staff in CBR number, contents, teaching methods, length of course, examination, evaluation (pre-course, after-course and follow-up) the effect of training course, etc.
- Changes happened in barrier-free facilities of road, buildings and house environment, etc.
- Changes happened in number of disabled persons in CBR program. Name, sex, age, type of disability, training activity and progress, etc.
- Changes of degree of disabilities. (slight, medium, severely).

The improvement rate of functional training for disabled persons, for instance, improvement in daily living care, behavior, communication, mobility, etc.

- Changes of schooling and education level; the rate of enrolment (or number) and the changes of individual in education level
- Changes of employment and income generation
- Changes in the role of family and participation in family life
- Changes of participation in social (community) life.

Keeping Evaluation Plans, Records and Reports

The evaluation plan should indicate the objectives, methods, contents, date and period, participants, results and suggestions. The evaluation report should contain: list of contents, acknowledgment, summary on the evaluation activities, general introduction on the CBR program, key discovery, analysis of results, conclusions and suggestions, appendix, references and footnotes.

A good evaluation report should following guidelines:

i. *Completeness:* It means the evaluation report should be detailed and comprehensive.
ii. *Preciseness:* It means the evaluation report should be accurate and no mistake.
iii. *Reliable:* It means the evaluation report should be real and objective.
iv. *Comparable:* It means the evaluation report can compare with the expecting goal of the CBR program or with other CBR program.

CHAPTER 5

Community Awareness and Communication

INTRODUCTION

Community awareness is essential tool of community health. The object of health awareness is to influence the people.

Health is defined as a state of complete physical, mental and social well-being and not merely absence of disease or infirmity so as to lead a socially and economically productive life.

Community participation and awareness is a process that informs, motivates and helps people to adopt and maintain healthy practices and lifestyles, advocates environmental changes as needed to facilitate this goal and conducts professional training and research to the same end.

OBJECTIVE OF THE COMMUNITY AWARENESS

Informing the People

- Disseminating scientific knowledge about prevention of disease and promotion of health
- Melts away barriers of ignorance, prejudice and misconceptions of the people
- Creates an awareness of health needs and problems and also responsibilities of the people.

Motivating the People

- To change their habits and ways of living
- Alteration of behavior in health practices which are detrimental to health, e.g. water pollution, outdoor defecation, alcoholism, smoking drug addiction, physical in activities.

Guiding into Action

- Encouraging people to use judiciously wisely the health services available to them.

APPROACHES TO COMMUNITY AWARENESS

- *Regulatory approach:* A legal approach to protect health of public through the enforcement of laws and regulations.
- *Service approach:* Provides facilities needed by the community, so that people use them to improve their health.
- *Educational approach:* Major means for achieving changes in health practices and recognition of health needs involve, motivation communication, decision making.

CONTENT OF COMMUNITY AWARENESS

- Human biology
- Nutrition
- Hygiene—personal and environmental
- Family health care
- Control of communicable and noncommunicable diseases
- Mental health
- Prevention of accidents
- Use of health service.

PRINCIPLE OF COMMUNITY AWARENESS

Community awareness bring together the art and science of the medicine and the principle and practice of general education

1. *Interest:* People are unlikely to listen those things which are not to their interest. People will listen to those things which are of their interest, meaningful and it should be their felt need, so educator find out their real health needs and educate. Then only the people will participate and the program become successful. Suppose the felt

need is not known to the people because of illiteracy. The educator should bring about the recognition of felt needs of the people.

2. *Participation:* Key word in community awareness based on the psychological principle of active learning better then passive learning. No health program will be successful without the participation of public. For that they must be motivated to participate by the health workers and social workers.
3. *Known to unknown:* That means the health education is given to the people from a level. Start where the people are and with what they know and understand and then proceeded to new knowledge, use existing knowledge as pegs on which to hang new facts which give insight into the problem. However, it is long process.
4. *Comprehension:* This means educating the people at a level they can understand and preferably in the same language they speak and avoiding difficult and strange words teaching should be done in mental capacity of the audience. Before educating the people must know the level of understanding, literacy and education of the people. Cut down barriers by sueing words that cannot be understood.
5. *Reinforcement:* This means repetition of the same message periodically, preferably in different ways, so that the audience can understand it better and remember longer. Otherwise they may go back to the preawareness state repetition at intervals is extremely useful.
6. *Motivation:* It is Awaking the fundamental desire among the people to learn.

   They can be motivated easily by giving incentives, which may be negative or positive. For example, if an obese woman is told to reduce her body weight because of the complication of coronary artery disease, it may have little effect. On the other hand if she is told that by reducing her weight she may look more beautiful and charming, she may accept with pleasure. Motivation is contagious. One motivated person may motivate an entire group of unvasectomized persons.
7. *Learning by doing:* An action process. This makes the person perfect. The Chinese proverb, " if I hear, I forget, if I see I remember and if I do, I know", illustrates the importance of learning by doing
8. *Good human relations:* Building good human relationship with the audience, makes the health education successful. Which is almost importance in learning?

9. *Leaders:* Leaders are agents of change. When they should be able to respect and regards. Understand needs and a demand of the community. Provides proper guidance, takes, initiative, receptive to the view and suggestions of the people. Identifies himself with the community, honest and impartial, possessing requisite skill and knowledge of eliciting cooperation and achieving coordination of various official and nonofficial organizations. Involvement of local leaders will make the education more easy and effective.

COMMUNICATION

Key element in the community awareness is the communication, communication is a complex process in which a source of information (sender) gives the information (Message) through various channels (Media) to the audience (receiver) and in turn gets the feedback to know the effect of the process (Fig. 5.1).

Sender

Sender is the communicator or originator of the message and should know the audience, the message to be given and the methods or channels to communicate.

The effect of communication depends upon the efficiency of the communicator.

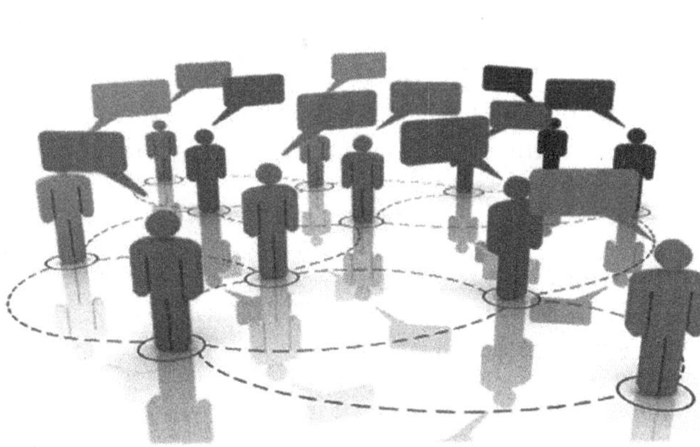

Fig. 5.1: Community network *(For color version see plate 1)*

Message

It is the "technical know- how" of the information being communicated to the audience. They should understand, accept and act upon the message should be clear, understandable, interesting, meaningful, related to the objective, specific, precise and acceptable by the audience.

Media, it is the channel bridges between the sender and the audience there are three **systems of media**

- *Interpersonal communication:* Face-to-face communication. It is very effective.
- *Mass media:* TV, radio, printed media and others. Advantage of this type of media is that large number of people can be reached. And disadvantage of this is that it is not very effective in bringing about the changes.
- *Traditional or folk media:* Drama, puppetry folk dance, song, Harikatha, Burakatha in AP, Nautanki in UP. These type are also close to cultural values and therefore they are very effective.

Audience

The receiver may be a single person or a group of people. If the audience is a homogenous group and have a common interest, it is called controlled audience, otherwise it is called uncontrolled or free audience.

Feedback

It is reverse flow of information or remarks made by the audience about the message to the sender, so that the sender can make modifications and improve the communication to make it more effective and acceptable to the audience.

TYPES OF COMMUNICATION

One-way Communication

It is also called *didactic methods.* In this type, the message flows in only one direction, i.e. from the communicator to the audience, e.g. delivering the lecture in a class room. The demerits are that:

- There is no participation from the receiver
- There is no feedback
- Information is imposed
- Learning is passive
- Less likely to influence the human behavior.

Two-way Communication

It is called *Socratic Method.* In this type, both the communicator and the audience take part. Audience may ask questions and they may give their own suggestions. thus the communication become active, effective and democratic. This method is more likely to influence the human behavior.

Verbal Communication

This is giving the information by talk, and not by showing written printed matter. It is more persuasive.

Nonverbal Communication

In this type, the message is communicated not by talk but body movement, posture facial expressions (smile, sorrow, staring, etc.) Often this is also effective.

Formal Communication

This consists of form like: toys, games, songs, etc.

Informal Communication

Information is given by rigid courses.

Visual Communication

Visual communication consists of charts, posters, pictures, graphs, tables, maps, etc.

Telecommunication and Internet

This is done by using electromagnetic instrument and the communication is done over distance. For example, radio, TV, internet, etc. Telephone, telex, telegraph are known as point-to-point telecommunication system. Launching of satellites is an advanced technology in the telecommunication system.

BARRIERS OF COMMUNICATION

There are certain barriers between the educator and the audience. Which will interface with the communication, these are:

Physiological Barriers

Difficulties in behavior and expression.

Psychological Barriers

Emotional disturbances, neurosis, low level of intelligence, language difficulties.

Environmental Registration

There are many environmental barriers like noise, overcrowding, invisibility.

Cultural Barriers

Cultural barriers are as follows:
Illiteracy, customs, beliefs, religion attitude, poverty, cultural difficulties between rural and urban, etc. to make communication successful, these barriers must be identified and removed.

COMMUNITY DEMAND ON PHYSIOTHERAPY SERVICES

Physiotherapy with its unique nonpharmacological exercise-oriented natural approach has assumed the role of a nonseparate entity factors like highly sedentary mechanical lifestyle and increased rate of trauma due to modernization industrialization and increased automobiles are the challenges faced by physiotherapists. The science of physical therapy has tremendous potential to face these goals due to its preventive therapeutic and restorative functions (Fig. 5.2).

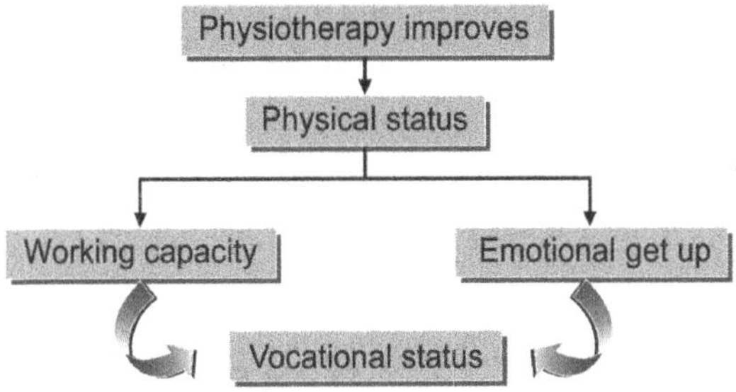

Fig. 5.2: Showing importance of physiotherapy

PHYSIOTHERAPY HELPS

- To corelate patient's problems daily routine and offers sounds advice on posture and movements detrimental to the problem.
- Guidance for simple home treatment program which may include easy methods of fermentation or cryotherapy for pain relief
- To provide guidelines to avoid recurrence.

Physiotherapy contributes not only for physical independence but also as a argumentive force to improve vocational professionals and psychological status to attain social security. Vocational placement of patients is directly depending on degree of restoration of physical independence and working capacity achievement of three aspects, i.e. physical, vocational and psychological aspects which ultimately lead to the social security.

CHAPTER

6

Self-help Group and Various Aspects

DEFINITION

Self-help group (SHG) is a small voluntary association of poor people, preferably from the same socioeconomic background. They come together for the purpose of solving their common problems through self-help and mutual help. The SHG promotes small savings among its members. The savings are kept with a bank.

Self-help group (SHG) is a village-based financial intermediary committee usually composed of 10–20 local women or men. A mixed group is generally not preferred. Most self-help groups are located in India, though SHGs can be found in other countries, especially in South Asia and Southeast Asia.

Members make small regular savings contributions over a few months until there is enough capital in the group to begin lending. Funds may then be lent back to the members or to others in the village for any purpose. In India, many SHGs are 'linked' to banks for the delivery of microcredit.

Self-help group is a successful strategy, which is now being used by both NGO's and government to get optimum community participation.

Self-help group—a useful strategy to get the community to Participate.

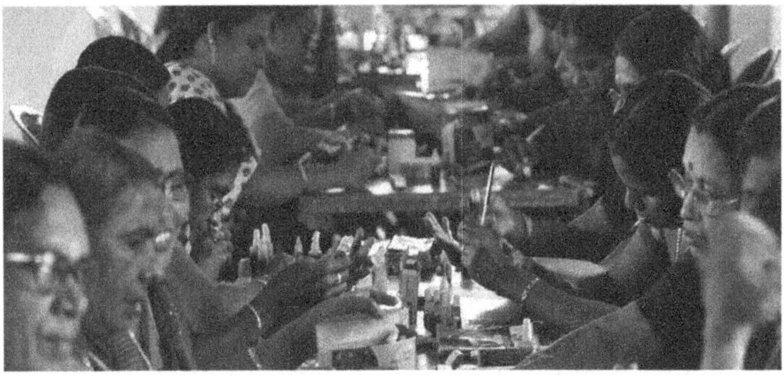

Fig. 6.1: Self-help group for women *(For color version see Plate 1)*

Self-help group is basically a strategy, which could be used in almost all areas of community development. Self-help groups are built on the strengths that are inherent in the families and the community. People of "common interests" form groups. SHG are heterogeneous because it can cut across caste/creed/and socioeconomic barriers. SHG consist of grassroots level workers who have firsthand knowledge about their problems. Since they are "Stake Holders" their participation is not only active but also very participatory.

SHG are also successful in creating simple employment opportunities for young people. These grassroots level people are adequately trained and rightly oriented to meet the needs of people in their own communities. Self-help groups are a strategy, which help people to move from charity to development perspective. Perspective to development and self-reliance through sharing community organization.

SHG is basically a strategy, which is used to address various issues in the community.

OBJECTIVES OF SELF-HELP GROUPS

Self-help groups provide a forum for people with disabilities in rural/ tribal areas.

The objectives of self-help groups (mutual support groups of people with disabilities) are:

- To provide a forum for sharing experiences and identification of needs concerning the individual and the community. It identifies strength and abilities and builds on them.

- To act as a nodal organization to meet the immediate needs of adults with disabilities.
- To facilitate mutual support in times of crisis.
- To promote self and group advocacy and networks with other advocacy groups.

PRINCIPLES OF SELF-HELP GROUP

The underlying principle of all self-help groups is same. They are:

1. Beneficiaries should be active participants in the project formulation and implementation
2. A feeling of sharing and mutual trust
3. A social responsibility to meet the needs of the community while meeting individual needs
4. Participation of people who are marginalized (women/people with disabilities/scheduled caste and schedule tribes)
5. To help each other in the times of crises
6. Flexibility in the approach
7. Social/cultural relevance
8. Absence of hierarchy and linear power structures. All are equal in self-help groups.

CHARACTERISTIC OF SELF-HELP GROUP

- Small size
- Identical interest/social heritage/common occupation, homogeneity, affinity
- Intimate knowledge of members intrinsic strength, needs and problems
- Flexible and responsive
- Democracy in operations
- Simple documentation
- Collective leadership, mutual discussion
- Group solidarity, self-help, awareness, social and economic empowerment.

Self-help Group Promoting Institutions (SHGPI)

- *NGOs:* NGOs are trust or societies which promote SHGs for bank linkage.

- *Banks:* Banks are themselves SHGPIs when branch staff themselves promote SHGs. From scratch, and then mobilize their savings and lend to them.
- *VVVs:* These are farmer's clubs which have been set up, usually with assistance from National Bank for Agriculture and Rural Development (NABARD). And initially to improve the credit culture in their community.
- *Government agencies:* It is a term which covers wide range of state and central government entities which have started to promote SHGs under various schemes.
- *Self-employed individuals:* They are people who promote SHGs not as employees or members of an institution but as individual.

KEY FEATURES OF THE SELF-HELP GROUP

Self-help/small saving credit groups are successfully implemented by NGO's.

It enables people to have access to small credit without going through the process of providing securities or guarantors. The self-help credit groups are very useful, to families from lower economic strata to get soft loans to start small enterprises. The SHG also provides technical training to its members to ensure the success of the entrepreneurship initiative. Since the members of SHG are the decision takers they plan and implement the project, which is locally relevant and sustainable by the community.

SHG for Women

SHG for women are able to address issues specifically concerning issues concerning women. SHG are finding local solutions to problems of child care crèche facilities of working women in villages, drinking water and sanitation issues, education of children, health of women and children and other issues concerning women. Some SHG members are trained in counseling skills and provide counseling service to women within the community.

Well-planned EDP programs/identification of jobs/market needs/ marketing of the produces/networking are some of the features of successful self-help groups.

SHG of Families with a Child with Disability

Families with a member with disability live in isolation and seclusion. They often go from one medical man to another in search of a quick cure. They go in search of miracle solution. It is always late in the day when they realize that they have been taken for a ride. Since families with a disabled member are scattered they do not get support from each other in the absence of self-help groups.

Many NGO's promote self-help for families with a member with disability. These Shags have four objectives. They are:

1. Meeting the special needs of the child (By transfer of simple rehabilitation skills to the families and community volunteers)
2. Helping each other in sharing the care of severely disabled children.
3. Helping each other in the times of crises
4. Self-help and group advocacy for positive community attitudes and policy makers. There are over 100 SHG, which are successfully managed by families/community in our country.

Self-help Groups of Adults with Disability

The purpose of any CBR program is to empower people with disabilities. The process of empowerment of adults with disability and families with a member with mental handicap essentially depends on well-defined plans and strategies to promote and sustain self-help groups in their own communities.

The advocacy groups are by and large based. But in reality, more than 80% of people with disabilities live in rural areas. That is why we need self-help groups in rural areas. Empowerment is an ongoing process, which enables an individual to fulfill his duties, responsibilities and protect her/his rights in the society.

CBR and Empowerment

Empowerment of people with disabilities is the ultimate goal of any CBR program. The road to empowerment compels the community to create and promote equal opportunities, so that people with disabilities get an access to: Health services, education, housing facilities, work placements, emotional security, family bonds, marriage, leisure/free personal time, recreation and other needs. And above all, the right to choose-full participation in decision-making on, issues concerning self, family, community. Adults with disability have specific needs. The SHG of adults with disabilities is a part of many CBR projects.

The objectives of these SHG are:

- Meeting ability-training needs of people with disabilities.
- Promoting self and group employment of people with disabilities.
- Meeting needs for active social integration (in sports/cultural activities/leisure activities, etc.)
- Arranging marriages of people with disabilities
- Self-help group advocacy for favorable public attitude and public policies.

SHG for Women with Disability

Women with disabilities are poorest of the poor in any community and they are most marginalized. The problems of women with disabilities are many fold. Lack of education/health/low status/poverty is some of the important issues.

SHG for women is slowly picking up the momentum in CBR projects. The objectives of these self-help groups are same as SHG for adults but with an additional focus on specific issues concerning women.

SHG for Senior Citizens

The population of geriatric group is fast increasing. By the end of 2000 in India, we will have over 12 million senior citizens. Old age homes segregate people away from the families and the community. The self-help groups of senior citizens are very useful, and this has been successfully tested by NGOs in India. These self-help/mutual aid groups have four objectives:

1. To assist senior citizens in the day-to-day life such as payment of bills/escort services/shopping assistance, etc.
2. To assist senior citizens who have vast knowledge and skills to participate in community development activities.
3. To assist senior citizens to get geriatric healthcare.
4. To assist senior citizens to avail benefits such as pensions/assistive devices.

How to promote self-help groups in CBR program:

1. Start in a known village.
2. Discuss with adults with disability (above 16 years).
3. What is a self-help group?
4. The need to start self-help groups
5. Explain the objectives of a self-help group.
6. Let the group meet once a week at a place convenient, which could be one of the homes of a disabled member. Let the group identify a facilitator for arranging meetings, sending information, documenting the proceedings, etc.
7. Organize together with them first level leaders advancement workshop with all members with disability.
8. Let the group identify and classify the needs and problems into individual, family and problems, which are common to all disabled people in the entire village. It is necessary on South Asian context for women with disabilities to meet exclusively and join the general group once a week. (The frequency of the meetings; weekly self-help group meetings is ideal).
9. Strategic plans to meet; the needs should be planned and implemented systematically with cooperative efforts of the members in the groups.
10. Self-help groups activities should flow like a river finding its own coarse. There is no Need to give formal set-up to self-help groups by giving labels, and designations should be avoided. The principle of equality within the group is likely to organize successful self-help groups.

    A core committee should not be formed but it should evolve as an outcome of selfless efforts of concerned people with commitments, who should consistently and collectively work, to find solutions to the problems of people with disability.

Some activities, which SHGs can take up in a village:

- Working collectively as a group to start self and small group employment agencies
- To start regular recreation groups
- To establish counseling centers
- Initiate distant education, braille and talking libraries, toy libraries, learning materials and other useful equipment

- Create an information center especially for government schemes
- Build-up pressure groups
- Promote trusts of families and members with disability with severely disabled members to find solutions to problems of care and support after their parents' death.

Resources for Self-help Groups/Mutual Support

- Voluntary services of adults with disabilities and families of members with disability
- Existing facilities available in the village community such as school building
- Community building, integrating recreation activities into the existing recreation center's
- Government's schemes for poverty alleviation to assist in self and group
- Employments, insurances for mentally handicapped persons, self-help group loans to the members
- Mobilizing family trades and local employers to generate employments for the disabled members is in the group.

Eligibility

All disabled adults above 16 years, parents and siblings can become members, if the member of their family with disability has severe mental handicap. People with mental handicap should be encouraged to participate in all the activities of self-help group and importance should be given to the opinions and suggestion that concerns their lives. At least 50% of the members should be women.

Panchayat Raj System is one example of decentralization of policy decision-making and implementation of all development programs.

Nongovernment organizations (voluntary organizations) have played an important role in creating public awareness, promoting self-advocacy/group advocacy, and implementing government development programs.

Advantages of Financing through SHGs

- An economically poor individual gains strength as part of a group
- Besides, financing through SHGs reduces transaction costs for both lenders and borrowers

- While lenders have to handle only a single SHG account instead of a large number of small-sized individual accounts, borrowers as part of an SHG cut down expenses on travel (to and from the branch and other places) for completing paper work and on the loss of workdays in canvassing for loans.
- Where successful, SHGs have significantly empowered poor people, especially women, in rural areas.

GENESIS OF SELF-HELP GROUPS

In India, Mahatma Gandhi emphasized the need for self-reliance and self-sustainable villages as early as the beginning of this century. The concept of self-help and Gram Swaraj are not foreign concepts to us.

The ancient village management system was also based on the principle of "sharing and caring".

Somewhere along the line, after independence, people started playing the role of "recipient of services and benefits" and became beneficiaries. This passive role of the community did not help in sustaining the projects.

Neither government nor the community can afford to start separate services for separate sets of people. Self-help mutual aid groups help to meet different needs of the community without disintegrating families from their communities.

There has been an increasing realization that the chances of sustaining programs without the community's participation at all levels of implementation are close to nil. The decentralization of power structures/increased number of grassroots NGO projects has strengthened the learning that community should be involved right from project conceptualization to implementation/evaluation stage.

Various project-planning skills such as rural appraisals/logical framework analysis, etc. were developed to ensure community participation in planning of projects.

The formation of self-help groups in almost all development programs addressing different issues and in varying degrees is one of the most important developments. This has resulted in a major shift

- From charity to development perspective
- From service providers to the role of facilitators/catalyst agents
- Transfer of skills to grassroots

- From role of passive beneficiary to active participant in the development process
- Preventing segregation and promoting integration
- Community ownership of projects is the key to sustainability

Projects did not develop into programs with community initiative as expected. Many evaluation reports of projects revealed that a prominent lacuna in the project was lack of community participation, as communities did not own these projects at all. In the middle of this, there was a new experimental trend by NGOs in which community not only participated, but also owned the entire project.

CHAPTER

7

Present Rehabilitation Services in India

INTRODUCTION

Alma Ata declaration on 1978 stated that comprehensive primary health care should include promotive, preventive, curative, and rehabilitative care. There are three approaches to rehabilitation, namely institution-based, outreach-based, and community-based. The major objective of community-based rehabilitation (CBR) is to ensure that people with disabilities are able to maximize their physical and mental abilities, have access to regular services and opportunities, and achieve full integration within their communities. CBR is a comprehensive approach at primary health care level used for situations where resources for rehabilitation are available in the community. In addition to transfer of knowledge related to skill development in various types of rehabilitation methods, community also will be involved in planning, decision making, and evaluation of the program with multisectoral coordination. Besides, referral system will be there for those disabled who cannot be managed at community level and referred to district, provincial, and national levels.

Disability limitation at early stage when they are amenable to preventive and rehabilitative measures, so that progression to severe disability can be minimized is a vital component in rehabilitation of disabled. It has shown that very few disabled people gets benefit from rehabilitation services in India. In general, of people with disability, 1/3 needs no rehabilitation, 1/3 can be helped through CBR alone and 1/3 needs specialized referral services. Basic principles of a CBR program for the disabled include inclusion, participation, sustainability, empowerment, and advocacy. These principles are overlapping, complementary, and interdependent and they cannot be addressed in isolation.

There are many measures initiated by Ministry of Social Justice and Empowerment and Health and Family Welfare in India.

DISTRICT REHABILITATION CENTER (DRC) PROJECT STARTED IN 1985

1. Four Regional Rehabilitation Training Centers (RRTC) have been functioning under the DRCs scheme at Mumbai, Chennai, Cuttack, and Luck now since 1985 for the training of village level functionaries and DRCs professionals, orientation and training of State Government officials, research in service delivery, and low cost aids. Apart from developing training material and manuals for actual field use, RRTCs also produce material for creating community awareness through the medium of folders, posters, audio-visuals, films, and traditional forms.
2. National Information Center on Disability and Rehabilitation
3. National council for Handicapped Welfare
4. National Level Institutes—National Institute for Mentally Handicaped (NIMH), National Institute for the Hearing Handicaped (NIHH), National Institute for the Visually Handicaped (NIVH), National Institute for the Orthopedically Handicaped (NIOH), Institute for the Physically Handicaped (IPH).
5. A new scheme District Disability Rehabilitation Center for persons with disabilities launched by the Honorable Minister of Social Justice and Empowerment, Government of India in Jan/Feb 2000 is a step towards providing rehabilitation services and implementation of Persons with Disability Act, 1995. The Government has decided to set up District Disability Rehabilitation Centers (DDRCs) in a phased manner. Presently, 199 DDRCs have been sanctioned and 100 new DDRCs are to be set up during the remaining two years of the 11th Plan. The DDRCs were established with the objective of providing comprehensive services to the persons with disabilities at the grass root level. The services

include awareness generation, survey, identification and early intervention, counseling, assessment of need for assistive devices, provision/fitment of assistive devices, and their follow-up/repair, therapeutic services like physiotherapy, occupational therapy and speech therapy, referral and arrangement for surgical correction through government and charitable institutions, facilitation of issue of disability certificates and bus passes, sanction of bank loans, and promotion of barrier-free environment.

6. The National Policy for Persons with Disability, 2005 is the recent development and welcome step by the Government of India.

SERVICE DELIVERY SYSTEM FOR COMMUNITY-BASED REHABILITATION

This will require coordinated efforts by ministries, local, district and provincial authorities, and nongovernmental organizations in the different sectors involved in rehabilitation. For the majority of the disabled (70%), interventions can be done effectively at the community level by local supervisors/school teachers. A recent study among mentally disabled adolescents showed that psychosocial intervention increases the quality of life and reduces the disability severity. Additional services should be set up in response to the needs of the community. At district or provincial level which caters around 20% of the disabled requires general physicians, intermediate level supervisors, orthopedic technicians, resource teachers and vocational trainers. National level professionals will be involved in delivery of complex rehabilitation services as well as training and supervision of personnel for district, provincial, and national levels. Disabled individuals in the community face many social problems. Improving the quality of life of people with different grades of various types of disabilities is a difficult and challenging task. Disabled individuals will be neglected in the community because of inaccessibility to services and lack of opportunities like health services, schools, vocational education programs, and jobs. In Chamarajnagar, Karnataka, a local nongovernmental organization (NGO) assisted people with disability and their families to construct accessible toilets. Besides, social segregation of disabled is common in the community. This is because of deep rooted fears and beliefs acquired from cultural and religious factors. Overall in reality, it is a social problem where the disabled becomes a liability to the society. For improving the quality of life of persons with disabilities, research will be supported on their socioeconomic and cultural context, cause of disabilities, early childhood education methodologies, development of user-friendly aids and appliances, and all matters connected with disabilities which will significantly alter the quality of their life and civil society's ability to respond to their felt needs.

BARRIERS TO ACCESSIBILITY FOR PEOPLE WITH DISABILITY

Barriers are obstacles. Barriers to accessibility are obstacles that make it difficult sometimes impossible for people with disabilities to do the things most of us take for granted things like going shopping, working, or taking public transit.

When we think of barriers to accessibility, most of us think of physical barriers like a person who uses a wheelchair not being able to enter a public building because there is no ramp.

The fact is there are many kinds of barriers. Some are visible. Many are invisible.

TYPE OF BARRIERS

Attitudinal

Attitudinal barriers are those that discriminate against people with disabilities.

Examples:

- Thinking that people with disabilities are inferior
- Assuming that a person who has a speech impairment cannot understand you.

Information or Communications

Information or communications barriers happen when a person cannot easily understand information.

Examples:

- Print is too small to read
- Websites that cannot be accessed by people who are not able to use a mouse
- Signs that are not clear or easily understood.

Technology Barriers

Technology barriers occur when a technology cannot be modified to support various assistive devices.

Examples:

- A website that does not support screen-reading software.

Organizational Barriers

Organizational barriers are an organization's policies, practices or procedures that discriminate against people with disabilities.

Examples:

- A hiring process that is not open to people with disabilities.

Architectural and Physical Barriers

Architectural and physical barriers are features of buildings or spaces that cause problems for people with disabilities.

Examples:

- Hallways and doorways that are too narrow for a person using a wheelchair, electric scooter or walker
- Counters that are too high for a person of short stature
- Poor lighting for people with low vision
- Doorknobs that are difficult for people with arthritis to grasp
- Parking spaces that are too narrow for a driver who uses a wheelchair
- Telephones that are not equipped with telecommunications devices for people who are deaf, deafened or hard of hearing.

CHAPTER

8

Needs of People with Disability

A thorough study of disabled people's needs should be the starting point of any plan for a rehabilitation program. In the past, few such studies were made in the developing countries. Instead, experts straightaway proposed technical solutions, construction of facilities and training of personnel. Services were supplied in accordance with conventional ideas rather than with realities. People's needs are manifold, and each society sees its priorities differently. The problems are many. Examples are lack of clean and safe water and basic sanitary conditions, proper nutrition, inadequate education, lack of jobs, poverty, difficulties in communication, access to health care, security concerns, and repression of human rights. These problems are not unique to disabled people, but are shared by other community members. Rehabilitation needs are specific to disabled people. In the developing countries, rural communities are often very well-organized, their members sharing the same values and traditions, with a close-knit network of social relations providing support and protection. This does not work to quite the same extent for marginal urban settlements, but even there one finds a local culture and a power structure, but far less social control. For anyone intending to study the needs of disabled people, it is essential to have an understanding of the social structures, the cultural traditions, the organization and the lines of authority prevailing in the communities where they live. This knowledge can only be acquired from people who have been living in the particular community for a long time, who share the culture, and who are familiar with local conditions.

Outsiders will need many years of experience, and to evaluate the specific needs of disabled people they must work with the local people. Where a rehabilitation program is to be managed by the community, utilizing its own resources, it is vital for it to be planned, structured and implemented in line with local customs and needs. This implies that any general rehabilitation program should be described in such a way as to allow both adaptations to local conditions and preservation of local influence. It should build on existing technology, allow for a service delivery system opted for by the community and apply a management system that fits into traditional approaches. This will facilitate the integration of programs designed to meet the specific needs of disabled people.

TYPES OF NEEDS

The term "needs" may be used in various ways. In this context, we will distinguish between three different types of needs.

(1) Felt needs (2) Expressed needs (3) Assessed needs

1. *Felt needs* are those verbalized directly or indirectly by the disabled person or his/her family or community or needs observed over a long-term period, preferably by a community member.
2. *Expressed needs* are those manifested by the disabled person and his/her family by the search for help in solving the particular problem. The help could come through traditional healers, religious or community leaders, or modern medicine or specialized facilities.
3. *Assessed needs* are the rehabilitation needs assessed by a person with professional training in rehabilitation. To be able to give a qualified opinion as to the likely outcome of rehabilitative measures undertaken in the disabled person carrying out this assessment must have experience from developing countries.

These needs should be studied before starting to design a technology. In the past, the "felt" and "expressed" needs tended to be neglected. Also, most experts (expatriates and nationals alike) did not take the trouble to visit homes and communities of disabled people when assessing needs and evaluating the likelihood of success of proposed interventions. Mostly, they based their views on studies of institutions for disabled people, of school populations, or of the working population, which are not very representative. In the text below, some experience of studies, observations and conclusions on the subject of needs will be presented.

The way people in the developing countries verbalize their needs is culture-dependent. Often, they employ specific words or expressions to indicate symptoms, difficulties and problems, many of which relate to the interpretations or ascribed causes made locally. Hence, direct answers to a list of Western medical or social questions may not tell the whole story. What is striking, however, is the very high proportion of people with health complaints and the long-term duration of those complaints.

When taking "expressed needs" into consideration, one has to understand how some of these have emerged through a sometimes-lengthy process. There is a risk that such expressions may be distorted by traditional attitudes and by frustration. They have to be evaluated with caution. It may prove advisable to analyze the initially "felt" needs instead and to start by designing individual rather than collective solutions. The identification of "expressed needs" is a positive sign. It shows that the disabled people themselves, their families and their organizations are taking an active part in the search for a solution.

Most commonly felt needs concerning disabled people in developing countries

Functional problems in daily life activities

- Self-care (eating, drinking, dressing, keeping clean)
- Mobility
- Communication, comprehension, ability to follow instructions
- Behavior
- Educational needs
- Ability training.

Needs for income-generating activities

- Participation in household duties, jobs, self-employment
- Lack of family and social integration
- Concerns relating to participation and representation in community affairs
- Security needs (protection against abuse, promotion of human and legal rights)
- Schooling.

DISABLED WOMEN

Although 70–80 percent of the disabled in developing countries, including those of Asia, live in rural areas, most of the programs for the disabled cater to the urban population. It is also evident that most of the program beneficiaries are men, in spite of the fact that many of them are 'gender neutral' and may even have a female bias in traditional terms. Most of the activities are related to self-employment or to employment in small and cottage industries (e.g. tailoring, cane furniture). For rural disabled women, there seems to be a considerable potential for small industrial activities.

There are a number of reasons to assume that disability causes more problems to women than to men. These are summarized in WPA as follows:

"The consequences of deficiencies and disablement are particularly serious for women. There are many countries where women are subjected to social, cultural and economic disadvantages, which impede their access to, for example, health care, education, vocational training and employment. If, in addition, they are physically or mentally disabled their chances of overcoming their disablement are diminished, which makes it all the more difficult for them to take part in community life. In families, the responsibility for caring for a disabled parent often lies with women, which considerably limits their freedom and their possibilities of taking part in other activities."

Seventy-seven recommendations of actions to take on behalf of disabled women have been taken by the participants of a Seminar on Women and Disability, held at UNCSDHA, at Vienna, in 1990. A few of these are reproduced below; these concern ethics and human rights.

Disabled women should be informed of their civil and human rights in order to be able to make their own decisions.

Appropriate legislation that guarantees the full exercise of the rights of women to decide on sexuality, pregnancy, new reproductive technology, adoption, motherhood and any other relevant issue should be adopted and implemented.

No medical decisions concerning a disabled woman should be made without her informed consent.

Measures should be adopted to protect women with mental or learning disabilities and information should be provided in a manner that they can easily understand. When appropriate, an advocate should be provided to facilitate the decision-making of such women.

Open and public discussions on topics such as sexuality, which are often considered too delicate to deal with, should be encouraged, with due respect to cultural norms, in order to increase the level of knowledge of disabled women, their families, professional staff and the general population.

In countries where cultural and religious traditions make access to medical, vocational, rehabilitative and other services and to employment for disabled women difficult, measures should be taken to ensure that these obstacles are removed, so that disabled girls and women can receive those benefits.

Development and application of new reproductive technologies to prevent disabilities should be seen in terms of ethical and human rights.

SPECIAL ISSUES CONCERNING DISABLED WOMEN

Dr Fatima Shah, President of the International Federation of the Blind, and herself blind, lists the "special issues" concerning disabled women, as follows:

a. Attitudes and prejudices of the public including family, community and even the government, which are stereotyped and negative towards disability.
b. Lack of mobility, isolation, confinement to the house. Socio-cultural patterns, and traditions stronger and more effective than legislation itself, are conducive towards creating this situation more acutely for females than males.
c. Lack of education and training. Generally, the percentage of literacy amongst women is lower than [amongst] men in most of the countries in this region. In the case of women with disability, it touches the lowest mark. Economic dependence on the male members of the family, lack of training and employment.
e. Lack of environmental adjustment, rendering mobility for the physically disabled very difficult.
f. Lack of equipment, necessary to cope with the disability, i.e. wheelchairs, prostheses, hearing aids, etc.
g. Poor health due to malnutrition, lack of activity, poverty and ignorance.
h. *Marriage:* This is a much greater problem for women with disability than it is for men, due to sociocultural patterns and the concept of a woman's physical image of marriage. This deprives her of her

traditional role and status as a wife and a mother, and combined with total economic dependence, she is relegated to the position of a non-person in the family and community.

i. *Motherhood:* If she is married and has children, she is not considered fit to look after them, which naturally deprives her of a role important for her emotional satisfaction and personal dignity.
j. *Severe frustration, inferiority complex:* Lack of opportunities and access to education and training for self-improvement and independence destroys the self-confidence, self-image and self-esteem due to the concept of her physical body image dominating the sociocultural pattern.
k. Noninvolvement in self-help movements at all levels.

AGING AND DISABILITY

At old age, many people suffering from a terminal disease have activity restrictions during a period before they die. For some this disability period lasts only a few days or weeks, but for others it is longer. It is not easy to draw a line and to decide who will be counted as a "newly disabled" person and will consequently be included in the annual incidence. For other people, the experience is that disability sets in gradually and may be seen as "normal ageing," "wear and tear," and the point at which a person enters the group of moderately and severely disabled people is not easy to decide. CBR programs should address the needs of senior citizens with disability.

CHAPTER

9

Community and Social Work Principles

COMMUNITY

Community is one of the concepts created by the social scientists for research. The word community is interpreted differently by different people. It is essential that we understand what differentiates society from community.

SOCIETY-COMMUNITY

Society is an organization set up to promote and sustain mutual human relations. When we talk of relations, we mean relations between individuals, relations between individuals and groups and relations between different groups. Social organization protects the freedom of the people and at the same time checks their licence. People live as per their traditions and behavioral patterns. Society is an ever changing set up.

Community is one of the manifestations of society. It is visible. Human settlements, village, town and even the entire world are the different forms of community.

Community has its own characteristics. They can be classified into physical and social. Physical characteristics decide the geographical boundaries of human settlements. Thus, community is a region where people live together carrying on their vocations for their living. Physical environment of the community consists of land, different forms of the mud, wild life forests, minerals, domestic animals, buildings, instruments used in industries.

Social environment includes people's economic, political, cultural, religious and mental activities. People living in a community live in social units like different religious groups, families; different communities with different characteristics mingle and bring about mutual influence on one another. Industrialization and modernization have blurred the boundaries between communities. In spite of the communities influencing one another, they have maintained their distinctive features.

Community living is a colorful variety. People of a community do not and need not depend on its internal resources for their wants. They go out of the community, mingle with others to eke out their livelihood. But still there is a sort of belonging and endearment with their own community believing that their community nurtured and nourished their forefathers.

COMMUNITY PRIDE (SENTIMENT)

The mere aggregate of physical and social environments do not constitute a community. People living in a community must have concern for others. They must respond to the joys and sorrows of others. Professor RM Mechiver and Professor CH Page, the social scientists have given their complementary reasons for having community sentiment. They are

1. The feeling of interdependence
2. The feeling of one's participation in social activities and
3. The feeling of oneness.

Right from the child to the old man everyone has to depend on others to meet his basic needs. He has to realize that without the cooperation of others he cannot survive. For this, he has to be grateful to the society at large. This feeling of indebtedness brings in him a feeling of pride towards the society.

Community living is an ancient one. It depends upon traditions. People of yore began to settle at one place after the advent of agriculture. Settling at one place developed in them the feeling for cooperation and friendliness. Community ensures the people their safety and well-being.

COMMUNITY TYPES

We can recognize communities based on population, prime occupation and administration. Villages and towns come under population, agricultural villages, fishermen villages, mining towns, steel towns come under prime occupation category. Village panchayats, municipalities and corporations form administrative communities. Sometimes, communities are formed based on caste and religion. Community organizer must acquaint himself with the different forms of communities, their structure and function and their handicaps. Arthur Dunham, an American Community organizer has given ten points formula for the organizer to follow for the development of the community, they are:

1. *Community planning:* What are the resources of the community? Are there any planned efforts to make the good use of them? Are there efficient transport systems and other facilities for a comfortable living.
2. *Housing facilities:* Are there sufficient housing facilities for all the community members?
3. *Government:* Are there any local popular self-governments and what are their relationships with the regional and central governments? Are there problems such as political unrest, corruption and red tapism.
4. *Economic life:* Are there any economic stability and satisfactory occupational opportunities.
5. *Education:* Is there any free education facility. Are there sufficient educational institutions for the members of the community?
6. *Health:* How is the public health system? How are the health services?
7. *Entertainment:* Are there healthy entertainment facilities for the community?
8. *Welfare services:* Are there facilities to treat physical, mental and socially handicapped persons?
9. *Religion:* How are different religions organized? Is there any freedom of religion? How are the interreligious relations?

10. *Community viewpoints:* Is there any freedom of speech in the community? Are the people free to organize associations? How are minorities treated? How do people involved in community activities? Is there unity in the community? In addition to these ten points, the social organize comes across many other points in the course of his service. He has to learn to cope with any problem that crops

SOCIAL WORK PRINCIPLES TO WORK WITH DISABLED PERSONS

1. *The values in social work practice*
   - *Belief in the basic dignity and worth of every human being:* There is a need to understand that however incapable people are they have a capacity to survive and thus one should give it importance that is itself the kind of dignity that one can to show to his fellow beings. Thus in a disability context one should respect the capability of the disabled person whatever may be the degree of his disability. One should give them the due recognition and worth as we do the rest of the societal members.
   - *Belief in the capacity for growth and change of every human being:* After one is able to give respect the capacity of a person, the next step would be that we, as social workers should have the belief that they also have the capacity to grow and progress in life and have the capacity to change to achieve certain position in the society.
   - *Belief in the right of every individual to equal opportunity social justice and social responsibility:* The underlying principle of social work is based on the principle that one should endeavor towards a society, which ensures opportunities to everyone without any kind of discrimination on any kinds of capabilities. Like there is feeling that severely disabled persons cannot always need support of others to run their day-to-day lives. But if one can provide training and an opportunity wherein they can perform their tasks and develop themselves.
   - *Belief in the right of every individual to make his own decisions concerning his life:* The other important thing, which is very important, is to respect the decision-making capabilities of individuals. Where it a social worker has to only facilitate and

give options to the individual but not decisions. For only when an individual takes his/her own decision then he/she shall feel confident and own the task.

- *Belief in the uniqueness of every human being:* It is very important that every person is unique in the sense that he has his own background and upbringing, which shapes his/her personality and so one cannot generalize that for a similar problem there shall be a similar solution.

2. *Purpose of social work*
   - Enhance problem-solving and coping capacities of people
     The steps involved in problem solving are
     - Exploration of the client's world
     - Identification of the problem area
     - Selecting-agreeing upon and committing work on a problem or a set of problems.
     - Translating the target problem into short-term and long-term goals.
     - Drawing up a contract
     - Problem Analysis
     - Formulating the tasks in problem resolution (actions required by both client and worker need to be identified)
     - Task modification of required problem
     - Client is to be helped to rehearsed performance of the task
     - Follow-up
     - Termination/evaluation.
   - Link people with systems that provide them with resources, services and opportunities
     - *Concept of human systems:* System is a structural organization of interacting units which endures over a period of time.
     - *Focus of social work practice:* Interactions between people and systems in the social environment. People are dependent on systems for help in obtaining material, emotional, spiritual resources and services and opportunities needed for coping with their life tasks.
     - Help taken from the three kinds of resource systems.
       a. Informal or natural resource systems
       b. Formal resource systems
       c. Societal resource systems

    - Inadequacies of these resource systems, e.g. reluctance to approach system; unaware of existence of a resource system; mechanisms or policies of a system may create a new problem or aggravate existing ones.
  - Promote the effective and humane operation of these systems
  - Contribute to the development and improvement of social policy.
  - Create new systems and alternatives.
3. *Social work frame of reference*
  - First concern with life tasks of people
  - People viewed in interaction with their network of resources systems. (Hence, not just, who has the problem, but what are the factors in interaction causing these problems)
  - Three types of interaction studied: among people within a resource systems; between people and resources systems.
4. *Art and science in social work practice*

   Social work practice is planned change

   Plan = purposeful, well thought out

   Change = movement

   Yet, intuition, spontaneity given due importance

   Units of interaction
  - Individuals
  - Families
  - Groups
  - Communities
  - Organizations.
5. *Methods of social work in relation to the units of intervention*

   Case work: Social case work is an enabling process through which the case worker helps the client through one-to-one relationship to take steps towards strengthening his own capacity to deal with his own problems and to achieve better adjustment to his/her environment by utilizing the resources available to the client, resources inherent in the strength of this personality, social system in which he/she lives or the social provisions supplied by the community including the agency through which he is receiving help.

   The problem may be within the individual or the environment or as is frequently of the person-situation interaction.

Principles of Case Work

a. Individualization—Every person is unique and has his/her own characteristics.
b. Acceptance-rejecting the behavior but accepting the person. It is very abstract.
c. Non-judgmental/Non-condemning.
d. Client's right to self-determination—Has to be done according to client's capacity to decide.
e. Client's participation.
f. Confidentiality.
g. Controlled emotional involvement.

Group work

The ten assumptions of group work are

1. There are different kinds of groups for different purposes at different times

   Purpose based:

   a. Remedial/rehabilitative/corrective
   b. Preventive/maintenance
   c. Developmental.

   Timebased:

   a. Open/Closed
   b. Short-term/Long-term.

2. Group work has certain advantages/disadvantages in comparison with working with individuals.

   Advantages

   a. Can reach many people at a specific time.
   b. Groups have built in support system.
   c. A nurturing environment within the group makes group members more willing to explore and try out new ways of thinking, feeling and behaving.
   d. Helps improve interpersonal skills and also works with specific problem areas.
   e. Vicarious learning and identification process through observing others are facilitated in groups.

   Disadvantages

   a. Potential problems seem directly proportional to the number of persons we attempt to help.
   b. Leader has less situational control than in individual counseling.

   c. Difficulties are more likely to develop if group leader cannot effectively balance the need for freedom v/s the need for structure.
   d. Confidentiality more difficult to mandate.
   e. Coercion and peer pressure may subtly shape individuals towards accepting norms and culture.
3. Groups can stifle autonomy, e.g.
   a. Cults and sects are proficient in group brainwashing.
   b. Responsibility diffused and multiple authorship of a decision. Groups tend to make collectively riskier decisions than they would alone—more spectatoring, self-judgment and self-evaluation occur in the presence of others.
4. Group membership can influence others groups are often conscious choice.
5. Members have equal status in a group. This needs to be emphasized by the group worker.
6. Many public fears and myths are associated with group work practice related to the need to belong and not to be isolated.
7. Associated with the group work is a specialized technology of intervention strategies which leads to planned change for the empowerment of the members.
8. If a group is considered to be a collectivity, there are successive and predictable stages in its development, i.e. initial, middle and termination.
9. Participation in groups involves personal risks related to potential life changes, e.g. members worry about confidentiality.
10. Groups are effective means for facilitating change.

– *Community organization*

  Basic values of community organization are—
  - Essential dignity and ethical worth of the individual
  - Possession of potential and resources by each individual to manage his/her own life
  - The importance of freedom to express one's individuality
  - The great capacity for growth within all social beings
  - The right of the individual to struggle and strive to improve his/her own life and environment
  - The need for a social climate suitable for individual growth and development

    - The right and responsibility of the individual to participate in the affairs of his/her own community
    - Consistent stand for the poor
    - Social development and justice.
  - *Basic assumptions*
    - Communities of people can develop the capacity to deal with their own problems
    - When people want to change they can change
    - People grow and fulfil themselves as they participate in the regulation of their own lives
    - Unless people so participate, they become entirely subjected to the whim of forces which leaves them socially and politically isolated and could make their lives meaningless
    - Without such participation, democracy has no life or vitality
    - Democracy requires cooperative participation and action in the affairs of the community and people must learn skills which make this possible
    - Changes in community living that are self-imposed or self-developed have a meaning and a permanence that imposed changes do not have.
    - A 'holistic approach' can deal successfully with problems, which a 'fragmented approach' will not.
6. *Multi-pronged approach to problem-solving, i.e. intervention in several units simultaneously.*
7. *Problem- solving techniques often cut across methods of social work.*
8. *Qualities of a social worker*
  - Good listener
  - Having less biased approach
  - Perseverance
  - Less of emotional involvement
  - Tolerance.
9. *Techniques of social work*
  - Supportive technique
    - Acceptance
      a. Our values, assumptions
      b. Knowledge of human growth and behavior
      c. Self-awareness of social worker's own feelings and attitudes.

    - Assurance
    - Facilitating of expression of feelings—sharing of feelings
    - Handling feelings which are over powering
    - Building of self-confidence
    - Encouragement and reassurance
    - Being with the client
    - Emotional support
    - Advocacy—Promoting the client's cause
- Technique of enhancing resources
    - Providing or procuring material help
    - Enhancing information and knowledge
    - Change in the physical environment
- Technique for changing the internal process
    - Reflective discussions
        a. Restating—Repeating back in single/full what the client stated.
        b. Paraphrasing—Rephrasing the clients views and showing their point of view.
        c. Summarizing—Longer paraphrasing, review the work.
    - Challenging
        a. To encourage the clients to review and question their current frame of reference in order to adopt difference and more empowering perspective
        Challenging the discrepancies of facts.

Contribution of Social Worker to Rehabilitation

Social worker in rehabilitation is basically educators, advocates, facilitators, and also act as a link between patients and family and community.

Educator: As educator they participate in teaching patients and their families in the nature of specific impairment, their implication; they conduct classes either in formal teaching settings and their conscious use of themselves. model reflecting adaptive attitudes and behavior thus by engaging patients and families in moving beyond the fear of disability.

Advocates: As advocate, they work with and on behalf of consumer to effect change through division on needed resources by making internal and external system more responsive to consumer needs and demands, they take active role in aggravating social policy. They act as advocate for patients and families with in the healthcare service system.

Collaborator: As collaborator utilize the knowledge of system to foster interdisciplinary collaboration and maintain therapeutic effect and treatment, they educate other team members about psychological issues both specific and general.

Specialist: As specialist, they provide consultancy on treatment.

The Social Work Role in Physical Rehabilitation

Social workers believe in the intrinsic worth and dignity of every human being. They are dedicated to the welfare of individuals and families and to the pursuit of social justice for all. Social workers are pledged to serve their clients without discrimination on any grounds. The values of acceptance, self-determination, and respect for the individual are fundamental to all forms of social work practice. The social worker in physical rehabilitation adheres to the Standards of Practice and Code of Ethics of their respective provincial governing bodies and of the Canadian Association of Social Workers.

Purpose of Social Work in Physical Rehabilitation

As a member of an inpatient or outpatient interdisciplinary team, the social worker facilitates the rehabilitation process to assist the patient in maximizing independence and autonomy in the various areas of his/her functioning. This process includes work with the patient, with his/her family, with the rehabilitation team, and with the community. Through assessment and interventions in the areas of psychosocial functioning and discharge planning, the social worker helps the client and the family move from a situation of uncertainty, anxiety, and dependency to one of increased confidence, hope, and autonomy.

Issues addressed by a rehabilitation social worker include:

1. Acknowledgment of diagnosis and need for intervention.
2. Adaptation to changes in the patient's role or relationships.
3. Modification in responsibilities and level of dependency.
4. Grief and adjustment to loss as a result of disability.
5. Dealing with altered self-image and expectations.
6. Adjustment to financial and social stressors related to disability.

7. Resource counseling for reintegration into employment and community; transportation; changes to home environment or choice of supervised care; funding of adaptive devices and other medical expenses.

Social workers in physical rehabilitation also have a responsibility to:

- Advocate on an individual and systemic level when gaps in service are identified.
- Initiate, conduct, and collaborate in research projects to enhance social work practice and to contribute to the body of knowledge associated with physical rehabilitation.
- Provide supervision and training to students developing their expertise in the field of physical rehabilitation.
- Act as a resource to community organizations by providing education, presentations, program development, and follow-up consultation.
- Maintain and develop expertise through participation in professional development activities in the hospital and community.

CHAPTER

10

Rural Rehabilitation and Extension Services

Rural Health Scheme emerged out of the recommendation of the Srivastava community and was introduced in 1977. It is based on a four system of services provided at the level of village, the subcenter, primary health center and community health center.

The theme of rural health scheme was ***"place public health in people's hand."***

1. *At village level:* There is a village health guide and trained traditional birth attendance who looks after the minor and basic ailments of people with guidance of the primary health center the village health guide will be a person from the community itself he is provided with a kit contains commons medications needed in community the target is to have one village health guide and a traditional birth attendant per village or 1000 population.
2. *The Subcenter Level:* There are health workers (Multipurpose worker) one male and one female at each subcenter to the population of about 5000 people. They are given the basic knowledge in all aspects of medicine in 18 months at the primary health center, he is supposed to visit 100–150 houses daily; health assistant (supervisor), they are supposed to look after the work of four health workers.

3. *Primary health center level:* Carries out preventive corrective and promotive aspect of health program including training of health program or village health guide.
    1. Health medicine care
    2. Mother and child health
    3. Family planning
    4. Training for health guide
    5. Safe water supply
    6. Education about health
    7. Collection of vital status
    8. Prevention and control local epidemic
    9. National health program
    10. Referral service.

It is located at the site of community development block to facilitate coordinated work. It carries out preventive, Curative, promotive aspects of health program including training of village health guide.

Community health center level (Regional): OHC should be opened by upgrading PHC in the block it consists of a 30-bed hospital preference is given to those areas without proper referral service in the vicinity, e.g. tribal, hilly areas.

EXTENDED CARE FACILITIES

If patients are not discharged from the hospital directly to their homes, they are most likely to be discharged to one of the 3 different types of extended care facilities:

1-*Skilled nursing facility (SNF):* which is commonly called a nursing home and usually provides special kind of care such as IV fluids and medicine.

INTERMEDIATE CARE FACILITY (ICF)

It is suitable if the patient's primary need is for help with the activities of daily living (Eating, bathing, gardening wearing cloths, lifting) unlike an SNF an ICE is not some nursing homes provides both skilled and intermediate levels of care.

A nursing home that specialized in providing terminal care, especially for patients with acquired immune deficiency syndrome.

Measurements in Epidemiology

Epidemiology measurement includes the following:

A. Measurement of mortality.
B. Measurement of morbidities.
C. Measurement of disability.
D. Measurement of nationality.
E. Measurement of presence, absence or distribution of the characteristic or attributes of the disease.
F. Measurement of medical needs, healthcare facilities civilization of health services and other health-related events.
G. Presence or absence or distribution in the environmental and other factors suspected of causing disease.

TOOLS OF MESUREMENTS

The epidemiology uses the basic tools for measurement such as rations and proportions the basic requirement of measurements are validity liability, accuracy sensibility and specificity

EXTENSION SERVICES AND MOBILE UNIT

Definition

Extension of the center-based rehabilitation activities to the unreached disabled population in the rural areas using mobile clinic van. Here a group of professional with necessary material goes to the community for intensive care of the disabled.

Need of Mobile Unit

1. Lack of awareness regarding rehabilitation services
2. Poverty
3. Condition of parent
4. No transport facility.
   Ultimately all these make main need of service to the community.

Team of Mobile Extension Service

Most of the extension service is concerned with physically disabled. The following professionals are mainly required in extension services:

1. Program manager/project incharge/supervisor
2. Physiotherapist
3. Occupational therapist
4. Speech and language therapist
5. Orthopedician
6. Prosthetic engineer
7. Social worker
8. Special educator.

Areas benefited by extension services most of the extension service activities are collaborated primary health center and hospital service are provided to

1. Primary health center
2. Hospital
3. Community itself.

Types of Work given by Extension Services

Hospital-based Service

a. Diagnostic screening, assessment of nature of disability of new case (Orthopedic diagnosis, speech and hearing assessment, assessing still for self-care, mobilizing, visual acuity, IQ).
b. Referring for surgical correction of polio, congenital, anomalies of limb.
c. Preoperative and postoperative care including X-ray hospitalization, medication, splinting, blood test.
d. Follow-up medical consultation.
e. Provision of mobility facility.

Community-based Services

- Membership training, leadership delivery, community-awareness motivation through exhibition, mass meeting, cultural program.
- *Skill training:* Here the disabled are trained in daily living skill, skill to general income generation.

Educational Services

School, notebook, other educational material placing disabled in special school, transporting the disabled in proper school and getting proper service, mental retardation, hearing or visual impairment.

Intervention: Intervention given through extension service is early intervention PT, OT, splint, language, education services, orthopedics management behavioral modification, counseling.

Advantages

1. No money collected
2. Decreased parent involvement.

Disadvantages

1. Money power
2. Man power.

CHAPTER

11

Geriatrics and Geriatric Rehabilitation

INTRODUCTION

Geriatrics or geriatric medicine is a specialty that focuses on health care of elderly people. It aims to promote health by preventing and treating diseases and disabilities in older adults. There is no set age at which patients may be under the care of a geriatrician or geriatric physician, a physician who specializes in the care of elderly people. Rather, this decision is determined by the individual patient's needs, and the availability of a specialist. It is important to note the difference between geriatrics, the care of aged people, and gerontology, which is the study of the aging process itself. The term geriatrics comes from the Greek geron meaning "old man", and iatros meaning "healer". However, geriatrics is sometimes called medical gerontology.

AGING

Aging is the process of becoming older. In the narrow sense, the term refers to biological aging of human beings, animals and other organisms. In the broader sense, aging can refer to single cells within an organism (cellular aging) or to the population of a species (population aging).

In humans, aging represents the accumulation of changes in a human being over time, encompassing physical, psychological, and social change. Reaction time, for example, may slow with age, while knowledge of world events and wisdom may expand. Aging is among the greatest known risk factors for most human diseases: of the roughly 150,000 people who die each day across the globe, about two-thirds die from age-related causes.

The causes of aging are unknown; current theories are assigned to the damage concept, whereby the accumulation of externally induced damage (such as DNA point mutations) may cause biological systems to fail, or to the programmed aging concept, whereby internal processes (such as DNA telomere shortening) may cause aging.

The discovery, in 1934, that calorie restriction can extend lifespan two-fold in rats, and the existence of species having negligible senescence and potentially immortal species such as Hydra, have motivated research into delaying and preventing aging and thus age-related diseases.

OSTEOPOROSIS

Osteoporosis is a disease where decreased bone strength increases the risk of a broken bone. It is the most common reason for a broken bone among the elderly. Bones that commonly break include the back bones, the bones of the forearm, and the hip. Until a broken bone occurs, there are typically no symptoms. Bones may weaken to such a degree that a break may occur with minor stress or spontaneously. Chronic pain and a decreased ability to carry out normal activities may occur following a broken bone. Osteoporosis may be due to lower than normal peak bone mass and greater than normal bone loss. Bone loss increases after menopause due to lower levels of estrogen. Osteoporosis may also occur due to a number of diseases or treatments including alcoholism, anorexia, hyperthyroidism, surgical removal of the ovaries, and kidney disease. Certain medications increase the rate of bone loss including some antiseizure medications, chemotherapy, proton pump inhibitors selective serotonin reuptake inhibitors and steroids. Not enough exercise and smoking are also risk factors. Osteoporosis is defined as a bone density of 2.5 standard deviations below that of a young adult. This is typically measured by dual-energy X-ray absorptiometry at the hip.

Prevention of osteoporosis includes a proper diet during childhood and efforts to avoid medications that cause the condition. Efforts to prevent broken bones in those with osteoporosis include a good diet, exercise, and fall prevention. Lifestyle changes such as stopping smoking and not drinking alcohol may help. Medication of the bisphosphonate type is useful in those with previous broken bones due to osteoporosis. In those with osteoporosis but no previous broken bones they are less effective. A number of other medications may also be useful.

Osteoporosis becomes more common with age. About 15% of white people in their 50s and 70% of those over 80 are affected. It is more common in women than men. In the developed world, depending on the method of diagnosis, 2 to 8% of males and 9 to 38% of females are affected. Rates of disease in the developing world are unclear. About 22 million women and 5.5 million men in the European Union had osteoporosis in 2010. In the United States in 2010 about eight million women and one to two million men had osteoporosis. White and Asian people are at greater risk. The word osteoporosis is from the Greek terms for "porous bones".

Prevention

Lifestyle prevention of osteoporosis is in many aspects the inverse of the potentially modifiable risk factors. As tobacco smoking and high alcohol intake have been linked with osteoporosis, smoking cessation and moderation of alcohol intake are commonly recommended as ways to help prevention.

In people with celiac disease adherence to a gluten-free diet decreases risk to develop osteoporosis. And increases bone density. It must ensure optimal calcium intake (of at least one gram daily) and measure vitamin D levels, and to take specific supplements if necessary.

Nutrition

Studies of the benefits of supplementation with calcium and vitamin D are conflicting, possibly because most studies did not have people with low dietary intakes. A 2013 review by the US preventive services task force (USPSTF) found insufficient evidence to determine if supplementation with calcium and vitamin D results in greater harm or benefit in men and premenopausal women. The USPSTF did not recommend low dose supplementation (less than 1 g of calcium and 400 IU of vitamin D) in postmenopausal women as there does not appear to be a difference in fracture risk. It is unknown what effect higher doses have. A 2015 review found little data that supplementation of calcium decreases the risk of fractures.

While some meta-analyses have found a benefit of vitamin D supplements combined with calcium for fractures, they did not find a benefit of vitamin D supplements alone.

While supplementation does not appear to affect the risk of death. there is an increased risk of myocardial infarctions, and stomach problems.

Vitamin K deficiency is also a risk factor for osteoporotic fractures. The gene gamma-glutamyl carboxylase (GGCX) is dependent on vitamin K. Functional polymorphisms in the gene could attribute to variation in bone metabolism and BMD. Vitamin K2 is also used as a means of treatment for osteoporosis and the polymorphisms of GGCX could explain the individual variation in the response to treatment of vitamin K supplementation may reduce the risk of fractures in postmenopausal women; however, there is no evidence for men.

Management

Weight-bearing endurance exercise and/or exercises to strengthen muscles improve bone strength in those with osteoporosis. Aerobics, weight bearing, and resistance exercises all maintain or increase BMD in postmenopausal women. Fall prevention can help prevent osteoporosis complications. There is some evidence for hip protectors specifically among those who are in care homes.

Sensory Impairment

Disability is the consequence of an impairment that may be physical, cognitive, mental, sensory, emotional, developmental, or some combination of these that result in restrictions on an individual's ability to participate in what is considered "normal" in their everyday society. A disability may be present from birth, or occur during a person's lifetime.

Disability is an umbrella term, covering impairments, activity limitations, and participation restrictions. Impairment is a problem in body function or structure; an activity limitation is a difficulty encountered by an individual in executing a task or action; while a participation restriction is a problem experienced by an individual in involvement in life situations. Thus, disability is a complex phenomenon, reflecting an interaction between features of a person's body and features of the society in which he/she lives.

—World Health Organization

Disability is a contested concept, with different meanings for different communities. On the one hand, it may be used to refer to physical or mental attributes that some institutions, particularly medicine, view as needing to be fixed (the medical model); it may refer to limitations on participation in social life imposed on people by the constraints of an ableist society (the social model); or the term may serve to name a social identity claimed by people with disabilities in order to mark their shared goals and politics.

The contest over disability's definition arose out of disability activism in the US and UK in the 1970s, which challenged how medical conceptions of human variation dominated popular discourse about disabilities and how these were reflected in common terminology (e.g. "handicapped", "cripple"). Debates about proper terminology as well as over appropriate models and their implied politics continue in disability communities and the academic field of disability studies. In many countries, the law requires that disabilities be clearly categorized and defined in order to assess which citizens qualify for disability benefits.

Types of Disability

The term "disability" broadly describes an impairment in a person's ability to function, caused by changes in various subsystems of the body, or to mental health. The degree of disability may range from mild to moderate, severe, or profound. A person may also have multiple disabilities. Disability can be measured objectively (observed) or subjectively (self-report).

Conditions causing disability are classified by the medical community as:

- Inherited (genetically transmitted);
- Congenital, meaning caused by a mother's infection or other disease during pregnancy, embryonic or fetal developmental irregularities, or by injury during or soon after birth;
- Acquired, such as conditions caused by illness or injury; of unknown origin.

Types of disability may also be categorized in the following way:

Physical Disability

Any impairment which limits the physical function of limbs, fine bones, or gross motor ability is a physical impairment, not necessarily a physical disability. The social model of disability defines physical disability as manifest when impairment meets a non-universal design or program, e.g. a person who cannot climb stairs may have a physical impairment of the knees when putting stress on them from an elevated position such as with climbing or descending stairs. If an elevator were provided, or a building had services on the first floor, this impairment would not become a disability. Other physical disabilities include impairments which limit other activities of daily living, such as severe sleep disorders.

A man with an above the knee amputation exercises while wearing a prosthetic leg.

Sensory Disability

Sensory disability is impairment of one of the senses. The term is used primarily to refer to vision and hearing impairment, but other senses can be impaired.

Vision Impairment

Vision impairment (or "visual impairment") is vision loss of a person to such a degree as to qualify as an additional support need through a significant limitation of visual capability resulting from either disease, trauma, or congenital or degenerative conditions that cannot be corrected by conventional means, such as refractive correction, medication, or surgery. This functional loss of vision is typically defined to manifest with best corrected visual acuity of less than 20/60, or significant central field defect, Significant peripheral field defect including homonymous or heteronymous bilateral visual, field defect or generalized contraction or constriction of field, or reduced peak contrast sensitivity with either of the above conditions.

Hearing Impairment

Hearing impairment or hard of hearing or deafness refers to conditions in which individuals are fully or partially unable to detect or perceive at least some frequencies of sound which can typically be heard by most people. Mild hearing loss may sometimes not be considered a disability.

Olfactory and Gustatory Impairment

Impairment of the sense of smell and taste are commonly associated with aging but can also occur in younger people due to a wide variety of causes.

There are various olfactory disorders:

- Anosmia—inability to smell
- Dysosmia—things do not smell as they "should"
- Hyperosmia—an abnormally acute sense of smell
- Hyposmia—decreased ability to smell
- Olfactory reference syndrome—psychological disorder which causes patients to imagine they have strong body odor
- Parosmia—things smell worse than they should
- Phantosmia—"hallucinated smell", often unpleasant in nature
- Complete loss of the sense of taste is known as ageusia, while dysgeusia is persistent abnormal sense of taste.

Somatosensory Impairment

Insensitivity to stimuli such as touch, heat, cold, and pain are often an adjunct to a more general physical impairment involving neural pathways and is very commonly associated with paralysis (in which the motor neural circuits are also affected).

Balance Disorder

A balance disorder is a disturbance that causes an individual to feel unsteady, for example when standing or walking. It may be accompanied by symptoms of being giddy, woozy, or have a sensation of movement, spinning, or floating. Balance is the result of several body systems working together. The eyes (visual system), ears (vestibular system) and the body's sense of where it is in space (proprioception) need to be intact. The brain, which compiles this information, needs to be functioning effectively.

Intellectual Disability

Intellectual disability is a broad concept that ranges from mental retardation to cognitive deficits too mild or too specific (as in specific learning disability) to qualify as mental retardation. Intellectual disabilities may appear at any age. Mental retardation is a subtype of intellectual disability, and the term intellectual disability is now preferred by many advocates in most English-speaking countries.

Mental Health and Emotional Disabilities

A mental disorder or mental illness is a psychological or behavioral pattern generally associated with subjective distress or disability that occurs in an individual, and perceived by the majority of society as being outside of normal development or cultural expectations. The recognition and understanding of mental health conditions has changed over time and across cultures, and there are still variations in the definition, assessment, and classification of mental disorders, although standard guideline criteria are widely accepted.

Pervasive Developmental Disorders

The diagnostic category of pervasive developmental disorders refers to a group of five developmental disabilities characterized by differences in the development of multiple basic functions including socialization and communication. The DSM-IV-TR listed the pervasive developmental disorders as autistic disorder, Asperger syndrome, Rett syndrome, childhood disintegrative disorder, and pervasive developmental disorder not otherwise specified (PDD-NOS). The DSM-5 does not describe individual diagnosis of any of the pervasive developmental disorders, replacing all of them with a unified diagnosis of autism spectrum disorder. The ICD-10 also includes the diagnosis of overactive disorder associated with mental retardation and stereotyped movements.

Developmental Disability

Developmental disability is any disability that results in problems with growth and development. Although the term is often used as a synonym or euphemism for intellectual disability, the term also encompasses many congenital medical conditions that have no mental or intellectual components, for example spina bifida.

Nonvisible Disabilities

Several chronic disorders, such as diabetes, asthma, inflammatory bowel disease, epilepsy, narcolepsy, fibromyalgia, and some sleep disorders may be counted as nonvisible disabilities, as opposed to disabilities which are clearly visible, such as those requiring the use of a wheelchair.

Disability and Aging

To a certain degree, physical impairments and diminishing mental states are almost ubiquitously experienced by people who are growing old. Aging populations are often stigmatized for having a high prevalence of disability. Kathleen Woodward, writing in "Key Words for Disability Studies" explains the phenomenon as follows:

Aging is invoked rhetorically-at times ominously—as a pressing reason why disability should be of crucial interest to all of us (we are all getting older, we will all be disabled eventually), thereby inadvertently reinforcing the damaging and dominant stereotype of aging as solely an experience of decline and deterioration. But little attention has been given to the imbrications of aging and disability.

Longevity

The word "longevity" is sometimes used as a synonym for "life expectancy" in demography —however, the term "longevity" is sometimes meant to refer only to especially long-lived members of a population, whereas "life expectancy" is always defined statistically as the average number of years remaining at a given age. For example, a population's life expectancy at birth is the same as the average age at death for all people born in the same year (in the case of cohorts). Longevity is best thought of as a term for general audiences meaning 'typical length of life' and specific statistical definitions should be clarified when necessary.

Reflections on longevity have usually gone beyond acknowledging the brevity of human life and have included thinking about methods to extend life. Longevity has been a topic not only for the scientific community but also for writers of travel, science fiction, and utopian novels.

There are many difficulties in authenticating the longest human life span ever by modern verification standards, owing to inaccurate or incomplete birth statistics. Fiction, legend, and folklore have proposed or claimed life spans in the past or future vastly longer than those verified by modern standards, and longevity narratives and unverified longevity claims frequently speak of their existence in the present.

A life annuity is a form of longevity insurance.

Malnutrition or Malnourishment

Malnutrition or malnourishment is a condition that results from eating a diet in which nutrients are either not enough or are too much such that the diet causes health problems. It may involve calories, protein, carbohydrates, vitamins or minerals. Not enough nutrients are called under nutrition or undernourishment while too much is called over nutrition. Malnutrition is often used specifically to refer to under nutrition where there is not enough calories, protein, or micronutrients. If under nutrition occurs during pregnancy, or before two years of age, it may result in permanent problems with physical and mental development. Extreme under nourishment, known as starvation, may have symptoms that include: a short height, thin body, very poor energy levels, and swollen legs and abdomen. People also often get infections and are frequently cold. The symptoms of micronutrient deficiencies depend on the micronutrient that is lacking.

Undernourishment is most often due to not enough high-quality food being available to eat. This is often related to high food prices and poverty. In some developing countries, over nutrition in the form of obesity is beginning to present within the same communities as under nutrition. Other causes of malnutrition include anorexia nervosa and bariatric surgery.

Efforts to improve nutrition are some of the most effective forms of development aid. Breastfeeding can reduce rates of malnutrition and death in children, and efforts to promote the practice increase the rates of breastfeeding. In young children, providing food (in addition to breast milk) between six months and two years of age improves outcomes. There is also good evidence supporting the supplementation of a number of micronutrients to women during pregnancy and among young children in the developing world. To get food to people who need it most, both delivering food and providing money so people can buy food within local markets are effective. Simply feeding students at school is insufficient. Management of severe malnutrition within the person's home with ready-to-use therapeutic foods is possible much of the time. In those who have severe malnutrition complicated by other health problems, treatment in a hospital setting is recommended. This often involves managing low blood sugar and body temperature, addressing dehydration, and gradual feeding. Routine antibiotics are usually recommended due to the high risk of infection. Longer-term measures include: improving agricultural practices, reducing poverty, improving sanitation, and the empowerment of women.

There were 793 million undernourished people in the world in 2015 (13% of the total population). This is a reduction of 216 million people since 1990 when 23% were undernourished in 2012, it was estimated that another billion people had a lack of vitamins and minerals. In 2013, protein-energy malnutrition was estimated to have resulted in 469,000 deaths—down from 510,000 deaths in 1990. Other nutritional deficiencies, which include iodine deficiency and iron deficiency.

Anemia, result in another 84,000 deaths. In 2010, malnutrition was the cause of 1.4% of all disability adjusted life years about a third of deaths in children are believed to be due to under nutrition, although the deaths are rarely labeled as such. In 2010, it was estimated to have contributed to about 1.5 million deaths in women and children, though some estimate the number may be greater than 3 million. An additional 165 million children were estimated to have stunted growth from malnutrition in 2013. Under nutrition is more common in developing countries. Certain groups have higher rates of under nutrition, including women—in particular while pregnant or breastfeeding—children under five years of age, and the elderly. In the elderly, under nutrition becomes more common due to physical, psychological, and social factors.

Nutrition and Aging

Essential nutrients are one of the main requirements of elderly care.

Malnutrition and being underweight are more common in the elderly than in adults of other ages. If elderly people are healthy and active, the aging process alone does not usually cause malnutrition. However, changes in body composition, organ functions, adequate energy intake and ability to eat or access food are associated with aging, and may contribute to malnutrition. Sadness or depression can play a role, causing changes in appetite, digestion, energy level, weight, and well-being. A study on the relationship between malnutrition and other conditions in the elderly found that malnutrition in the elderly can result from gastrointestinal and endocrine system disorders, loss of taste and smell, decreased appetite and inadequate dietary intake. Poor dental health, ill-fitting dentures, or chewing and swallowing problems can make eating difficult. As a result of these factors, malnutrition is seen to develop more easily in the elderly.

Rates of malnutrition tend to increase with age with less than 10 percent of the "young" elderly (up to age 75) malnourished, while 30 to 65% of the elderly in home care, long-term care facilities, or acute hospitals are malnourished. Many elderly people require assistance in eating, which may contribute to malnutrition. Because of this, one of the main requirements of elderly care is to provide an adequate diet and all essential nutrients. In Australia, malnutrition or risk of malnutrition occurs in 80% of elderly people presented to hospitals for admission. Malnutrition and weight loss can contribute to sarcopenia with loss of lean body mass and muscle function. Abdominal obesity or weight loss coupled with sarcopenia lead to immobility, skeletal disorders, insulin resistance, hypertension, atherosclerosis, and metabolic disorders. A paper from the Journal of the American Dietetic Association noted that routine nutrition screenings represent one way to detect and therefore decrease the prevalence of malnutrition in the elderly.

Elderly Care

Elderly care, or simply eldercare (also known in parts of the English speaking world as aged care), is the fulfillment of the special needs and requirements that are unique to senior citizens. This broad term encompasses such services as assisted living, adult day care, long-term care, nursing homes (often referred to as residential care), hospice care, and home care. Because of the wide variety of elderly care found nationally, as well as differentiating cultural perspectives on elderly citizens, cannot to be limited to any one practice. For example, many countries in Asia use government-established elderly care quite infrequently, preferring the traditional methods of being cared for by younger generations of family members.

Elderly care emphasizes the social and personal requirements of senior citizens who need some assistance with daily activities and health care, but who desire to age with dignity. It is an important distinction, in that the design of housing, services, activities, employee training and such should be truly customer-centered. It is also noteworthy that a large amount of global elderly care falls under the unpaid market sector.

Depression

Depression is a state of low mood and aversion to activity that can affect a person's thoughts, behavior, feelings and sense of well-being.

People with a depressed mood can feel sad, anxious, empty, hopeless, helpless, worthless, guilty, irritable, ashamed or restless. They may lose interest in activities that were once pleasurable, experience loss of appetite or overeating, have problems concentrating, remembering details or making decisions, and may contemplate, attempt or commit suicide. Insomnia, excessive sleeping, fatigue, aches, pains, digestive problems or reduced energy may also be present. Depressed mood is a feature of some psychiatric syndromes such as major depressive disorder, but it may also be a normal reaction to life events such as bereavement, a symptom of some bodily ailments or a side effect of some drugs and medical treatments.

Geriatric Rehabilitation

Geriatric rehabilitation covers three areas—normal aging due to disuse and deconditioning, cardiovascular problems like vascular disease and stroke, and skeletal problems including osteoporosis and osteoarthritis conditions such as knee and hip replacements. Physical medicine physicians use rehabilitation to work toward the goal of returning the patient to a preinjury quality of life and may use physical, occupational, and speech therapies (Fig. 11.1).

With increased age, patients often face many physical and emotional changes that can affect level of function and well-being. Rehabilitation maintains functional independence in the elderly. Rehabilitation of

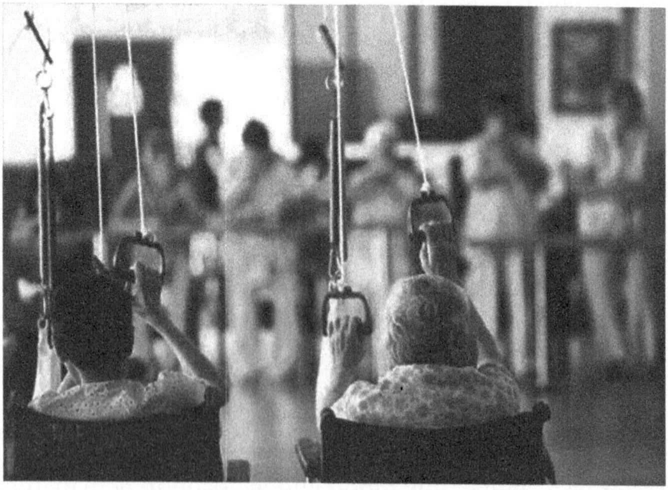

Fig. 11.1: Geriatric rehabilitation *(For color version see Plate 2)*

geriatric patients is imperative for the patients' well-being and for society, so that we can thrive socially and economically. Essential to geriatric rehabilitation is communication, specifically improving any sensory impairment, including those related to vision and hearing. The prevention of falls and osteoporosis can improve the patient's health and longevity. Addressing malnutrition can promote healing and vitalize the patient to participate in a formal rehabilitation program. Depression is common in the older population if a functional loss of mobility and an inability to perform activities of daily living (ADLs) predominates. Cognitive impairment, such as delirium and dementia, can affect the patient's rehabilitation goals and outcomes. Finally, a driver's evaluation for an appropriate elderly candidate is an underutilized part of rehabilitation that has a considerable impact on society.

Geriatric rehabilitation also have a role in intermediate care, where patients are referred by a hospital or family doctor, when there is a requirement to provide hospital-based short-term intensive physical therapy aimed at the recovery of musculoskeletal function, particularly recovery from joint, tendon, or ligament repair and, or, physical medicine and rehabilitation care when elderly patients get out of sync with their medication resulting in a deterioration of their personal health which reduces their ability to live independently.

Finally, geriatric rehabilitation has a large influence on the growing life expectancy around the globe. The American Physical Therapy Association (APTA) surveyed 556 adults over 65 years old in order to gain an understanding on the factors that affect adherence to an exercise program. Adherence to an exercise program influences frailty, speed, ability to live independently, and best of all, life expectancy. The study compared 2 factors: (1) exercise barriers, and (2) motivation. The study concluded that exercise barriers play the largest role in determining adherence to a Home Exercise Program (HEP). According to APTA, motivators include self-efficacy, the ability to control behavior, and outcome expectation, the belief that consequences follow certain actions. APTA describes barriers as: insufficient time, lack of social support, no place to exercise, limited finances, no transportation, and the fear of falling. Researchers recently found that depression, stress levels, increased age, decreased health status and lack of pleasure while exercising contribute to exercise adherence.

CHAPTER 12

Vocational Evaluation and Assessment Methods

VOCATIONAL EVALUATION

Vocational evaluation is an educational process in which a client obtains greater self and work knowledge through participation in work activities designed to evaluate vocational skills, interests, and abilities. Clients learn about the functional impact of their disability in relation to their career options.

Vocational evaluation is a process to assist individuals with disabilities, injured or displaced workers identify and explore their career interests, aptitudes, and skills and formulate immediate and long-term work/career goals.

Vocational assessment is the process of determining an individual's interests, Abilities and aptitudes and skills to identify vocational strengths, needs and career potential. Vocational assessment may use a variety of standardized techniques (e.g. tests) or non-standardized approaches (e.g. interviews, observing people). Vocational assessment is part of the vocational guidance process and usually results in recommendations for training or employment.

An operational definition of vocational evaluation distinguishes it as a profession and a process. Vocational evaluation is highly specialized, requiring the ability to administer and interpret testing instruments that are not usually found in other testing center inventories. Generally, the evaluator has a background in vocational rehabilitation and specialized training in vocational evaluation. Those who have been certified and/or have certain recognized competencies may use the title. The definitions which follow provide a broad range of interpretations and may include one or more of these interpretations.

- Of observing behaviors and interpreting them against some criterion;
- The process of assessing what an individual does and how well it is done;
- One function of a personalized service delivery system in which information is obtained and synthesized to assist individuals to identify and plan for appropriate occupations; A comprehensive process that systematically uses work, real or simulated, as the focal point for assessment and vocational exploration, the purpose of which is to assist individuals in vocational development (CCWAVES, 1987).

GOALS OF VOCATIONAL EVALUATION

Typical outcomes or goals are:

- Determine eligibility for rehabilitation services
- Identify training and job options
- Job placement and/or personnel selection
- Counseling and personal development
- Vocational guidance and exploration
- Predict an individual's behavior in a job-related setting
- Determination of disability benefits
- Test development and research.

EVALUATION METHODS

There are several testing methods used in vocational evaluation. The procedure used by the evaluator will depend upon the size of the evaluation unit, the population served, and needs of referral sources. Generally, vocational evaluation involves a combination of at least two or more of the methods described below:

- *Psychological tests:* An objective and standardized measure of a sample of behavior (cognitive, psychomotor, or affective trait) considered important to general or specific job functioning.

- *Work sample:* An actual or simulated job which is administered and observed under a standard set of conditions.
- *Situational assessment:* A systematic procedure for observing, recording, and interpreting work behavior in a real (though controlled) work situation where, under close supervision, the participant works with others on contract jobs for real wages (Dunn, 1973).
- *Occupational exploration:* Used when more occupational information is needed in order to make a choice among several types of work.

COMMON ERRORS MADE DURING EVALUATION

Errors made during test administration threaten the overall accuracy of the evaluation. The following statements represent the most common errors committed by evaluators.

- Failure to consider the client and his/her needs
- Overuse of certain tests
- Insufficient use of certain tests
- Use of tests with questionable validity and reliability checks
- Use of tests normed on groups differing markedly from those being tested
- Overemphasis on the initial interview
- Rushing the assessment process
- Paraphrasing instructions
- Failure to check for inconsistencies between test results and recommendations
- Failure to individualize service, training, and job recommendations
- Failure to write to the reader and answer the referral questions completely
- Poor use of grammar and sentence structure
- Incomplete evaluation
- Lack of familiarity with a particular test
- Lack of objectivity in writing the report
- Creating a "halo effect" by attributing highly positive characteristics or abilities to a client despite test results or other significant data.

TYPES OF TESTS USED IN VOCATIONAL EVALUATION

Testing instruments are designed to measure certain behavioral characteristics. Multifactor batteries such as the General Aptitude Test

Battery (GATB) measure more than one aptitude (e.g. general learning ability, verbal ability, dexterity). It is important, therefore, to understand and define the particular trait or behavior that is being measured.

Intelligence

The capacity to meet novel situations, or to learn to do so, by new adaptive responses. Also, the ability to think rationally, act purposefully and to deal effectively with one's environment (Wechsler, 1980). The most common measure is the ability to survive in a learning environment and to think abstractly.

Aptitude

Specific aspects of intelligence which relate to an individual's potential for learning certain skills. A combination of abilities whether native or acquired, that are indicative of an individual's ability to learn or develop proficiency in some particular area if appropriate education or training is provided.

Interest

A preference for certain work, school, or leisure activities. Most measures relate the individual's preference patterns to certain occupational groups and/or classifications.

Personality

Tests which relate to the affective or emotional aspects of a person. Includes likes, attitudes, self-concepts and general view of one's environment. Generally classified as projective (subjectively scored) and paper and pencil (objectively scored).

Dexterity

Measures speed and accuracy in performing simple manual activities as well as eye-hand coordination.

Special

Types of tests that do not fit within other categories. For example, the McCarron-Dial Work Evaluation System.

TESTS USED IN VOCATIONAL EVALUATION

Achievement

Apticom AS—Achievement Section Kaufman Test of Educational Achievement (KTEA) Peabody Individual Achievement Test-Revised (PIAT-A) Peabody Picture Vocabulary Test (PPVT) Test of Nonverbal Intelligence (TONI) Wide Range Achievement Test-Revised {WRAT-R) Woodcock-Johnson Psycho-Educational Battery {W-J).

Interest

Apticom AS—Interest Section California Occupational Preference System (COPS) Geist Picture Interest Inventory Becker Reading Free Vocational Interest Inventory (RFVII) Minnesota Importance Questionnaire (MIQ) Occupational Aptitude and Interest Schedule (OASIS) Strong-Campbell Interest Inventory (SCII) Wide Range Interest-Opinion Test (WRIOT).

Aptitude

Apticom AS—Aptitude Section Bennett Mechanical Comprehension Test Career Ability Preference System (CAPS) Detroit Tests of Learning Ability (DTLA) Occupational Aptitude Survey and Interest Schedule (OASIS).

Dexterity

Bennett Hand Tool Test Crawford Small Parts Test Minnesota Rate of Manipulation Test O'Connor Fine Motor Pennsylvania Bi-Manual Purdue Pegboard.

Work Samples

Singer Evaluation System Valpar Vocational Information and Work Evaluation System (VIEWS) Vocational Interest, Temperament, and Aptitude System (VITAS).

Intelligence

Peabody Picture Vocabulary Test (receptive language) Ravens Standard Progressive Matrices (Abstract Reasoning) Revised Beta Stanford-Binet Test of Nonverbal Intelligence (TONI).

Specialized Tests

McCarron-Dial Work Evaluation System (MDWES) Microcomputer Evaluation Systematic Assessment (MESA) Social and Prevocational Information Battery (SPIB) Vocational Transit.

Differences between Vocational Assessment of Person with Disability and Nondisabled Persons

Vocational assessment for people with disabilities should make use of the assessment procedures that are widely used in other assessment settings, such as schools, employment service and psychological settings. Sometimes, these procedures need to be adapted for disabled persons. Additionally, specialized techniques and strategies have been developed for people with disabilities who seek employment or rehabilitation services.

Vocational assessment should focus on identifying abilities and strengths that can be used in training and work situations. It should compare these to viable job requirements and make recommendations. For people with disabilities, the recommendations may also include the need for support services, assistive devices, job accommodations or address other disability-specific issues that will further the person's training or job success.

ILO Standards about the Vocational Assessment

ILO Convention 159 concerning vocational rehabilitation and employment (disabled persons), 1983 and the related Recommendation 168 require that competent authorities should provide vocational guidance.

Recommendation 99 concerning vocational rehabilitation of the disabled spells out the following ten steps as part of the vocational guidance process:

1. An interview with a vocational guidance officer.
2. Examination of record of work experience.
3. Examination of scholastic or other records relating to education or training received.
4. Medical examination for vocational guidance purposes.
5. Appropriate tests of capacity and aptitude and, where desirable, other psychological tests.

6. Ascertainment of personal and family circumstances.
7. Ascertainment of aptitudes and development of abilities by appropriate work experiences and trail and other similar means.
8. Technical trade tests, either verbal or otherwise, in all cases where such seem necessary.
9. Analysis of physical capacity in relation to occupational requirements and the possibility of improving that capacity.
10. Provision of information concerning employment and training opportunities related to the qualifications, physical capacities, aptitudes, preferences and experience of the person concerned and to the needs of the employment market.

Vocational Assessments Team

In many settings, vocational assessment is carried out by a multidisciplinary team that may include, depending on the setting and person's disability, specialists from fields such as occupational therapy, rehabilitation medicine or psychiatry, psychology, social work, vocational guidance, education and rehabilitation. Employers or specialists from a technical field may also be involved.

In some countries or settings (such as a vocational rehabilitation facility), a especially trained vocational evaluator, knowledgeable a variety of disciplines related to assessment, conducts a vocational evaluation. Such evaluations are usually supplemented by assessments done by a psychologist, medical personnel or others depending on the person's disability.

Vocational assessment personnel should be knowledgeable about the labor market, job and training opportunities, so that the recommendations they make are realistic.

The person with a disability should be kept fully informed about the processes and their purposes. Family members, employers, trainers or others may also be involved in the process.

Criteria of Vocational Assessment

In the narrowest sense, vocational assessments are usually concerned with the correlation between a person's abilities and skills and job requirements. However, since many issues other than skills and aptitudes influence job success, most vocational assessments take a more holistic approach.

The following is assessed as part of a comprehensive vocational assessment (assuming a medical or psychiatric assessment has already taken place):

- History, education, employment, background, etc.
- Psychosocial strengths and development
- Independent living skills
- Literacy
- Knowledge of the world of work
- Abilities/aptitudes
- Technical/job skills
- Generic work behaviors (social, communication, etc.)
- Job seeking skills
- Job readiness
- Special needs.

The Techniques or Methods Used in Vocational Assessment

Vocational assessment includes a variety of methods and assessment techniques. Some are standardized and some are non-standardized, that is are less formal and more subject to individual bias or educated judgment. As noted, standardized methods include various tests or work samples that have norms or averages form the general population against with the person's score or outcome is based. Non-standardized methods may include observation of a person working. Non-standardized methods are important and a mix of approaches will produce the best assessment.

Vocational assessment includes the following techniques and tools:

- Background information and reports of other professionals and the individual
- Interviews with the person with a disability and perhaps his/her family, former teachers, employers or others
- Checklists (for use by professionals or the individual being assessed)
- Vocational exploration and counseling to clarify goals and help direct the process
- Paper and pencil tests, including a variety of standardized psychometric and psychological tests (some which must be administered by a trained psychologist)

- Work samples (work tasks that require individuals to perform work and compares his/her performance to that of others)
- Situational assessment (observing people in work or training settings)
- Job tryouts.

Work Samples

Work samples are real or simulated work tasks that are used for both assessment and job exploration processes. By engaging in such tasks, the individual tests his/her ability to complete the tasks against a norm (collected data about the average performance of a certain population or normative group).

Through direct experience, the individual confronts his or own abilities and skills in relation to the task. The evaluator, through observation and a comparison to norms is able to make some assessment and judgment about the person's capabilities.

Work samples are commercially available and developed. For example, a company named Valpar produces work samples in tasks such as sorting color tiles. Work samples can also be developed in response to assessment needs to local jobs. For example, an evaluator may develop a work sample related to filing, sorting, assembling a computer, using a sewing machine or sweeping a floor and so forth.

Situational Assessment

Situational assessment involves placing the person in an actual work situation to assess their performance. Situation assessments are commonly used in rehabilitation facilities that have workshops and typically used to assess work behaviors, work tolerance, ability to follow instructions, work with others, etc. However such assessments can also be used to assess specific work skills and abilities. If a situational assessment is coordinated with specific job analysis (a checklist of sorts that outlines all the requirements of a particular job) it can be most effective in determining a person's ability to use a job.

Training centers and individual's classroom or experiential activities can provide a venue for situation assessment as well as vocational exploration.

A job tryout is like a situational assessment, but it is usually at the end of the assessment process when the individuals is fairly certain about what he/she wants to do and seems to have all the requisite aptitudes, abilities and skills. The evaluator arranges for a short job tryout to determine if the person can do the job and if it is a good fit.

The Methods used in Assessment

A skilled and experienced evaluator will use the variety of methods noted, such as reviewing background information, interviewing, providing vocational exploration experiences, using tests and checklists as well as work samples, situational assessment, job tryouts and even individually tailored assignments to help a person determine the career potential and direction. The following are general approaches for each of the major areas of assessment.

Assessment Relevant Psychosocial Issues

Psychosocial factors refer the behaviors, attitudes and lifestyle conditions that can contribute to the individual's success in training or on-the-job. Some of these factors include:

- Motivation
- Self-esteem
- Social and communication skills
- Family situation
- Social life
- Personal stability and strengths
- Personality characteristics
- Problem solving skills
- Life goals
- Economic and financial situation, etc.

Many of these factors and their significance to the workplace will be culturally determined. However, they can be crucially important to success in the workplace.

These can be assessed by use of:

- Interviewing techniques
- Checklists (commercially available or designed to suit needs)
- Personality tests and inventories
- Psychological and aptitude tests
- Review of background information.

Note that many personality or psychological tests are culture bound and require administration by a trained psychologist.

Assessment of Independent Living Skills

It is important to have some assessment of a person's independent living skills, such as:

- Self-care
- Grooming
- Ability to tell time and time management
- Ability to handle finances
- Ability to use transportation
- Ability to maintain a home

These can be assessed through various methods:

- Interviewing
- Checklists
- Paper and pencil tests
- Especially designed experiences
- Observation.

Assessment of Literacy Level

Literacy levels, including math, reading/language and if needed, computer and foreign language literacy.

Tests are usually used to determine literacy level. Use whatever tests are commonly used in the country for the general population. Consult employers, schools and computer companies for tests related to computer or foreign language literacy.

Assessment of Interest

Interests refer to what a person wants to do.

Several methods exist for measuring interests:

- Interviewing
- Interest inventories
- A variety of vocational exploration activities
- Work samples
- Situation assessment
- Job tryouts.

Interview techniques can be used to determine vocational interests. Many people who have not had experience or are not familiar with job opportunities will have limited exposure to the world of work to know what they would like to do. Interview techniques will have to include questions about past work and school work, hobbies, work experience both formal and informal to try to get at what interests the individual.

Many countries have interest inventories which are used to determine interest levels. Some are picture inventories for those who are illiterate; others are paper and pencil tests that ask individuals to respond to items.

As part of assessing interests and helping a person with a disability make career decisions, they need to understand the options available to them. Many may have not have had the experiences of learning about jobs or the world of work, or may assume that they cannot do certain types of jobs. As a result, it may be necessary to conduct some vocational exploration and counseling as part of the assessment process.

Why is vocational exploration part of the process?

People need occupation information in order to make career choices or to know what they want to do. Their interests may point in the direct of career possibilities, however many disabled people have lacked the experiences that might expose them to the world of work and the possibilities that are available to them. For this reason, the evaluation process in some countries includes a process called vocational information.

There are many ways to assess a person's knowledge about jobs (interviews, checklists, etc.) and to help them explore jobs opportunities. The best thing to do is to determine what career guidance tools are used in schools and employment settings for a general population. Another is to use situational assessment, job tryouts, guided activities like having the person with a disability interview someone with a job they think they might like, arrange visits to training centers and work sites, e.g. outside speakers and mentors can assist with the vocational exploration process. Job shadowing (the individual spends time just observing someone do a job that might interest them) is another technique. Many require employer support.

Without some knowledge of the possibilities the person with a disability will have difficulty in knowing about possibilities and what they want to do.

Types of abilities and aptitudes need to be measured

Abilities and aptitudes refer to natural talents or capacities, whereas skills refer to what a person has learned to do. Success in learning a skill is dependent on aptitudes and abilities. Some examples of aptitudes include intelligence and cognitive abilities, verbal, numerical, spatial, form and clerical perception, motor-coordination, finger dexterity, manual dexterity, eye-hand-foot coordination, color discrimination, etc. Physical abilities, tolerance and stamina refers to another set of capacities.

- *Intelligence* is typically measured through Intelligence Quotient or IQ tests. Psychologists usually administer these tests. Other cognitive abilities such as learning ability, memory, concentration, and reasoning may require a psychologist or neuropsychologist for proper assessment if there appears to be significant loss in these areas of functioning.
- *Aptitude* is typically measured by a battery of paper and pencil tests, although some aptitudes can be measured through work samples and other means.
- *Dexterity,* coordination and manual abilities refer to a variety of aptitudes that require the use of body and are necessary for tasks such as use of the equipment, handicrafts, etc. They can be measured through tests such as the Purdue Peg Board which times the individual's completion of a manual task and compares it to a group norm. Many dexterity tests and work samples are commercially available. Others can be constructed locally.
- *Physical capacity* or functioning refers to an individual's ability to perform a range of physical functions such as sitting, standing, bending, lifting, range of motion for arms, etc.). Such assessments are needed for people with certain types of disabilities and are conducted by physical therapists, physicians, or in some cases by trained evaluators using commercially available work samples.
- *Work tolerance* refers to how long and at what level of physical intensity a person can work. For example, can they work a full 8-hour day? This type of assessment is usually done by a skilled physiotherapist or in a situational assessment, such as a sheltered workshop, where people work and their capacity to perform and sustain work is measured.

Measurement of Skills

Skills refer to what a person has learned to do. Successful skill development is often based on the existence of particular abilities and on successful training or life experiences. Specific technical or occupational as well as generic work and life skills are needed to success on the job. The types of occupational skills that are measured will usually be determined by the person's abilities, the outcome of the assessment to date and the type of job or career that interests them.

Skills as well as the knowledge of the process of how to apply skills (e.g. describe how you would fix a broken engine) can be measured in a variety of ways. These include:

- Interviewing
- Checklists
- Paper and pencil tests
- Trade tests
- Work sample
- Performance-based tasks
- Situational assessment
- Job tryouts.

Many companies have skill tests to determine if a person is skilled in the job duties. A typing test is an example of a simple skills test. Trade tests may also be available from associations, apprenticeship programs, employers or other to evaluate capacity in a particular trade.

Work samples can also be designed to compare a person's performance to that of the average worker in the job. An easy example is piece rate in a textile situation. The performance of a person with a disability can be compared to that of the average worker to determine the level of his/her skill development. You might consider developing some work samples or tests that relate to specific and common jobs in the country, such as sewing machine operation, computer operator, etc.

- In evaluating, the capacity of a person to do a specific job, it is worthwhile to conduct a job analysis. On-the-job assessments with employers can be very useful for skills that are more difficult to assess in a testing situation such as cooking, meeting high-demand public situation, etc., and in many ways, this is the best way to determine if a person can do a job. In such cases, you should provide the employer with a checklist or assessment, based on a job analysis. On the job assessment are also useful for assessing a person's generic or job readiness skills.

Measurement Job-seeking Skills

Job-seeking skills refers to all those skills needed to find a job, such as identifying job leads, making contact with employers, completing job application and interviewing to name a few.

Knowledge of these skills can be determined through:

- Interviewing
- Paper and pencil tests
- Observation
- Results of actual job searching.

Proficiency and competency in these skills can only be determined through situation assessment and observation through role-play and real-life experience and interviewing for job seeking skills.

Job Readiness

Job readiness refers to a series of criteria that may be culturally determined or dependent upon the availability on the job support services, which determine if an individual is ready for employment. These criteria could include things like:

- Has are a realist job goal?
- Has transportation?
- Is able to manage money?
- Had good work habits and generic work skills?
- Understands the work of work
- Has appropriate generic work habits and skills?

Many organizations create checklists to assess job readiness. Aspects of job readiness are then determined through interviews, situational assessment, observation and the entire assessment process that can culminate in a job tryout.

Assessment for Special Needs

Before and throughout the assessment process, those involved in working with the disabled person should work with that person to determine what types of assistive devices or technology they need for independent living, training and employment. Once a specific job is identified or type of work, specific job modifications, support services or assistive devices can be identified with the evaluator or job placement specialist working with the disabled person and the employer to make the necessary determinations and adjustments.

Are there specific methods for assessing different types of disabled persons?

For people who have limited intellectual capacities or verbal skills, paper and pencil tests, or interviewing may not yield the necessary information. Work samples, situation assessments and task and job tryouts may be most useful.

CHAPTER 13

Vocational Rehabilitation

INTRODUCTION

Vocational rehabilitation is a process which enables persons with functional, psychological, developmental, cognitive and emotional impairments or health disabilities to overcome barriers to accessing, maintaining or returning to employment or other useful occupation.

Vocational rehabilitation can require input from a range of health care professionals and other non-medical disciplines such as disability employment advisers and career counselors. Techniques used can include:

- Assessment, appraisal, program evaluation and research
- Goal setting and intervention planning
- Provision of health advice and promotion, in support of returning to work
- Support for self-management of health conditions
- Making adjustments to the medical and psychological impact of a disability
- Case management, referral, and service coordination
- Psychosocial interventions
- Career counseling, job analysis, job development, and placement services
- Functional and work capacity evaluations.

BASIC STEPS TO VOCATIONAL REHABILITATION

- Referral and application
- Initial interview
- Evaluation/assessment
- Eligibility
- Planning
- Services
- Employment
- Successful rehabilitation—Employed.

Step 1–Referral and Application

To apply for VR services, contact the rehabilitation service office nearest to where you live. You should be prepared to give the following information:

- Name
- Disability
- Telephone number
- Address
- Date of birth
- Social security number.

A VR counselor will schedule an initial interview.

Prior to client interview, he should notify his counselor of any special accommodations he may need.

Step 2–Initial Interview

During client initial interview, VR counselor will review and/or complete his application for VR services with him. Counselor will ask him many questions about his disability, education, family, and work history to determine his eligibility for services.

To speed up the eligibility process, client should bring the following during the Initial interview:

- Medical reports regarding clients disability
- Transcripts and/or grades from high school, college/vocational technical school
- Reports from other professionals who have provided services to him
- A description or resume of his work history if he has work experience.

Sometimes additional medical exams are needed. VR counselor may arrange additional examinations including a general physical/ specialist evaluation, psychological, and/or a vocational evaluation. All evaluations; medical, psychological, and vocational are provided to him. Client with his VR counselor may also discuss his career plans and possible VR services. Client may be eligible for that would help him to reach his goal of employment.

Step 3–Evaluation/Assessment

Vocational rehabilitation counselor uses the medical information to evaluate the effects of client disability on his ability to prepare for, get, and keep a job. A vocational evaluation consisting of a series of tests, activities, and interest inventories is used to learn more about clients abilities, skills, interests, and the kinds of jobs that would be best suited for him. All his medical and vocational information helps him.

VR counselor determines whether you qualify for VR services and what types of services you will need to reach your employment goal.

Step 4–Eligibility

VR counselor will determine if client is eligible for services. A decision should be reached for VR services.

Eligibility for VR Services

Someone have a physical, mental, learning, or emotional disability; and he has a problem getting or keeping a job because of his disability; and he need VR services to help him prepare for, get, and/or keep a job.

Trial Work Period

When there is a question about clients employability because of the severe nature of his disability, he is allowed a trial work period. During the trial work period, he and his VR counselor will decide which vocational rehabilitation services client will need to evaluate his ability to get or keep a job. If he cannot participate in trial work, he may be placed into extended evaluation. At any time during the trial work period or extended evaluation, if needed, his counselor can make a decision to determine his eligibility for VR services.

SSI/SSDI Recipients

- An individual who has a disability or who is blind as
- Determined pursuant to Title II or Title XVI of the Social
- Security Act (42 USC 401 et. seq. and 1381 et seq.)
- Shall be: Considered to be an individual with either a significant disability or a most significant disability; and presumed to be eligible for vocational rehabilitation services, provided that the individual intends to achieve an employment outcome.
- The VR counselor can find an SSDI or an SSI recipient ineligible for services if the counselor can demonstrate by clear and convincing evidence through the use of trial work experiences that the severity of the individual's disability prohibits the individual from benefiting from VR services in terms of an employment outcome.
- For providing vocational rehabilitation services.
- This means eligible individuals with the most significant
- Disabilities are given first priority for services.
- If client is not eligible for vocational rehabilitation services, his counselor will explain why and discuss other resources in the community that may help him.

Step 5–Planning

Once determined eligible for services, client and his VR counselor work together to plan and develop a vocational rehabilitation program designed just for him. Deciding on his career goals and the VR services he need to reach this goal is the most important part of his VR program. Client should be prepared to give a great deal of thought and planning into making this decision.

During the planning stage, he will be asked to provide documentation regarding his financial status, including verification of his income, assets, and checking and saving accounts. He will also need to provide verification of any disability related expenses he may have. His VR counselor will complete a budget analysis. Based on his income, he may be required to pay a portion of the cost of services.

In deciding his career goals, he has the option of choosing to develop his own plan or having VR counselor help him to develop his plan. This plan is called the *"Individualized Plan for Employment."* It identifies client's employment goal, time frames for services, and approved service providers necessary for his vocational rehabilitation.

The plan also outlines his financial participation in services. This is an important document. The services outlined on the plan are conditioned on the approval and signatures of client, The VR counselor, the district supervisor and, if required, any other Agency approval(s), Clients and his VR counselor will review the IPE at least annually. If your situation changes, the IPE is updated.

Step 6–Services

VR services are provided to help persons who are disabled prepare for, enter, and/or keep employment. Client and his VR counselor determine the specific kind and number of services he might need. Services are based on his individual needs; therefore, the types of services he receive may differ from services that other individuals receive. Not everyone requires the same or every service.

To achieve his employment goals, VR can provide a wide range of services:

- Medical examinations (general physical, psychological, or other specialist examinations)
- Vocational evaluation of interests, skills, and abilities for future work
- Vocational guidance
- Career counseling.

Physical or mental restoration services that could include mental health counseling, speech therapy, physical therapy, etc.

Training: Universities, colleges, technical schools, apprenticeship programs, on-the-job training, supported employment, etc.

Rehabilitation devices: Medical equipment necessary for employment (wheelchairs, prosthesis, glasses, self-help devices, etc.)

Rehabilitation engineering: Assistance with job site modifications (changing lighting, adapting a telephone, a computer, or a tool, etc.); and training on the use of the modified equipment.

Job Placement

Follow-up after employment to ensure job success.

Step 7–Employment

- All VR services are geared to prepare client for a job. After successfully completing his planned services, he is ready for employment. Finding a job takes a lot of work, but together he and VR counselor can match his skills with a job. He may discover that this is the most difficult part of the whole process. It is very important that he actively look for a job.

- VR counselor and/or a rehabilitation employment specialist will help client with his job search. These are some examples of how they can help you:
  - Complete application forms
  - Develop a resume
  - Prepare for an interview
  - Conduct your job search
  - Find job leads.

Step 8–Successful Rehabilitation—Employed

Once he is employed, VR counselor will continue to work with him for an additional 90 days. During this 90 day period, VR counselor will meet with him and, if he approve, his employer to determine his job satisfaction.

Sometimes, unforeseen problems can occur that put he at risk of losing his job. If this happens, contact VR counselor immediately for assistance. Often, his counselor can help him work out the problem and/or provide services he might need to maintain his job.

Once his case has been closed as successfully rehabilitated, but he find that he need additional short-term services to help he maintain his current employment, he should ask to VR counselor about post-employment services.

Post-employment services are available to meet any simple, short-term rehabilitation need(s).

Rights of Client

Client has certain rights under the vocational rehabilitation program. It is important that he know and understand his rights. He has the right to: Apply for vocational rehabilitation services.

- Be treated with respect.
- Be evaluated fairly and completely to have your eligibility determined.
- Receive a determination of eligibility for vocational rehabilitation services within 60 days of application or agree to extend this period of time.

- Know why he is considered ineligible for services.
- Be referred to other agencies and facilities as appropriate.
- Appeal any decision or denial of vocational rehabilitation service through either an administrative review and/or a fair hearing.
- Receive an explanation of the help available through the Client Assistance Program (CAP).
- Receive an assessment of his need for post-employment services.

Responsibilities of Rehabilitation Team

VR program; is a "team" effort. To make clients rehabilitation a success, client and his VR counselor must work together.

Vocational rehabilitation works better If VR program in-charge.

- Take an active part in planning and making decisions
- Ask questions anytime clint do not understand something
- Stay in regular contact with the people working with him
- Follow through with all the agreed upon activities
- Keep his counselor advised of anything that changes clients ability to complete his VR program
- Ask counselor for any help in-charge need during any part of VR program
- Actively seek employment when client is job ready
- Tell his counselor when he gets a job.

Program in-charge is responsible for making sure that the rehabilitation plan developed by him and VR.

Counselor meets their needs.

Confidentiality

VR counselor will ask client to provide personal information about himself to understand his disability, determine his eligibility, and plan VR program. A case record is developed to keep all clients information together. All case record information is confidential.

RS will not share clients information with other individuals and/or agencies without his signed consent to release the information. The only exception would be to protect client or others if client are a threat to his own safety or the safety of others.

Client Assistance Program

Client can request help from the Client Assistance Program (CAP) at any time to resolve problems or misunderstandings that occur during your vocational rehabilitation program. CAP is independent of RS, and provides advocacy and information free of charge.

If you are eligible, some of the services include:

- Counseling—to help you adjust to your disability
- Personal care attendant—someone to assist you with your daily living needs
- Home modifications—a ramp, grab bars, etc.
- Rehabilitation devices—prostheses, wheelchairs, lifts, etc.
- Interpreter and reader services
- Other services that may help you live independently or become eligible for vocational rehabilitation services
- These centers provide information on topics of concern or interests regarding persons with disabilities and refer consumers to appropriate resources to meet their inquiries and needs.

CHAPTER

14

Legislations for Rehabilitation Services and PWD Act

DISABILITY

Disability is the consequence of an impairment that may be physical, cognitive, mental, sensory, emotional, developmental, or some combination of these. A disability may be present from birth, or occur during a person's lifetime.

A disability is an umbrella term, covering impairments, activity limitations, and participation restrictions. Impairment is a problem in body function or structure; an activity limitation is a difficulty encountered by an individual in executing a task or action; while a participation restriction is a problem experienced by an individual in involvement in life situations. Thus, disability is a complex phenomenon, reflecting an interaction between features of a person's body and features of the society in which he/she lives.

Types of Disability

The term "disability" broadly describes an impairment in a person's ability to function, caused by changes in various subsystems of the body, or to mental health. The degree of disability may range from mild to moderate, severe, or profound. A person may also have multiple disabilities. Disability can be measured objectively (observed) or subjectively (self-report).

Conditions causing disability are classified by the medical community as:

- Inherited (genetically transmitted);
- Congenital, meaning caused by a mother's infection or other disease during pregnancy, embryonic or fetal developmental irregularities, or by injury during or soon after birth;
- Acquired, such as conditions caused by illness or injury;
- Of unknown origin.

Types of disability may also be categorized in the following way:

Physical Disability

Any impairment which limits the physical function of limbs, fine bones, or gross motor ability is a physical impairment, not necessarily a physical disability. The social model of disability defines physical disability as manifest when impairment meets a non-universal design or program, e.g. a person who cannot climb stairs may have a physical impairment of the knees when putting stress on them from an elevated position such as with climbing or descending stairs. If an elevator were provided, or a building had services on the first floor, this impairment would not become a disability. Other physical disabilities include impairments which limit other activities of daily living, such as severe sleep disorders.

A man with an above the knee amputation exercises while wearing a prosthetic leg.

Sensory Disability

Sensory disability is impairment of one of the senses. The term is used primarily to refer to vision and hearing impairment, but other senses can be impaired.

Vision Impairment

Vision impairment (or "visual impairment") is vision loss of a person to such a degree as to qualify as an additional support need through a significant limitation of visual capability resulting from either disease, trauma, or congenital or degenerative conditions that cannot be corrected by conventional means, such as refractive correction, medication, or surgery. This functional loss of vision is typically defined to manifest with best corrected visual acuity of less than 20/60, or significant central field defect, Significant peripheral field defect including homonymous or heteronymous bilateral visual, field defect or generalized contraction or constriction of field, or reduced peak contrast sensitivity with either of the above conditions.

Hearing Impairment

Hearing impairment or hard of hearing or deafness refers to conditions in which individuals are fully or partially unable to detect or perceive at least some frequencies of sound which can typically be heard by most people. Mild hearing loss may sometimes not be considered a disability.

Olfactory and Gustatory Impairment

Impairment of the sense of smell and taste are commonly associated with aging but can also occur in younger people due to a wide variety of causes.

There are various olfactory disorders:

- Anosmia—inability to smell
- Dysosmia—things do not smell as they "should"
- Hyperosmia—an abnormally acute sense of smell
- Hyposmia—decreased ability to smell
- Olfactory reference syndrome—psychological disorder which causes patients to imagine they have strong body odor
- Parosmia—things smell worse than they should
- Phantosmia—"hallucinated smell", often unpleasant in nature
- Complete loss of the sense of taste is known as ageusia, while dysgeusia is persistent abnormal sense of taste.

Somatosensory Impairment

Insensitivity to stimuli such as touch, heat, cold, and pain are often an adjunct to a more general physical impairment involving neural pathways and is very commonly associated with paralysis (in which the motor neural circuits are also affected).

Balance Disorder

A balance disorder is a disturbance that causes an individual to feel unsteady, for example when standing or walking. It may be accompanied by symptoms of being giddy, woozy, or have a sensation of movement, spinning, or floating. Balance is the result of several body systems working together. The eyes (visual system), ears (vestibular system) and the body's sense of where it is in space (proprioception) need to be intact. The brain, which compiles this information, needs to be functioning effectively.

Intellectual Disability

Intellectual disability is a broad concept that ranges from mental retardation to cognitive deficits too mild or too specific (as in specific learning disability) to qualify as mental retardation. Intellectual disabilities may appear at any age. Mental retardation is a subtype of intellectual disability, and the term intellectual disability is now preferred by many advocates in most English-speaking countries.

Mental Health and Emotional Disabilities

A mental disorder or mental illness is a psychological or behavioral pattern generally associated with subjective distress or disability that occurs in an individual, and perceived by the majority of society as being outside of normal development or cultural expectations. The recognition and understanding of mental health conditions has changed over time and across cultures, and there are still variations in the definition, assessment, and classification of mental disorders, although standard guideline criteria are widely accepted.

Pervasive Developmental Disorders

The diagnostic category of pervasive developmental disorders refers to a group of five developmental disabilities characterized by differences in the development of multiple basic functions including socialization and communication. The DSM-IV-TR listed the pervasive developmental disorders as autistic disorder, Asperger syndrome, Rett syndrome, childhood disintegrative disorder, and pervasive developmental disorder not otherwise specified (PDD-NOS). The DSM-5 does not describe individual diagnosis of any of the pervasive developmental disorders, replacing all of them with a unified diagnosis of autism spectrum disorder. The ICD-10 also includes the diagnosis of overactive disorder associated with mental retardation and stereotyped movements.

Developmental Disability

Developmental disability is any disability that results in problems with growth and development. Although the term is often used as a synonym or euphemism for intellectual disability, the term also encompasses many congenital medical conditions that have no mental or intellectual components, for example spina bifida.

Nonvisible Disabilities

Several chronic disorders, such as diabetes, asthma, inflammatory bowel disease, epilepsy, narcolepsy, fibromyalgia, and some sleep disorders may be counted as nonvisible disabilities, as opposed to disabilities which are clearly visible, such as those requiring the use of a wheelchair.

DISABILITY ACT

The person with disability (Equal Opportunities, Protection of Rights and Full Participation) Act, 1995.

PURPOSE OF THE ACT

The purpose of this Act which was made law in 1996 (Gazette number 1 of 1996) is to fix responsibilities on the Central and State Government to the extent of their resources permit, to provide services, create facilities and give support to people with disabilities in order to enable them to have equal opportunities in participating as productive and contributing citizens of this country to the fullest extent their abilities. It fixes its responsibilities on the Governments (Center and State) to ensure that disabilities do not prevent individual citizens of this country from living a full life and making full contribution each in accordance with his/her ability.

This Act provides a frame within which specific demands can be made by the disabled people in order to ensure that the promises made in this Act are honored by the Government.

Chapter I: Preliminary

In chapter 1, legal definitions of the terms used in the Act are given. Disability means blindness, low vision, leprosy-cured, hearing impairment, locomotor disability, mental retardation and mental illness.

1. *Blindness:* No vision at all.
2. *Low vision:* Person capable of execution of a task with appropriate assistive devices.
3. *Leprosy cured:* Cured but loss of sensation in hands or feet as well as loss of sensation and paresis in the eye and eye lid OR manifest deformity, but sufficiently mobile to do normal economic activity or extreme physical deformity and cannot do any gainful occupation.
4. *Hearing impairment:* Loss of 60 decibels or more in the conversational range of frequencies.
5. *Locomotor disability:* Disability of the bone joints or muscles leading to substantial restriction of limb movements or any of cerebral palsy.
6. *Mental illness:* Any mental disorder other than mental retardation.
7. *Mental retardation:* Condition of arrested or incomplete development of the mind of a person.

A person with disability has to be certified by a medical authority that he/she is suffering from not less than 40% of the disability.

Chapter II: The Central Coordination Committee

In the purpose of this Act, the Central Government shall constitute a Central Coordination Committee (CCC), headed by the Minister of Social Justice and Empowerment.

The Central Coordination Committee consists of 39 persons, 34 will be official members and five nominated by the government, will represent NGOs and associations concerned with disabilities. Among the five, inclusion of at least one women and one person from SC or ST is envisaged. The term of all the members will be for three years.

The committee shall meet once every six months and the committee shall have a Central Executive Committee which shall carry out the decision of the Central Coordination Committee. The Executive Committee shall meet every three months.

Central Executive Committee (CEC)

Central Executive Committee will consist of 23 persons, including 5 nominated by the government, with a composition as laid down in CCC for the group.

The function of the Central Coordination Committee shall be the following:

1. Review and coordinate the activities of government, governmental and non-governmental organizations, which are dealing with matters relating to persons with disabilities.
2. Develop a national policy.
3. Advice the central government on the formulation of policies, programs, legislation and projects with respect to disability.
4. Advocacy with national, international organizations with a view to provide for schemes and projects for the disabled in the national and international plans and programs.
5. Review donor funding policies from the perspective of their impact on persons with disabilities.
6. To ensure barrier free environment
7. Monitor and evaluate the impact of policies and programs designed for achieving equality and full participation of persons with disabilities.
8. To perform such other functions as may be prescribed by the central government.

The Central Coordination Committee will be bound by such directions in writing as the central government may give it,

Chapter III: The State Coordination Committee

Identical to the Central Coordination Committee, each state shall appoint a State Coordination Committee, consisting of 23 official and 5 non-official members.

The State Executive Committee will be akin to (similar to) its central counterpart with 13 official and 5 non-official members.

The terms and conditions governing the State Committees shall be the same as those of the Central Coordination Committee, and the functions shall also be the same.

The State Coordination Committee shall be bound by such directions in writing as the Central Coordination Committee or as state government may give it.

Chapter IV: Prevention and Early Detection of Disabilities

Within the limits of their economic capacity and development, the appropriate governments and the local authorities, with a view to preventing the occurrence of disabilities, shall:

a. Undertake or cause to be undertaken surveys, investigations and research concerning the cause of occurrence of disabilities.
b. Promote various methods of preventing disabilities.
c. Screen all the children at least once in a year for the purpose of identifying at-risk cases.
d. Provide facilities for training to the staff at the primary health centers.
d. Sponsor or cause to be sponsored awareness campaigns and disseminate or cause to be disseminated information for general hygiene health and sanitation.
e. Take measures for prenatal, perinatal, and postnatal care of mother and child.
f. Educate the public through the preschools, primary health centers, village level workers and Anganwadi workers.
g. Create awareness amongst masses through television, radio and other mass media on the causes of disabilities and the preventive measures to be adopted.

Chapter V: Education

The central and state governments and local authorities shall ensure that every child with disability has access to free and adequate education till the age of 18, integrate students with disabilities into normal schools, set up special schools in government and private sectors for those in need of special education and equip these special schools with vocational training facilities for children with disabilities.

The local authorities shall also introduce schemes for non-formal education of children with disabilities who have discontinued their education after 5th class. Conduct special part time classes for functional literacy for children with disabilities in the age group of 16 and above, and provide each child with disability, free of cost, special books and equipments needed for his/her education, including in open schools and universities.

The government shall set up adequate number of teacher training institutions, capable of training teachers specialized in disabilities and adequate in number, in order to run both special schools and integrated schools for children with disabilities.

The government shall provide transport facilities to children with disabilities, remove architectural barriers from schools, colleges and other institution imparting vocational training and education to students with disability, provide books uniform and other materials to children attending schools, grant scholarships to students with disabilities, restructure curriculum for the benefit of students with disabilities.

Government shall promote research for assistive devices to give a child disability equal opportunities in education.

Chapter VI: Employment

Government shall identify posts which can be reserved for persons with disabilities. These reservations shall not be less than 3% of which 1% will be reserved for each of the below mentioned disabilities.

1. Blindness or low vision
2. Hearing impairment
3. Locomotor disability or cerebral palsy.

Special employment exchange will be the nodal agency for the purpose of employment. If in any year, any of the above vacancy cannot be filled then people with other disabilities can be given employment, and finally, if there is no person with disability who can fill the vacancy, then a person other than a person with disability can be given employment.

Appropriate governments and local authorities shall formulate schemes for ensuring employment of persons with disability and this shall include training of persons with disabilities. All government educational institutions and those receiving aids from the government shall reserve not less than 3% seats for persons with disabilities. Not less than 3% of all poverty alleviation schemes shall be reserved for persons with disabilities. Government shall within their economic capacities, give incentives to employers in public and private sectors to ensure that 5% of the work force is composed of persons with disabilities.

Chapter VII: Affirmative Action

The government shall provide aids and appliances to persons with disabilities and shall provide land at concessional rates for allotment to persons with disabilities for housing, business, special recreation centers, special schools, research centers and factories by entrepreneurs with disabilities.

Chapter VIII: Nondiscrimination

Government transport shall take special measures to adopt their facilities and amenities, so that they permit easy access to persons with disabilities, inclusive of persons on wheel chairs.

Government and local authorities shall also within their capacity, provide auditory signals along red lights, crossing constructions shall be designed for wheel chair users and engraving on zebra crossing for blind people. Warning signals shall be provided at appropriate places for the people with disabilities, etc. Building and toilets shall be constructed with ramps and other features, so that wheel chair users can have access to them. No employer shall terminate an employee who acquires a disability during service. No employer shall also deny promotion to an employee on grounds of disability, but provide for circumventing this, based on the type of work.

Chapter IX: Research and Manpower Development

Government and local authorities shall promote and sponsor research in order to prevent disability, rehabilitate the disabled, develop assistive devices, identify jobs for disabled and develop predisabled structural features in factories and offices.

Chapter X: Recognition of Institutions for Persons with Disabilities

Within six months of this Act being passed, persons running establishments or institutions for persons with disability shall apply under this Act, for a certificate or registration of the institution. This certificate shall be issued by a competent authority of the state government and shall remain in force for such period as granted by the state government. It shall be renewed through an application of renewal to be submitted not less than 60 days before the expiry of the certificate, the certificate can be denied or revoked for valid reasons and with a proper hearing granted to the applicant. The state government is the final appellate authority. Government institutions are immune from the provisions of this chapter.

Chapter XI: Institution for Persons with Severe Disabilities

Person having 80% or more of one or more disabilities are considered persons with severe disability. Governments shall establish and maintain institutions for them. Where private institutions exists, which meet government standards, they shall be recognized as institutions fit for persons with severe disabilities.

Chapter XII: The Chief Commissioner and Commissioners for Persons with Disabilities

The central government shall appoint a Chief Commissioner for persons with disabilities for the implementation of this Act. The Chief Commissioner shall coordinate the work of the Commissioners, monitor the utilization of funds given by the central government for persons with disabilities, ensure that rights and facilities made available to persons with disabilities are protected, and submit an annual report to the central government on the implementation of this Act.

Commissioner shall have similar responsibilities at the state level. The Chief Commissioner and the Commissioner shall take up any complaint regarding deprivation of rights of persons with disabilities and non-implementation of laws, rules, orders, instructions issued by the government or local authorities for the welfare and protection of rights of persons with disabilities.

The Chief Commissioners have the same powers as are vested in a court under the Code of Civil Procedure, 1908 for summoning and enforcing attendance of witness, receiving evidence on affidavits, etc.

The Chief Commissioners shall prepare an annual report giving full account of his activities during the previous financial year to the central government and this report shall be laid before each house of parliament. Similarly, the Commissioner shall submit an annual report to the state government.

Chapter XIII: Social Security

The government shall within their economic limits, undertake rehabilitation of all persons with disabilities and grant financial assistance to NGOs undertaking rehabilitation programs for persons with disabilities. Where possible, give unemployment allowance to persons with disabilities registered with the special employment exchange for more than 2 years, and would could not be placed in any gainful occupation. Insurance schemes for the unemployed, and if needed, insurance schemes for non-employed by the government is also mentioned.

Chapter XIV: Miscellaneous

Whoever attempts to commit fraud and avail of benefits for persons with disabilities shall be punished upto two years imprisonment and upto ₹ 20,000/- fine.

The government shall have the authority to make all rules and regulations necessary for carrying out the provisions of this Act. These rules and regulations shall be issued in the form of Government Orders (GO's) which shall have approval of both houses of parliament.

The Chief Commissioner, the Commissioners, Officers and staff provided to implement this Act shall be deemed to be public servant within the meaning of Section 21 of IPC, no suit, prosecution or other legal proceedings shall be allowed against the government and local authorities and the officers in respect of anything which was done in good faith or intended to be done in pursuance of this Act, and any rules or orders made there under.

The Act is in addition to and not in derogation of any other law, rules order, and instruction currently in force. Ministry of Social Justice and Empowerment have initiated action of implementation of "The Persons with Disabilities" (Equal Opportunities, Protection of Rights and Full Participation) Act, 1995 in the right earnest.

Several measures have been taken for the creation of necessary institutional arrangements which includes, notification of rules, constitution of Central Coordination Committee and constitution of Central Executive Committee for ensuring the implementation of the provision of the Act. Five core groups of experts for recommending suitable schemes of people with disabilities in various areas viz.

1. Prevention, early detection and intervention.
2. Education including preschool education.
3. Barrier free environment.
4. Women, children and aged with disabilities.
5. Vocational training and employment have been set up. Three core groups have since submitted their reports and action is in hand.

The "National program for Rehabilitation of People with Disabilities" has prepared for setting up suitable delivery system for people with disabilities especially in the rural areas. All the central ministries/departments, state governments and UT administrations have been impressed upon time and again to initiate appropriate action for implementation of the provisions of the Act. Due to the efforts of the Ministry of Social Justice and Empowerment, a greater understanding on the approach of multi-sectoral collaborative action for people with disabilities under which each sectoral ministry have to play a greater role for including the concerns of the disabled persons in their mainstream policies has got wider appreciation.

Efforts have also been made to have linkages with the National Open School to accredit the special study centers for people with disabilities. An Inter-Ministerial Committee set up under the chairmanship of Additional Secretary, Ministry of Social Justice and Empowerment is keeping a regular watch over the implementation of the Act.

CHAPTER

15

Facilities Available to the Persons with Disabilities in India

Concessions offered by the central government to the persons with disabilities.

TRAVEL CONCESSIONS FOR THE DISABLED

By Train

As per the order of Ministry of Railways, Government of India, the following concessions are available for the disabled.

Blind Person

The blind person traveling alone or with an escort, on production of a certificate from government doctor or a registered medical practitioner, is eligible to get the concession as below:

Element of concession

Class of reservation	First class	Second class	Sleeper class	Season ticket	
				Class first	Class second
Percentage of concession	75	75	75	50	50

The concession certificate may be issued by the Station Master on collection of the concession certificate may be issued by the Station Master on collection of the certificate form and the copy of original certificate duly attested by a Gazetted Officer, MP, MLA, etc. may be produced while collecting the ticket. The blind person may not be present at the station for purchase of the ticket.

Orthopedically Handicapped Person

The orthopedically handicapped person traveling with an escort, on production of a certificate from a government doctor to the effect that the person concerned is orthopedically handicapped and cannot travel without the assistance of an escort, is eligible for getting concession.

Element of concession

Class of reservation	First class	Second class	Sleeper class	Season ticket	
				Class first	Class second
Percentage of concession	75	75	75	50	50

All categories of orthopedically handicapped persons/patients.

Accompanied by escort, when traveling for admission or on discharge from hospital where the OH persons are treated or for consultation with medical expert, on production of a certificate from a government doctor/orthopedic surgeon that the person is a bonafide OH person and he cannot travel without an escort for availing concession.

Deaf and Dumb Person

A deaf and dumb person traveling alone (both afflictions together in the same person) on production of a certificate from a government doctor is eligible for the concession.

Element of concession

Class of reservation	First class	Second class	Sleeper class	Season ticket	
				Class first	Class second
Percentage of concession	75	75	75	50	50

Notes: (i) A deaf person is allowed 50% concession in railway fare both in first and second class, but concession is not available for the escort. (ii) A deaf and dumb person is permitted to travel by 2 -tier AC sleeper on payment of concessional fare for first class and full surcharge for 2-tier AC sleeper).

Mentally-retarded Person

A Mentally-retarded (MR) person, accompanied by an escort, on production of a certificate in the prescribed form, from a government doctor, is eligible to get the concession.

Element of concession

Class of reservation	First class	Second class	Sleeper class	Season ticket	
				Class first	Class second
Percentage of concession	75	75	75	50	50

Note: Mentally-retarded person is permitted to travel by 2-tier AC sleeper on payment of concessional fare for first class and full surcharge for 2-tier AC sleeper. Facility of issue of concessional return ticket will also be available in one month from the date of commencement of outward journey. MR person should be given preference in allotment of coupe on reservation in first class, if required. Free ticket for one escort is available for every two persons in the same class of carriage whether they hold adult or half ticket. All the concessional fares shall be calculated on the basis of the basic railway fare for the journey. No person/party will be allowed more than one concession at one time.

The holder of a concession ticket will not be permitted to change the ticket to a higher class by paying the difference except in the case of TB and cancer patient, leprosy patient, etc. The break-up journey shall not be allowed on a concession ticket for a specific journey, for example, students traveling for an examination center, patient traveling to/from a hospital, professor traveling from/to a conference, etc. The break journey will be allowed only if it is a natural event. During break journey, the passenger has to endorse the ticket along with Station Master's initial, date and station code. Refund of the untraveled journey on such tickets will not be allowed.

By Air

Blind Persons

The Indian Airlines Corporation allows 50% concessional fare to blind persons on single journey or single fare round trip journey on all domestic flights. To avail this facility (for blind persons) they have to produce a certificate from a medical practitioner. Air Hostess/Steward will look after the blind persons not accompanied by escorts in flight. The Public Relation Officer or the Traffic Officer In-charge at the airport will tender necessary assistance to such infirm passengers at the airport. Escorts are to pay full fare. This concession cannot be combined with any other concessional fare allowed by the Indian Airlines.

Locomotor Disability

Locomotor disabled persons (80% and above) are allowed following concessions in Indian Airlines:

a. About 50% of normal economy class INR fare or point-to-point fare. Full Inland Air Travel Tax and Passenger Service Fee applicable.
b. About 50% of INR fare applicable to foreigners resident in India for travel on domestic sectors. Full Inland Air Travel Tax and Passenger Service Fee applicable.

COMMUNICATION

Postage

Payment of postage, both inland and foreign, for transmission by post of Blind Literature packets are exempted if sent by surface route only. If packets are to be sent by air, prescribed air mail charges should be paid.

The relevant rule from the Post Office Guide is reproduced below:

Exemption from Postal Fees

1. 'Blind Literature' packets are exempted from the payment of postage and also for (i) registration fee, (ii) fee for acknowledgment, and (iii) fee for the attested copy of the receipt.
2. Postage free 'Blind Literature' packets will be transmitted by surface route only, and if they are to be sent by air, the air mail charge as prescribed for packets has to be paid.

Contents and Conditions of Posting

Papers any kind, periodicals and books printed in Braille or other special type for the use of the blind may be transmitted by post as 'Blind Literature' packets provided that they are posted in accordance with the following conditions:

Plates bearing the characters of writing, sound records for the use of the blind, and disks, films, tapes and wires on which spoken message for the blind have been recorded, when sent by, or addressed to, an officially recognized institution for the blind, shall also be treated as 'Blind Literature'.

a. The packets shall consist only of articles specially impressed as described above for the use of the blind, and shall not contain any communication either in writing or printed in ordinary type, except the title and table of contents of the book or periodical and any key to, or instructions for the use of special type, or any enclosure except a level for the return of the packet.
b. The packet shall bear on the outside the inscription 'Literature for the Blind' and the written or printed name and address of the sender.
c. The packet shall be posted without a cover, or in cover open at both ends, which can easily be removed for the purpose of examination.
d. No 'Blind Literature' packet may weigh more than 7 kg.
e 'Blind Literature' packets are subject to the same limits of dimensions as printed papers.

Penalty for Breach of Condition

Should any of the conditions mentioned above be infringed? The packet (Unless it is admissible as an ordinary packet) will be charged on delivery with letter or parcel postage, whichever may be less.

Rule 304, 305 and 306 in regard to definition of 'Blind Literature' conditions and exemption from postal fees in respect of foreign postage are the same as prescribed in rule 129 and 130 in regard to Inland Postage. However, the penalty for breach of conditions in respect of foreign postage is specified under rule 307—Penalty for Breach of Conditions: 'Blind Literature' packets which contain any note or document having the character of actual and personal correspondence, or which are not made up in such a manner as to admit of easy examination of the contents, or which contain postage stamps, form of pre-payment whether obliterated or not or paper representing any value, or which infringe any of the foregoing conditions will not be forwarded, but will be returned to the sender and will be charged on delivery with letter or parcel postage at the internal postage rate whichever is applicable. If the sender wishes to report the article after complying with the necessary conditions, he may do so. It is permissible in such cases to use the original wrapper, but the use of a fresh wrapper is preferable and is recommended.

Telecommunication

Concessional Telephone Connection to Blind Persons

It has been decided to provide telephone facility to blind persons on concession and priority basis on the following terms:

- Rental rebate—50 percent of the normal rental.
- Advance rental—50 percent of the annual advance rental and bimonthly rental as applicable to a private subscriber. This facility is available in non-OYT (S) category only.
- (c) Preference in allotment of STD/PCO to handicapped persons
- Educated unemployed persons are eligible for allotment of STD/ PCOs.
- The educational qualification for the applicant is:
  - VIIIth or Middle School Pass for rural areas.
  - At least matriculation or high school for urban areas.

CUSTOMS CONCESSIONS

Individuals

(Notification number 105/86 dated 17.2.86 Annexure issued by the Department of Revenue, Ministry of Finance)

The central government exempts goods specified below, when imported into India by a handicapped or disabled person for his personal use, from the whole of the duty of customs and the additional duty subject to the condition that the importer produces to the Assistant Collector of Customs, at the time of importation, a certificate from the Civil Surgeon of the District, Medical Officer or the Administrative Medical Officer or the Director of Health Services of the concerned state or a specialist in the concerned specialty attached to a government hospital or a recognized medical college to the effect that the importer suffers from the particular handicap or disability and that the imported goods in respect of which the exemption is claimed are essential to overcome the said handicap or disability.

1. Braille writers and Braille writing equipment
2. Hand writing equipment, Braille frames, slates, writing guides, Braille erasers, script writing guides.
3. Canes, electronic aids like the Sonic guide.
4. Optical, environmental sensors.
5. Arithmetic aids like the Taylor Frame (Arithmetic and Algebra types) Cubarythm, speaking or Braille calculator.
6. Geometrical aids like combined graph and mathematical demonstration board, Braille protractors, scales compasses and spar wheels.
7. Electronic measuring equipment, such as calipers, micrometers, comparators, gauges, blocks levels, and yard sticks.
8. Drafting drawing aids, tactile displays.
9. Specially adapted clocks and watches.
10. Orthopedic appliances falling under heading 90.21 of the first schedule to the said Tariff Act.
11. Wheel chairs falling under heading number 87.13 of the said First Schedule.
12. Artificial electronic Larynx and Spares thereof. Institutions

    As per notification CSR No. 550 (E) dated 10.11.1978 issued by the Department of Revenue, Ministry of Finance, Government of India, the Institutions (including Registered Cooperative Societies) for the Blind and the Deaf are permitted to import equipment and apparatus as below, being bonafide gifts to, as purchased out of donations received in foreign exchange by such institutions from (i) the whole of the duty of customs leviable thereon under the first schedule to the Customs Tariff Act, 1975 (51 of 1975); (ii) the whole of the auxiliary duty of customs leviable under subsection (I) section 35 of the Finance Act; and (iii) the whole of the additional duty leviable thereon under section 3 of said Customs Tariff Act at the time of importation of such goods into India:

    a. All tangible appliances for the blind.
    b. Hearing aids and other audio-visual aids for the education of the deaf.
    c. Vocational aids for the blind and the deaf.
    d. Articles including instruments, apparatus, appliances, machinery and spares or component parts of accessories

thereof required by such institution for the purpose of giving training or imparting instructions to the blind and the deaf.

Instructions

Where any such institution is scheduled to begin function only after the importation of the goods specified above the exemption shall not apply in respect of the goods imported by that institution, unless an undertaking in writing is given by the President or Secretary of that institution that it will begin to function within a period of six months from the date of importation of the goods. Provided that in any particular case, the aforesaid period of six months may, on sufficient cause being shown, be extended by the Collector of Customs concerned such further period as, he may deem fit. Where goods have been purchased out of donations received abroad in foreign exchange, the institution has been permitted to maintain an account abroad by the Reserve Bank of India for the purpose of receiving funds donated overseas.

Exemption for Braille Paper

Ministry of Finance (Department of Revenue) vide their Notification dated 1st March, 1981, has exempted Braille paper, falling under item number 17 of the First Schedule to the Central Excise and Salt Act, 1994 (1 number of 1994) from the whole of the duty of excise leviable thereon subject to the condition that such paper is supplied direct to a school for the blind or to a Braille press against an indent placed by the National Institute for the Visually Handicapped, Dehradun, Uttarakhand, India.

Import of Audio Cassettes

Ministry of Finance (Department of Revenue) vide their Notification number 379/86-Customs (F-14-839/86 C) dated 3rd July, 1986, has exempted audio cassettes, falling within Chapter 85 of the First Schedule to the Customs Tariff Act, 1975 (51 of 1975) newspapers or magazines for the blind when consigned by an organization and imported into India by an organization:

1. The whole of the duty of customs leviable thereon, which is specified in the said First Schedule,
2. The whole of the additional duty leviable thereon under Section 3 of the said Customs Tariff Act subject to the conditions that:

a. The audio cassettes so imported shall be re-exported within one year from the date on which these are imported into India or a such extended period as the Assistant Collector of Customs may allow,
b. The importer executes an undertaking binding himself to pay an amount equal to the duty leviable on the audio cassettes at the time of import to the Assistant Collector of Customs in the event of failure to re-export the said audio cassettes within the period specified or, as the case may be, such extended period as may be allowed; and
c. The importer produces the audio cassettes before the proper officer for identification before re-export.

CONVEYANCE ALLOWANCE

In accordance with the revised Orders number F.19029/2/86-E.IV and F. 19029/1/89-E.IV dated 16.5.87 and 12.9.89 respectively, issued by the Ministry of Finance, Department of Expenditure, the Central Government employees who are on regular establishment (including work charged staff) and who are blind or orthopedically handicapped (with disability of upper or lower extremities) are to be granted conveyance allowance at 5% of basic pay subject to a maximum of Rs. 100 per month subject to the following conditions:

- An orthopedically handicapped employee will be eligible for conveyance allowance only if he/she has a minimum 40% permanent/partial disability of either upper or lower limbs or 50% permanent/partial disability of both upper and lower limbs together.
- Conveyance allowance will be admissible to the orthopedically handicapped employee on the recommendation of the head of Orthopedic Department of a Government Civil Hospital.
- In the case of a blind employee, the allowance will be admissible on the recommendation of the head of Ophthalmological Department of a Government Civil Hospital.
- Conveyance allowance is also applied to central government employees suffering from spinal deformity (generally known as hunch back disability) at the same rate as available to other physically handicapped persons. The allowance will not be admissible during leave (except casual level), joining time or suspension.

CHILDREN'S EDUCATIONAL ALLOWANCE

As per Office Memorandum number 21011/21/88-Estt (Allowances) dated 17.10.88, issued by the Ministry of Personnel Grievances and Pensions (Department of Personnel and Training), grant of children educational allowance, reimbursement of tuition fee, etc., to central government employees will be governed by the Central Civil Services (Educational Assistance) Orders, 1988. Under this order, the reimbursement of tuition fee in respect of physically handicapped and mentally retarded children of the central government employee has been enhanced to Rs. 100 per month (from class I to XII) in comparison with general category where it restricts only to Rs. 40 per month. The disabled children will however, get other assistance under this scheme as per rates prescribed for the other children.

SCHEME OF INTEGRATED EDUCATION FOR THE DISABLED CHILDREN

This scheme is a Centrally Sponsored Scheme and was launched in 1974 by the then Department of Social Welfare. The scheme has however been transferred to the Department of Education since 1982. Under the scheme, handicapped children are sought to be integrated in the normal school system. About 100% assistance is provided to the States/UTs for education of the children suffering from certain mild handicaps in common schools with the help of necessary aids, incentives and especially trained teachers.

The following types of disabled children are covered under this scheme:

a. Children with locomotor handicaps (OH)
b. Mildly and moderately hearing impaired.
c. Partially sighted children.
d. Mentally handicapped-educable group (IQ 50–70).
e. Children with multiple handicaps (blind and orthopedic, hearing impaired and orthopedic, educable mentally retarded and orthopedic, visual impaired and mild hearing handicap).
f. Children with learning disabilities.
    1. The handicapped children are provided the following allowances and facilities under this scheme:
        a. Books and stationery allowance of Rs. 400 per annum.
        b. Uniform allowance of Rs. 50 per annum.

   c. Transport allowance of Rs. 50 per month (if a disabled child admitted under the scheme resides in a hostel of the school within the school premises, no transportation charges would be admissible).
   d. Reader allowance of Rs. 50 per month in case of blind children after class V.
   e. Escort allowance for severely handicapped children with lower extremity disabilities @ Rs. 75 per month.
   f. Actual cost of equipment subject to a maximum of Rs. 2,000 per student for a period of five years.
2. In the case of severely orthopedically handicapped children, it may be necessary to allow one attendant for 10 children in a school. The attendant may be given the standard scale of pay prescribed for Group 'D' employees in the States/UTs concerned.
3. Disabled children residing in school hostels within the same institution where they are studying may also be paid boarding and lodging charges as admissible under the state government rules/schemes. Where there is no State Scheme of Scholarships to hostellers, the disabled children, whose parents income does not exceed Rs. 3,000 per month, may be paid actual boarding and lodging charges subject to a maximum of Rs. 200 per month.
4. Severely orthopedically handicapped children residing in school hostels may need the help of a helper or an ayah, a special pay or Rs. 50 per month is admissible to any employee of the hostel willing to extend such help to children in addition to his/her duties.
5. In a school in rural areas where at least 10 handicapped children are enrolled, capital cost for purchase of school rickshaw for free use of these children and expenses for rickshaw puller Rs. 300 per month will be provided under the scheme. In such cases, no transport allowance will be payable to the students.

INCOME TAX CONCESSIONS

Relief for the Handicapped

Section 80 DD: Section 80 DD provides for a deduction in respect of the expenditure incurred by an individual or HUF resident in India on the medical treatment (including nursing) training and rehabilitation, etc., of handicapped dependants. For officiating the increased cost of such maintenance, the limit of the deduction has been raised to Rs. 41,000.

Section 80 V: A new Section 80 V has been introduced to ensure that the parent in whose hands, income of a disabled minor has been clubbed under Section 64, is allowed to claim a deduction upto Rs. 40,000 in case of an individual who is suffering from a permanent disability (including blindness) or is subject to mental retardation.

Section 88 B: This Section provides for an additional rebate from net tax payable by a resident individual who has attained the age of 65 years, has been amended and a tax rebate of Rs. 10,000 has been allowed. In his budget speech on 15th March, 1995, Mr Manmohan Singh, Finance Minister, Government of India made the following announcements: Deductions from the total income of handicapped persons under Section 80 V of the Income Tax Act has been raised from Rs. 20,000 to Rs. 40,000.

AWARD OF DEALERSHIPS/AGENCIES BY OIL COMPANIES

Award of Retail Outlet, 2/3 Wheeler Outlet, Kerosene-LDO Dealerships and LPG Distributorships.

Ministry of Petroleum and Natural Gas has reserved 7½% of all types of dealership agencies of the public sector oil companies for physically handicapped/Government personnel (other than defense personnel) disabled on duty/widows of government personnel (other than defense personnel who die in the course of duty). The oil industry appoints its dealers/distributors through an advertisement in one English daily and one regional daily newspaper having maximum circulation in the district in which the dealership/distributorship is to be located.

Eligibility Criteria

1. Indian National.
2. Age group (between 21 and 30 years).
3. Educational qualification (Matriculation or equivalent).
4. Physically handicapped persons should produce a certificate from Civil Surgeon/CMO or Superintendent of a Government Hospital that he/she is OH to the extent of minimum 40% permanent, partial or either upper or lower limb or both upper and lower limbs together.

Partially HH candidates are also eligible. Totally blind persons are eligible to apply for retail outlet/kerosene/LDO dealership. They are however not eligible for LPG distributorship.

Income

The candidate's income should not be more than Rs. 50,000 PA. Income for this purpose would include the income of the candidate, his/her spouse, dependent children put together. In case of dependent, his/her parents income would also be taken into consideration.

Application Form

Standard formats can be obtained from divisional/regional area office of the concerned oil companies.

RESERVATION OF JOBS AND OTHER FACILITIES FOR THE DISABLED PERSONS

Three Percent Reservations in Grade 'C' and 'D' Posts

As per the order of Government of India reservation of 3% in jobs have been made in Grade 'C' and Grade 'D' posts for the PH persons. The category of handicapped persons benefitted are the blind, the deaf and the orthopedically handicapped (OH) persons, as given below:

Category of handicapped percent of reservation

1. The blind 1
2. The deaf 1
3. The OH 1.

For effective implementation of the reservation, it has been advised to maintain a roaster of vacancies arising in Grade 'C' and Grade 'D' posts from year-to-year. The 34th vacancy may be earmarked for the blind. Similarly the 67th vacancy and 100th vacancy would be reserved for the deaf and the OH respectively in a cycle of 100 vacancies.

Definitions of Disabled for the Purpose of Reservation

1. *The blind:* The blind are those who suffer from either of the following conditions:
   a. Total absence of sight.
   b. Visual acuity not exceeding 6/60 or 20/200 (Snellen) in the better eye with correcting lenses.

   c. Limitation of the field of vision subtending an angle of 20 degrees or worse.

2. *The deaf:* The deaf are those in whom the sense of hearing is nonfunctional for ordinary purposes of life. They do not hear and understand sounds at all events with amplified speech. The cases included in this category will be those having hearing loss more than 90 decibels in the better ear (profound impairment) or total loss of hearing in both ears.
3. *The orthopedically handicapped:* The orthopedically handicapped are those who have a physical defect or deformity which causes an interference with the normal functioning of the bones, muscles and joints.

Identification of Jobs

In order to implement these reservation, without loss of productivity some posts are identified disability wise. To ensure sufficient recruitment of blind persons, separate list has been identified for the blind and partially blind persons.

Posting of Handicapped Candidates

As per the decision of Government of India Grade 'C' and Grade 'D' posts recruited on regional basis and who are physically handicapped may be given posting as far as possible near to their native place within the region subject to administrative constraints. PH employees may be given preference in transfer case near to their native place.

Relaxation of Ban Order on Recruitment to Vacancies Earmarked for PH Persons

As per the government order regarding ban on filling-up of non-operational vacant posts will not be applicable in case of reserve vacancies to be filled-up for PH person.

Carry Forward of Vacant Posts Under Reserve Category

As per the government order if a reserve category of person is not available or the nature vacancy in an office is such that the given category of person cannot be employed then the post may be carried forward for a period of three subsequent years.

Appointment of VI Persons as Caner in Government Department

As per the decision of Government of India it has been instructed that Recaning of chairs in government offices should be done by blind persons as far as possible when the volume of work require a full time chair caner then a suitable post may be created in consultation with the finance department. For the purpose of recaning the chairs in government offices, Vocational Rehabilitation Centers and Special Employment Exchange for the PH persons may be contacted.

Instruction to Appointing Authority for Intimating Vacancies Reserved for Handicap

As per the existing instruction of the government, all the vacancies in Grade 'C' and 'D' irrespective of their nature and duration are to be notified to the Employment Exchange and also to be filled through the agency unless filled through UPSC/SSC. It has also been decided that all the appointee should send their request to Employment Exchange/ Special Employment Exchange/nearest Vocational Rehabilitation Center for PH for nominating suitable handicapped persons.

Grant of Age Concession to PH Persons

As per the Government order, it has been decided to extend the age concession of 10 years in favor of handicap persons to recruitment to posts filled through the SSC and through Employment Exchange in Grade 'C' and Grade 'D' posts.

Relaxations in Typing Qualifications

As per the order PH persons who are otherwise eligible for appointment to posts of LDC but cannot be so appointed for being unable to satisfy the typing qualifications due to their disability may be exempted from the typing qualification for appointment.

Consideration for Confirmation in Job for Blind Persons

It has been instructed to all the Ministries/Departments of Government of India that there should not be any delay in confirmation of officers including blind persons on account of administrative delay. Ministry/ Department should ensure, especially in which blind persons are employed that confirmation is made without delay and at appropriate time.

Reservation for PH Persons in Posts Filled by Promotion

As per the order handicapped persons may be promoted to Grade 'C' From 'D' and within Grade 'C' against the identified post if they are capable of being filled/held by the appropriate category of PH.

Exemptions from Payment of Examinations Fee

As per the order PH persons recruited to Grade 'B' and Grade 'C' posts advertised by the UPSC and SSC will be exempted from the payment of Applications and examination fee as prescribed by UPSC/SSC.

SPONSORSHIP POWER TO NATIONAL INSTITUTIONS

The Ministry of Labor in consultation with the Ministry of Social Justice and Empowerment and Department of Personnel and Training has decided to grant co-sponsoring power to the national level rehabilitation institutes as given below:

1. National Institute for the Visually Handicapped, Dehradun, Uttarakhand, India.
2. National Institute for the Mentally Retarded, Secunderabad, Telangana, India.
3. Ali Yavar Jung National Institute for the Hearing Handicapped, Mumbai, Maharashtra, India.
4. National Institute for the Orthopedically Handicapped, Kolkata, West Bengal, India.
5. National Institute for Rehabilitation Training and Research, Cuttack, Odisha, India.
6. The Institute for the Physically Handicapped, Delhi, NCT of Delhi, India.

ECONOMIC ASSISTANCE

A Note containing this Scheme has been Forwarded by the Department of Economic Affairs Vide DO No F 301/89-SCT (B), dated 8.9.89 to the Ministry of Social Justice and Empowerment.

Public Sector Banks

Under the Scheme of Public Sector Banks for Orphanages, Women's Homes and Physically Handicapped Persons the benefits of the differential rate of interest are available to physically handicapped persons as well as institutions working for the welfare of the handicapped. The details of the scheme are as under.

Eligibility (For Individuals)

Physically handicapped persons are eligible to take loans under the scheme, if they satisfy the following conditions:

- Should be pursuing a gainful occupation
- Family income from all sources should not exceed Rs. 7,200 PA in urban or semi-urban areas or Rs. 6,400 PA in rural area
- Should not have land holding exceeding 1 acre if irrigated, and 25 acres if unirrigated
- Should not incur liability to two sources of finance at the same time
- Should work largely on their own and with such help as other members of their family or some joint partners may give them and should not employ paid employees on a regular basis.

Eligibility (For Institutions)

Institutions for the physically handicapped persons pursuing a gainful occupation are also eligible to take benefit under this scheme. The institutions are exempted from income criteria. However, these institutions could utilize the funds for productive purposes only and not for meeting their normal administrative and establishment expenses.

*Public Sector Banks refer to Nationalized Banks, the State Bank of India and its subsidiaries.

Assessment

The quantum of loan, both for working capital and for acquisition of fixed assets, will be determined on the basis of the needs of institutions/individuals in a scientific method to ensure that all their legitimate financial requirements are met in Toto.

Amount of Loan

The amount of loan will depend on the particular scheme proposed to be financed. It should be adequate to enable the borrower to finance his requirements without having to borrow funds from other sources. The normal limit will be Rs. 6,500 for working capital loan and Rs. 5,500 for a term loan. In exceptional cases, particularly for institutions, etc., higher amounts are allowed. Both the working capital and term loan are admissible in accordance with the specific requirement of the borrower.

In the case of small scale industries, village artisans, etc., in decentralized sector advances under the scheme may be granted upto Rs. 6,000 without making any distinction between working capital and term loan by way of composite loan.

Repayment

Term for the acquisition of fixed assets are normally allowed for five years, including a grace period not exceeding two years on the repayment of principal. The repayment schedule will be worked out in each case having regard to the nature of the activities of the borrower and the economics of the scheme. In assessing the surplus for the payment of interest and principal, due allowance is made for the sustenance requirements of the borrower himself.

Security

The borrower may or may not be able to offer tangible security to secure the loan. The viability or the potential viability of a project will be the main criteria for the grant of advance. However, the assets purchased with the loan may be hypothecated to the bank. In addition, in appropriate cases of loans to a homogeneous group of borrowers group guarantee may be accepted.

Margin

In the case of borrowers belonging to the weakest strata of society who may not be in a position to furnish margin money, requirements of margin money will not be insisted upon.

Rate of Interest

Keeping in view the social objective the interest will uniformly be charged @ 3% per annum, Physically handicapped persons including blind eligible under DRI Scheme are also given loans for purchasing of artificial limbs, hearing aids, wheel chair, etc., subject to maximum of Rs. 2,500 per borrower provided such assistance is given along with the advances for productive activities and self-employment ventures and all other requirements under DRI scheme are fulfilled.

Under the scheme of 'Financing Small Scale Industries' a special provision has been made to allow concession of 1/2% in the rate of interest to the physically handicapped availing working capital limit above Rs. 25,000 and upto Rs. 2 lakhs. Repayment Medium Term Loan: 5 to 7 years including moratorium period of 6 to 12 months Old machinery other than generator set 36 months New generator set 42 months Old generator set 30 months.

Interest for Working Capital

With aggregate advance upto Rs. 25,000 12.5%

Above Rs. 25,000 upto Rs. 2 lakh 13.5%.

Subsidy to Handicapped under the Integrated Rural Development Program (IRDP)

Under the IRDP, 3% quota is earmarked for the physically handicapped persons. The government has now decided that per family subsidy limit under the IRDP be raised from:

- Rs. 3,000 to Rs. 4,000 in normal areas.
- Rs. 4,000 to Rs. 5,000 in drought prone areas and desert development Program areas. — Rs. 5,000.

DETAILS OF BUS CONCESSION AVAILABLE IN DIFFERENT STATES OF INDIA

Delhi

Free for blind and 50% for escorts. Delhi Transport Corporation (DTC) has been issuing free traveling passes to physically handicapped persons.

Uttar Pradesh

Free travel facility is available to any physically handicapped person whose disability according to the certificate provided by the CMO is 40% or more in ordinary buses. One co-passenger can travel free of charge with them, the same is not applied for hearing and speech impaired.

Maharashtra

State Road Transport is giving 75% concession in bus fares to blind, deaf and orthopedically handicapped persons and 50% concession to their attendants.

Andhra Pradesh

The disabled persons are entitled to free bus journey in the city and in the suburban buses with escorts. In other buses, they get 50% concession.

Gujarat

Gujarat State Transport Corporation has given 100% concession to the blind and their escorts in state buses. Other categories of disabled are also provided 100% concession and 50% concession to their escorts.

Odisha

Free bus travel is provided to those OH and blind persons whose disability is 50% and above and 50% concession to their escorts. 50% concession is given to those OH and blind persons whose disability is 40 to 50% without escort. Two seats are reserved for the disabled. The mentally retarded persons are given 100% concession along with an escort with 50% concession.

Karnataka

Free travel facility is provided to blind persons in government buses.

Kerala

Free travel facility is provided to blind on bus and boat. Physically handicapped persons with 50% disability and above are eligible for 75% concession in State Buses. In private buses, 70% concession to travel upto 40 km are allowed to physically handicapped persons having 50% disability or above.

Madhy Pradesh

i. Visually impaired persons get 75% concession in fare in state level transport buses.
ii. Locomotor impaired persons get 75% concession in fare in state level transport buses, if the person is traveling alone. In case of the escort, 100% concession is given to the impaired person, while there is no concession for the escort.

Nagaland

Free bus travel facility to PH persons. Blinds with escorts also get free transport facility in State Transport Buses.

Puducherry

Free bus passes are issued to all disabled persons having a minimum of 40% disability and income not exceeding Rs. 30,000/- PA for traveling in State Government owned transport corporation buses as well as private buses plying within the union territory.

Punjab

Free travel concession is allowed to the blind persons in the buses of Punjab Roadways and Punjab Road Transport Corporation (PRTC) and 50% concession is allowed to attendant accompanying the blind persons. Other handicapped persons are allowed 50% concession in the fare.

Rajasthan

Free bus travel is provided to physically and mentally handicapped persons in Rajasthan State Roadways Corporation.

Sikkim

Free travel facility to the blind is available in the state owned buses.

Tamil Nadu

Visually handicapped persons are allowed free travel in state owned transport corporation buses from any place to any place within the district in which they reside. Mentally retarded/Mentally ill persons are provided free travel facility with one escort. The speech and hearing disabled and locomotor disabled persons are also given free travel concession to go to schools/colleges/work spots, etc.

Tripura

Free bus pass for the blind and other types of disabled persons are given for the State Transport Buses.

West Bengal

Free bus and tram journey facility is available to following types of physically handicapped persons (i) persons who are blind in both eyes, (ii) persons whose visual impairment is 40% or above, (iii) persons who are unable to move on their own because of disease of long duration or congenital defects, (iv) deaf and dumb persons including students.

Chandigarh

Free bus travel for blind and 50% concession is admissible to other categorise of physically handicapped persons in CTU buses.

Goa

Free for disabled students in private and government buses and 50% concession for escorts. 50% concession is available to other handicapped persons, other than students. (Director, Social Welfare Department, Goa issue photo identity card to the handicapped for availing this facility.).

Himachal and Manipur

- Free bus travel facility is available for the disabled person
- Concession rates, rules and regulations are subject to change from time-to-time.

CHAPTER 16

Disability Survey and Disability Evaluation

DISABILITY SURVEY

- Provides evidence for accountability and decision-making
- Disability survey consensus in the global human rights, development and health communities demands action to improve the health and well-being of people with disability, and to reduce the barriers that hinder their participation in society on an equal basis with others. Effective policy-making in this area requires reliable, detailed data on all aspects of disability—impairments, activity limitations, participation restrictions, related health conditions, environmental factors information that is lacking in most countries. The Model Disability Survey (MDS) is designed to address these data gaps.

DEFINITION

The disability survey is a general population survey that provides detailed and nuanced information on the lives of people with disability. It allows direct comparison between groups with differing levels and profiles of disability, including comparison to people without disability. The evidence resulting from the disability survey (DS) will help policy-makers identify which interventions are required to maximize the inclusion and functioning of people with disability.

The DS is grounded in the International Classification of Functioning, Disability and Health (ICF) and represents an evolution in the concept of disability measurement. It explores disability as an Outcome of interactions between a person with a health condition and various environmental and personal factors, rather than focusing only on a person's health or impairments. This gives a more complete understanding of the lived experience of people with disability and provides a better approximation of the true size of the population with disability.

NEED OF DISABILITY SURVEY

There is no standardized instrument for data collection on disability that provides

- Comprehensive and systematic documentation of all aspects of functioning in a population
- Existing data focus mainly on impairment or activity limitation and do not provide the evidence base needed for effective public policy that improves the well-being of people with disability
- To implement the Convention on the Rights of Persons with Disabilities (CRPD, 2008), countries need reliable data and evidence. The CRPD therefore requires governments to collect statistical and research data to identify and address barriers faced by people with disability, to formulate and implement policies, and to help assess progress implementing States Parties obligations under the Convention (CRPD, Article 31)
- Both the UN High-Level Meeting of the United Nations General Assembly on Disability and Development (2013) and the UN High-Level Panel of Eminent Persons on the Post-2015 Development Agenda (2013) call for radical improvements in disability data collection, analysis and monitoring
- The world report on disability, the most recent World Health Assembly resolution on disability (A66/12, 2013) and the draft WHO global disability action plan 2014–2020 (2014) urge WHO Member states to establish and strengthen monitoring and evaluation systems for disability that include information on needs and unmet needs, costs, barriers and quality of life.

GUIDING PRINCIPLES

- People with disability have a right to participation in society on an equal basis with others
- Disability is an outcome of the interaction between a person with a health condition and contextual factors. It is not merely an attribute of the person
- Disability is a continuum, a matter of degree. The experience of disability is diverse
- Disability measurement should consider societal or environmental barriers that can have a strong disabling effect, as well as an individual's impairments and health condition
- Questions that focus on the respondents' lived experience and real-life environment will yield a better understanding of how disability affects people's daily lives, and what can be done to improve their lives
- Cross-national relevance and standardization of the questionnaire are essential. A modular format allows it to be used as a stand-alone survey or incorporated into other national surveys.

USES OF DISABILITY SURVEY'S DATA

- The understanding of how people live their lives and the identification of key barriers to full participation are crucial to helping governments actualize their CRPD obligations, and to determine what actions are required to promote and protect the human rights of people with disability
- The DS provides for more robust prevalence estimates for tracking national trends and making international comparisons
- Analysis of the interaction between health conditions and environmental factors will facilitate more effective policy in many areas, e.g. assistive devices and accessible environments
- Sufficiently detailed analysis facilitates monitoring the situation of people with disability, to make sure they are not left behind in the wake of development progress, and to identify ways to include disability in national development agendas. These are priorities of the Post-2015 Development Agenda
- DS data can be used in intersect oral policy-making, e.g. national poverty reduction strategies, and in sector-specific policies, e.g. to monitor the reach of universal health coverage and to plan

improvements in health service policy and delivery, to maximize the likelihood that people with disability may obtain the health services they need without suffering financial hardship.

DISABILITY SURVEY DEVELOPMENT PROCESS

The World Health Organization and the World Bank have developed the MDS questionnaire in collaboration with the Washington Group on Disability Statistics, Statistics Norway, and a diverse range of other stakeholders, including the International Disability Alliance. Throughout the process, steps have been taken to insure comparability with existing instruments. This work is funded by the Governments of Australia, Germany and Norway.

The MDS draws on questions from 179 disability surveys, which have been analyzed and mapped to the ICF. Drafts of the questionnaire have been reviewed in expert consultations. The revised questionnaire is undergoing cognitive testing to evaluate whether the questions perform as intended. Results from the first round of cognitive testing are highly favorable. The concept of the MDS is fully supported by organizations representing people with disabilities. Pilot studies and the first national survey are planned for 2014. The final questionnaire and supporting.

Materials are expected to be made freely available on the WHO website. Planning has begun for a Multi-Country Study on Disability, and for providing support for data collection, analysis and utilization.

DISABILITY EVALUATION

The Universal guidelines for assessment and certification of the following:

Disabilities were finalized by group of experts and were notified by the Ministry of Social Justice and Empowerment, GOI in June 2001.

1. Visual impairment
2. Locomotor disability
3. Speech and hearing
4. Mental retardation
5. Multiple disabilities.

Guidelines for certification were framed.

According to the Persons with Disabilities (Equal Opportunities, Protection of Rights and Full Participation) Rules, 1996 notified on

31.12.1995 by the Central Government in exercise of the powers conferred by sub-section (1) and (2) of section 73 of the Persons with Disabilities Act, 1995, the empowered persons to give disability certificate, will be a Medical Board, consisting of at least three members, out of which at least one shall be a specialist in the particular field for assessing locomotor/visual including low vision/hearing and speech disability, mental retardation and leprosy cured as the case may be, duly constituted by the Central and State Government. Specified tests as indicated in guidelines should be conducted by the medical board and recorded before a certificate is given. The certificate would be valid for a period of five years for those whose disability is temporary, while in permanent disability the validity is life-long. The Director General of Health Services, Ministry of Health and Family Welfare will be the final authority, should there arise any controversy/doubt regarding the interpretation of the definitions/classifications/evaluations/tests, etc.

The minimum degree of disability should be 40% in order to be eligible for any concession/benefit.

As per PWD Act and in its compliance, various benefits and concessions are to be provided to the 'persons with disability'.

'Person with disability' means a person suffering from not less than 40% of any disability as certified by a medical authority;

"Medical authority" means any hospital or institution specified for the purposes of this Act by notification by the appropriate Government.

The 'Disability' under PWD act means:

i. Blindness,
ii. Low vision,
iii. Leprosy-cured,
iv. Hearing impairment,
v. Locomotor disability,
Vi. Mental retardation,
vii. Mental illness.

Broad Principles of Disability Assessment

Following guiding principles to assess disability, required before issue of disability.

Certificate, should be known to doctors/members of board with additional inputs related to disability of their concerned specialty.

The specialist from the ares of locomotor, vision, speech and hearing and mental retardation should also have broad knowledge on multiple disability.

Functional loss: It is assessment of functional loss based on some uniform test, resulting from permanent physical impairment caused due to congenital or acquired conditions (traumatic or post-disease). In case of amputees, the percentage is calculated directly depending on the level of the part that is lost and additional weightage. Individual Function requirement: The functions assessed are in relation to standard desired functions of anatomical part irrespective of individuals age, sex, nature of work, job, social status, requirement of specific part to him/her.

Personal opinion: There is no scope of personal opinion or to refer tests other than mentioned in guidelines notified.

Where to decide percentage on extent of function/activity.

Wherever a limit to percentage disability (like each activity of ten activities to coordination in upper limb, nine activities to test stability and additional weightage, a certain percentage limit may be given, the specialist need to use his conscience with full satisfaction. It is advised to be uniform and unbiased, such range may be divided into three group as:

a. No loss: Activity can be performed normally without assistance.
b. Partial loss: Activity can performed partly or with assistance.
c. Total loss: Activity cannot be performed even with assistance.

Trick movement: In case where specialist feel that particular group of muscle/part required to perform the function and said function should be performed in the event of involvement, despite this the individual is able to perform function due to trick movement or some part synergistic to it, this should be taken as function performed and percentage of PPI be calculated accordingly.

Authority: As per the act, authorities to give disability certificate will be a Medical Board duly constituted by the Central and State Government. The Medical Board should consist of at least three members. Out of which one shall be a specialist in the concerned disability subject.

Testing Tools and Guidelines

The standard guidelines and tools mentioned in the notification have to be used in evaluation of disability for proper certificate.

When to assess: For purpose of certification, disability should be assessed when the specialist is satisfied that further medical treatment/intervention is not like to reduce the extent of impairment. Normally, a period of six months is considered in such medical conditions.

Certification in condition of deformity, which is likely to be modified by surgery.

In cases of conditions which can be corrected by surgical procedures, no strict mention is given. Ideally the assessment should be done only after best possible correction but the benefit is also given in favor of individual.

Validity of certificate: The certificate would be valid for a period of five years in case of temporary disability means that PPI may change to some extent, but no way it means that disability will be cured or significantly reduced. For example, after traumatic amputation, the percentage may change due to improvement in additional factors as pain, neuroma, scar infection, etc. For permanent disability, certificate once issued is permanent and life-long. If disability percentage is changed after surgery: before issue of permanent disability certificate, the board ensures that improvement in medical condition has reached to its maximum and not likely to improve further. In case if an individual get his disability due to deformity get corrected by surgery, the percentage of disability if assessed in changed condition may vary. For example, in case of polio with contracture if get himself operated, contracture relieved and function improvement occurred due to tendon transfer, the percentage of disability will be less in postoperated as compared to preoperated stage. Can he use his earlier disability certificate to avail benefit/concession?

Whether certificate issuing doctor be responsible?

Ideally, before issue of disability certificate all options to reduce/correct disability should have been tried but in view of practical difficulty and resource constraints and taking a holistic view, certificate cannot be denied for want of medical intervention suggested. The percentage disability in the certificate was based on the condition on the day of assessment, when there were no chances of improvement by usual treatment. In case where further specific medical/surgical intervention done afterward, the percentage disability mentioned in the certificate, earlier shall not be valid. Such note may be mentioned if issuing authority apprehend, case-to-case basis. Appeal—In case of controversy arises on percentage of disability given by a board, the individual can appeal to the same board to reassess his/her disability. The board is authorized to consider and reassess the individual and modify its certificate with reasons. In case of further controversy, the individual can approach to higher state government medical authority to get reassessed by board/designated authority. The Director General Health Services, Government of India shall be final appellate authority.

Disability

- *'Locomotor Disability'* means disability of the bones, joints or muscles leading to substantial restriction of the movement of the limbs or any form of cerebral palsy;
- *'Cerebral Palsy'* means a group of non-progressive conditions of a person characterized by abnormal motor control posture resulting from brain insult or injuries occurring in the prenatal, perinatal or infant period of development;
- *'Leprosy cured person'* means any person who has been cured of leprosy but is suffering from:
  - Loss of sensation in hands or feet as well as loss of sensation and paresis in the eye and eye-lid but with no manifest deformity
  - Manifest deformity and paresis but having sufficient mobility in their hands and feet to enable them to engage in normal economic activity
  - Extreme physical deformity as well as advanced age which prevents him from undertaking any gainful occupation, and the expression "leprosy cured" shall be construed accordingly;
    'Blindness' refers to a condition where a person suffers from any of the following conditions, namely—
  - Total absence of sight; or visual acuity not exceeding 6/60 or 20/200 (snellen) in the better eye with correcting lenses; or
  - Limitation of the field of vision subtending an angle of 20 degrees or worse.

'Person with low vision' means a person with impairment of visual functioning even after treatment or standard refractive correction but who uses or is potentially capable of using vision for the planning or execution of a task with appropriate assistive device;

'Hearing Impairment' means loss of sixty decibels or more in the better ear in the conversational range of frequencies;

'*Mental Illness*' means any mental disorder other than mental retardation;

'*Mental Retardation*' means a condition of arrested or incomplete development of mind of a person which is especially characterized by subnormality of intelligence;

'*Rehabilitation*' refers to a process aimed at enabling persons with disabilities to reach and maintain their optimal physical, sensory, intellectual, psychiatric or social functional levels;

Multiple disabilities: (In case of more than one disability).

Multiple disabilities means a combination of two or more disabilities as defined in Persons with Disabilities (Equal Opportunities, Protection of Rights and Full Participation) Act, 1995, namely:

1. Locomotor disability including leprosy cured
2. Blindness/Low vision
3. Speech and hearing impairment
4. Mental retardation
5. Mental illness.

A specialist, authorized to make assessment of disability in a disabled individual and issue disability certificate through duly constituted medical board (disability), need to understand how to add disabilities assessed by him/her, or the disabilities given by other experts in the concerned area/areas. The final certificate is sum of various disabilities, as per guidelines, using a telescopic sum formula. In assessing disability (PPI) and giving percentage of disability, there is hardly any scope of personal opinion, individual's, age, sex, profession, nature of work, race, religion or importance of function impaired for that individual or society. But there is scope to bring such instances into notice and to be get clarifications/considerations, whenever review/modification of existing guidelines is made in future. In case of multiple disabilities, the subject specialist from the area with higher percentage may sign the final certificate. In case two areas are having the same percentage, either of specialists may sign the certificate.

Guidelines for Evaluation

In order to evaluate the multiple disability, the same guidelines shall be used as have been developed by the respective subcommittees of various single disability, viz mental retardation, locomotor disability, visual disability, and speech and hearing disability, and recommended in the meeting held on 29.2.2000 under the Chairmanship of Dr SP Agarwal, Director General of Health Services, Government of India, with reference to Order No. 16- 18/96-NI.I, dated 28th August, 1998 and communicated to Ministry of Social Justice and Empowerment, Government of India, vide letter No. S-13020/4/98-MH, dated 16th March, 2000.

However, in order to arrive at the total percentage of multiple disability the combining formula a + b (90 – a), as given in the "Manual for Doctors to 90.

Evaluate Permanent Physical Impairment developed by Expert Group meeting on Disability Evaluation", shall be used, where "a" will be the higher score and "b" will be the lower score.

However, the maximum total percentage of multiple disabilities shall not exceed 100%.

Procedure for Certification of Multiple Disabilities

The procedure will remain the same as has been developed by the respective subcommittees on various single disabilities and finalized in a meeting under the Chairpersonship of Dr SP Agarwal held on 29.2.2000. The final disability certificate for multiple disability will be issued by Disability Board which has given higher score of disability by combining the score of different disabilities using the combining format, i.e.

$$\frac{a + b(90 - a)}{90}$$

In case where two scores of disability are equal, the final certificate of multiple disabilities will be issued by any one of them as decided by local authority.

FORMAT STANDARD OF THE CERTIFICATE (FOR OH/VH/SP AND HG)

(Name and Address of the Institute/Hospital: (Issuing the Certificate)

Certificate No. Date

CERTIFICATE FOR THE PERSONS WITH DISABILITIES

This is to certify that Shri/Smt/Km/.. Son/wife/daughter of Shri ....Age .... years old male/female, Registration No...is a case of physically disabled/visual disabled/speech and hearing disabled and has .... % (..............................percent) permanent (physical impairment/visual impairment/speech and hearing impairment) in relation to his/her...

Note:

1. This condition is progressive/non-progressive/likely to improve/ not likely to improve.
2. Re-assessment is not recommended/recommended after a period of .... months/years.

   Strike out which is not applicable.

Sd/-	Sd/-	sd/-
Doctor	Doctor	Doctor
Seal	seal	Seal

Signature/Thumb impression of the patient:

Countersigned by the

Medical Superintendent/CMO/Head of Hospital (with seal)

Recent Attested Photograph showing the disability

LOCOMOTOR DISABILITY

Definition

1. Impairment: Impairment is any loss or abnormality of psychological, physiological or anatomical structure or function in a human being.
2. Functional limitations: Impairment may cause functional limitations which are partial or total inability to perform those activities necessary for motor, sensory or mental function within the range or manner of which a human being is normally capable.
3. Disability: A disability is any restriction or lack (resulting from an impairment) of ability to perform an activity in the manner or within the range considered normal for a human being.
4. Locomotor disability: Locomotor disability is defined as a person's inability to execute distinctive activities associated with moving

both himself and objects, from place to place and such inability resulting from affection of musculoskeletal and/or nervous system.

Categories of Locomotor Disability

The categories of locomotor disabilities are enclosed in subsequent paragraph.

Process of Certification

A disability certificate shall be issued by a Medical Board of three members duly constituted by the Central and State Government Out of which, at least, one member shall be a specialist from either field of Physical Medicine and Rehabilitation or Orthopedics. Two specimen copies of the disability certificate for mental retardation and others (visual disability, speech and hearing disability and locomotor disability) are enclosed at Annexure. It was also decided that whenever required the Chairman of the Board may co-opt other experts including that of the members constituted for the purpose by the Central and the State Government.

On representation by the applicant, the Medical Board may review its decision having regard to all the facts and circumstances of the case and pass such order in the matter as it thinks fit. Variables-in assessing locomotor disability (PPI).

In locomotor disability following variables need to be taken into consideration while assessing function loss resulting permanent physical impairment (disability).

1. Strength of muscle (MRC scale)
2. Range of joint motion
3. Coordination
4. Stability
5. Limb length discrepancy
5. Hand functions (prehension, sensation and strength)
6. Sensation
7. Deformity, etc.
8. Complications like pain, infection, etc.
9. Extremity dominant or non-dominant.

The PPI (disability) due to amputation/congenital loss of limb, neurological conditions, post-stroke.

GUIDELINES FOR EVALUATION OF PERMANENT PHYSICAL IMPAIRMENT (PPI)

Upper Limb

1. The estimation of permanent impairment depends upon the measurement of functional impairment and not expression of a personal opinion.
2. The estimation and measurement should be made when the clinical condition has reached the stage of maximum improvement from the medical treatment.
   Normally, the time period is to be decided by the medical doctor who is evaluating the case for issuing the PPI certificate as per standard format of the certificate.
3. The upper limb is divided into two components; the Arm Component and 'Hand Component.'
4. Measurement of the loss of function of 'Arm Component' consists of measuring the loss of motion, muscle strength and coordinate activities.
5. Measurement of loss of function of Hand Component consists of determining the prehension, sensation and strength. For estimation of prehension—opposition, lateral pinch cylindrical grasp, spherical grasp and hook grasp have to be assessed as shown in Hand Component of Form-A (Assessment Performa for Upper Extremity).
6. The impairment of the entire extremity depends on the combination of the functional impairments of both components.

Arm Component

Total value of Arm Component is 90%.

Principles of evaluation of 'Range of Motion' (ROM) of Joints

1. The value of maximum ROM in the Arm Component is 90%.
2. Each of the three joints of the Arm is weighed equally (30%).

Example:

The intra-articular fractures of the bones of right shoulder joint may affect Range of Motion even after healing. The loss of ROM should be calculated the each arc of Motion as envisaged in the Assessment Form-A (Assessment Performa for Upper Extremity).

Arc of ROM	*Normal value*	*Active ROM*	*Loss of ROM*
Shoulder Flexion	0–220	110	50%
Rotation	0–180	90	50%
Abduction-Adduction	0–180	90	50%
Hence the mean loss of ROM of shoulder will be (50 + 50 + 50)/3 = 50%			

Shoulder movements constitute 30% of the Motion of the Arm Component; therefore the loss of Motion for Arm Component will be 50 × 0.30 = 15%. If than one joint of the Arm is involved the loss of percentage in each joint is calculated separately as above and then added together.

Principles of Evaluation of Strength of Muscles

1. Strength of muscles can be tested by manual method and graded from 0–5 as advocated by Medical Research Council (MRC) of Great Britain depending upon the strength of the muscles.
2. Loss of muscle power can be given percentages as follows:

Manual muscle strength grading	*Loss of strength in percentage*
0	100%
1	80%
2	60%
3	40%
4	20%
5	0%

3. The mean percentage of loss of muscle strength around a joint is multiplied by 0.30.
4. If loss of muscle strength involves more than one joint the mean loss of percentage in each joint is calculated separately and then added together as has been described for loss of motion.

Principles of Evaluation of Coordinated Activities

1. The total value for coordinated activities is 90%.
2. Ten different coordinated activities should be tested as given in Form A.
3. Each activity has a value of 9%.

Combining Values for the Arm Component

The total value of loss of function of 'Arm Component' is obtained by combining the value of loss of ROM, muscle strength and coordinated activities, using the combing

$$\text{Formula} = \frac{a + b \times (90 - a)}{90}$$

Where a = higher value, b = lower value

Example

Let us assume that an individual with an intra-articular fracture of bones of shoulder joint in addition to 16.5% loss of motion in arm has 8.3% loss of strength of muscles and 5% loss of coordination. These values should be combined as follows:

a. Loss of strength of muscles—8.3%,
b. Loss of ROM—16.5%
c. Loss of coordination—5%
d. To add above (a and b) $= \frac{16.5 + 8.3 \times (90 - 16.5)}{90}$
$= 23.33\%$
e. Now to add loss of coordination (d and c) $= \frac{23.3 + 5(90 - 23.3)}{90}$
$= 27.0\%$

So total value of loss of functions in arm component 27.0%

Hand Component

1. Total value of Hand Component is 90%
2. The functional impairment of hand is expressed as loss of prehension, loss of sensation and loss of strength.

Principles of Evaluation of Prehension

1. Total value of prehension is 30%. It includes:
   a. Opposition—8%
   Tested against
      - Index finger—2%
      - Middle finger—2%
      - Ring finger—2%
      - Little finger—2%
   b. Lateral pinch—5%
   (Tested by asking patient to hold a key between thumb and lateral side of index finger).

c. Cylindrical grasp—6%
   tested for
   i. Large object of 4" size (diameter)—3%
   ii. Small object of 1" size (diameter)—3%
d. Spherical grasp—6%
   tested for
   i. Large object of 4 inches size—3%
   ii. Small object of 1 inch size—3%
e. Hook grasp—5%
   tested by asking the patient to lift a bag.

Principles of Evaluation of Sensation

1. Total value of sensation in hand is 30%
2. It should be assessed according to distribution as below:
   i. Complete loss of sensation
      Thumb ray—9%
      Index finger—6%
      Middle finger—5%
      Ring finger—5%
      Little finger—5%.
   ii. Partial loss of sensation: Assessment should be made according to percentage of loss of sensation in thumb/finger(s).

Principles of Evaluation of Strength

1. Total value of strength—30%
2. It includes:
   i. Grip strength—20%
   ii. Pinch strength—10%.

   Strength of hand should be tested with 'Hand Dynamometer' or by clinical method (grip method).

   Additional weight age: A total of 10% additional weightage can be given to following accompanying factors, if they are continuous and persistent despite treatment.
   1. Pain
   2. Infection
   3. Deformity
   4. Malalignment
   5. Contractures
   6. Cosmetic disfiguration

7. Dominant extremity—4%
8. Shortening of upper limb—First 1"weightage, for each 1" beyond first 1"-2% disability.

   The extra points should not exceed 10% of the total arm component and total PPI should not exceed 100% in any case.

Combining Values of Hand Component

The final value of loss of function of hand component is obtained by summing up values of loss of prehension, sensation and strength.

Combining Values for the Extremity

Values of impairment of arm component and impairment of hand component should be added by using combining formula.

$$\frac{a + b\,90 - A}{90}$$

a = higher value

b = lower value

Example: Impairment of arm - 27%, impairment of hand—64%
Total of upper limb (by combining formula)

$$= \frac{64 + 27\,(90 - 64)}{90} = 71.8\%$$

The total value can also be obtained by using the 'Ready Beckoner Table' for combining formula (Annexed).The total value can also be obtained by using the 'Ready Beckoner Table' for combining formula (Annexed).

GUIDELINES FOR EVALUATION OF PPI (DISABILITY) IN LOWER LIMB

The measurement of loss of function in lower extremity is divided into two components: Mobility and stability components.

Mobility Component

1. Total value of mobility component is 90%
2. It includes range of movement (ROM) and muscle strength.

Principles of Evaluation of Range of Movement

1. The value of maximum range of movement in mobility component is 90%.
2. Each of three joints, i.e. hip, knee and foot-ankle component is weighted equally—30%.

Example:
A fracture of right hip joint bones may affect range of motion of the hip joint. Loss of ROM of the affected hip is different and should be assessed as given in Form B.
(Assessment Performa for lower extremity).
Affected joint—right hip:

Arc of movement	*Normal ROM*	*Active ROM*	*Loss in %age*
a. Flexion-Extension	0–1400	700	50
b. Abduction-Adduction	0–900	600	33
c. Rotation	0–900	300	66

Mean loss of ROM of Rt Hip = (50+33+66)/3 = 50%

Since the hip constitutes 30% of the total mobility component of the lower limb, the loss of motion in relation to the lower limb will be 50 × 0.30 = 15%.

If more than one joint of the limb is involved, the mean loss of ROM in percentage should be calculated in relation to individual joint separately and then added together as follows to calculate the loss of mobility component in relation to that particular limb.

For example:
Mean loss of ROM of right hip—50%
Mean loss of ROM right knee—40%
Loss of mobility component of right lower limb will be (50 × 0.30) + (40 × 0.30) = 27%.

Principle of Evaluation of Muscle Strength

1. The value for maximum muscle strength in the limb is 90%.
2. Strength of muscles can be tested by manual method and graded 0–5 as advocated by MRC of Great Britain depending upon the residual strength in the muscle group.

3. Manual muscle grading can be given percentage like below:

Grade of muscle strength	*Loss of strength in %age*
0	100
1	80
2	60
3	40
4	20
5	0

4. Mean percentage of muscle strength loss around a joint is multiplied by 0.30 to calculate loss in relation to limb.
5. If there has been loss of muscle strength involving more than one joint the values are added as has been described for loss of ROM.

Combining Values for Mobility Component

1. The values of loss of ROM and loss of muscle strength should be combined with the help of combining formula

$$= \frac{a + b\,90 - a}{90}$$

(a = higher value, b = lower value)

Example: Let us assume that the individual with a fracture of right Hip bones has in addition to 16% loss of motion, 8% loss of muscle strength also. To combine, motion-16% and strength 8% 16 + 8 (90 - 16).

$$\text{Combined value} = \frac{16 + 8\,(90 - 16)}{90} = 22.6$$

Stability Component

1. Total value of the stability component is 90%.
2. It should be tested by clinical method as given in 'Form B' (Assessment Performa for lower extremity). There are nine activities, which need to be tested, and each activity has a value of 10%. The percentage value in relation to each activity depends upon the percentage of loss of stability in relation to each activity.

Extra Points

Extra points have been given for pain, deformities, contractures, loss of sensation and shortening maximum points to be added are 10% (excluding shortening). Details are as following:

1. Deformity
    a. In functional position—3%
    b. In non-functional position—6%.
2. Pain
    a. Severe (grossly interfering with function)—9%
    b. Moderate (moderately interfering with function)—6%
    c. Mild (mildly interfering with function)—3%.
3. Loss of sensation
    a. Complete loss—9%
    b. Partial loss—6%
4. Shortening
    First" Nil
    (For every additional ½" shortening—4%
5. Complications
    a. Superficial complications—3%
    b. Deep complications—6%.

GUIDELINES FOR EVALUATION OF PERMANENT PHYSICAL IMPAIRMENT OF TRUNK (SPINE)

Basic Guidelines

1. As permanent physical impairment caused by spinal deformity tends to change over the years, the certificate issued in relation to spine should be reviewed as per the standard format of the certificate given at Annexure.
2. Permanent physical impairment should be awarded in relation to spine and not in relation to whole body.
3. Permanent physical impairment due to neurological deficit in addition to spinal impairment should be added by combining formula.

    The local effects of the lesions of the spine can be conventionally divided into 'Traumatic and non-traumatic.' The percentage of PPI in relation to each situation should be valued as follows:

Traumatic Lesions

Cervical spine injuries	*Percentage of PPI in relation of spine*
i. 25% or more compression of one or two adjacent vertebral bodies with no involvement of posterior elements. No nerve root involvement. Moderate neck rigidity and persistent soreness	20
ii. Posterior element damage with radiological evidence of moderate partial dislocation/sub-luxation including Whiplash injury a. With fusion healed, No permanent motor or sensory changes b. Persistent pain with radiologically demonstrable instability	10
iii. Severe dislocation: a. Fair to good reduction with or without fusion with no residual motor or sensory involvement b. Inadequate reduction with fusion and persistent radicular pain	25 10 15

Cervical intervertebral disk lesions	*Percentage of PPI in relation to spine*
i. Treated case of disk lesion with persistent pain and no neurological deficit	10
ii Treated case with pain and instability	15
Thoracic and thoracolumbar spine injuries	
i. Compression of less than 50% involving one vertebral body with no neurological manifestation	10
ii. Compression of more than 50% involving single vertebra or more with involvement of posterior elements, healed, no neurological manifestations persistent pain, fusion indicated	20
iii. Same as (b) with fusion, pain only on heavy use of back	15
iv. Radiologically demonstrable instability with fracture or fracture dislocation with persistent pain	30

Lumbar and lumbosacral spine: Fracture	
a. Compression of 25% or less of one or two adjacent vertebral bodies, No definite pattern or neurological deficit	15
b. Compression of more than 25% with disruption of posterior elements, persistent pain and stiffness, healed with or without fusion, inability to lift more than 10 kg	30
c. Radiologically demonstrable instability in low lumbar or lumbosacral spine with pain	35
Disk lesion	
a. Treated case with persistent pain	15
b. Treated case with pain and instability	20
c. Treated case disk of disease with pain activities of lifting moderately modified	25
d. Treated case of disk disease with persistent pain and of heavy weight stiffness; aggravated by lifting of heavy weight, necessitating modifications of all activities requiring heavy weight lifting	30

Nontraumatic Lesions

Scoliosis

- Basic guidelines—following modification is suggested.
- The largest structural curve should be accounted for, while calculating the PPI and not the compensatory curve or both structural curves.

Measurement of Spine Deformity

Cobb's method for measurement of angle of curve in the radiograph taken in standing position should be used. The curves have been divided into following groups depending upon the angle of major structural scoliotic deformity.

Group	*Cobb's angle*	*PPI in relation to spine*
I	0–20	Nil
II	21–50	10%
III	51–100	20%
IV	101 and above	30%

Torso Imbalance

In addition to the above, PPI should also be evaluated in relation the torso imbalance. The torso imbalance should be measured by dropping a plumb line from C7 spine and measuring the distance of plumb line from gluteal crease.

Deviation of plumb line	*PPI*
Up to 1.5 cm	4%
1.5–3.0 cm	8%
3.1–6.0	16%
6.1 cm and more	32%

Head Tilt over C7 Spine PPI

Upto 15	4%
More than 15	10%

Cardiopulmonary Test

Incases with scoliosis of severe type cardiopulmonary function tests and percentage deviation from normal should be assessed by one of the following method whichever seems more reliable clinically at the time of assessment. The value thus obtained may be added by combining formula

a. Chest expansion	*PPI*
4–5 cm	Normal
Less than 4 cm reduction	5% for each cm chest expansion
No expansion	25%
b. Counting in one breathe	
Breathe count	*PPI*
More than 40	Normal
0–40	5%
0–30	10%
0–20	15%
0–10	20%
Less than 5	25%

Associated Problems: To be Added Directly but the Total Value of PPI in Relation to Spine should not Exceed 100%

a. Pain	
Mildly interfering with ADL	4%
Moderately restriction ADL	6%
Severely restriction ADL	10%
b. Cosmetic appearance	
No obvious disfiguration with clothes on	Nil
Mild disfigurement	2%
Severe disfigurement	4%
c. Leg length discrepancy	
First ½ shortening	Nil
Every ½ beyond first ½	4%
d. Neurological deficit: Neurological deficit should be calculated per established method of evaluation of PPI in such cases. Value thus obtained should be added telescopically using combining formula	

Kyphosis

Evaluation should be done on the similar guidelines as used for scoliosis with the following modifications:

Spinal deformity	*PPI*
Less than 20	Nil
21–40	10%
41–60	20%
Above 60	30%

Torso Imbalance

Plumb line dropped from external ear normally falls at ankle level. The deviation from normal should be measured from ankle anterior joint line to the plumb line.

Less than 5 cm in front of ankle	4%
5–10 cm in front of ankle	8%
10–15 cm in front of ankle	16%
More than 15 cm in front of ankle (Add directly)	32%

Miscellaneous conditions

Those conditions of the spine which cause stiffness and pain, etc. are rated as follows:

Conditions Percentage	*PPI*
a. Subjective symptoms of pain, no involuntary muscle spasm, not substantiated by demonstrable structural pathology	0%
b. Pain, persistent muscles spasm and stiffness of spine, substantiated by mild radiological change	20%
c. Same as B with moderate radiological changes	25%
d. Same as B with severe radiological changes involving anyone of the regions of spine	30%
e. Same as D involving whole spine	40%

GUIDELINES FOR EVALUATION OF DISABILITY (PPI) IN NEUROLOGICAL CONDITIONS MAY/MAY NOT BE ASSOCIATED WITH SPINE

Basic Guidelines

1. Assessment in neurological conditions is not the assessment of disease but the assessment of its effects, i.e. clinical manifestations.
2. These guidelines should only be used for central and upper motor neuron (UMN) lesions.
3. Performa (form A and B) will be utilized for assessment of lower motor neuron lesions, muscular disorders and other locomotor conditions.
4. Normally any neurological assessment for the purpose of certification has to be done six months after the onset of disease however exact time period is to be decided by the medical doctor who is evaluating the case who has to recommend the review of the certificate as given in the standard format of certificate.
5. Total percentage of physical impairment in any neurological condition should not exceed 100%.
6. In mixed cases, the highest score will be taken into consideration. The lower score will be added telescopically to it by the help of combining formula.
7. Additional weightage of 4% will be given for dominant upper extremity.

8. Additional weightage upto 10% can be given for loss of sensation in each extremity but keeping a total 100%.

Neurological status	*Physical impairment*
Altered sensorium	100%

Intellectual Impairment (to be Assessed by Psychiatrist/Clinical Psychologist)

Degree of mental retardation impairment	*IQ range*	*Intellectual*
Borderline	70–79	25%
Mild	50–69	59%
Moderate	35–49	75%
Severe	20–34	90%
Profound less than	20	100%

Speech Defect

Speech defect	*PPI*
Mild dysarthria	Nil
Moderate dysarthria	25%
Severe dysarthria	50%

Cranial Nerve Disability

Type of cranial nerve	*Physical impairment*
Involvement	
Motor cranial nerve	20% for each nerve
Sensory cranial nerve	10% for each nerve

Motor System Disability—Hemi Paresis

Neurological involvement	*Physical impairment*
Mild	25%
Moderate	50%
Severe	75%

Sensory System Disability

Anesthesia	Upto 10% for each limb
Hypoesthesia	Depending upon % of loss of sensation
Paresthesia	Loss of sensation upto 30% depending
Hands/feet sensory loss	Depends upon % of loss of sensation

Bladder Disability due to Neurogenic Involvement

Bladder involvement	*Physical impairment*
Mild (Hesitancy/Frequency)	25%
Moderate (precipitancy)	50%
Severe (occasional but recurrent incontinence)	75%
Very Severe (Retention/total incontinence)	100%

Post-head Injury Fits and Epileptic Convulsions

Frequency/Severity of convulsions	*Physical impairment*
Mild-occurrence of one convulsion only	Nil
Moderate 1–5 convulsions/month on adequate medication	25%
Severe 6–10 convulsions/month on adequate medication	50%
Very Severe more than 10 fits/month on adequate medication	75%

Ataxia (Sensory or Cerebellar)

Severity of ataxia	*Physical impairment*
Mild (detected on examination)	25%
Moderate	50%
Severe	75%
Very severe	100%

GUIDELINES FOR EVALUATION OF PPI IN CASES OF SHORT STATURE/DWARFISM

Basic Guidelines

1. Recumbent length or longitudinal height below 3rd percentile or less than 2 standard deviation from the mean is considered to have 'Short Stature.'

2. The evaluation of 'Short Statured' person should be considered only when it is of disproportionate variety and is accompanied by underlying pathological conditions, e.g. Achondroplasia, Spondyloepiphyseal dysplasia, Mucopolysaccharidosis, etc.
3. The Indian Council of Medical Research (ICMR) norms as enclosed should be taken as guidelines for the height.
4. Every 1 inch vertical height reduction should be valued as 4% Permanent Physical Impairment (PPI).
5. Associated skeletal deformities should be evaluated separately and total percentage of both should be added by combining formula.

ICMR Norms for Indian Population Standing Heights for Indian Population (Inches) Mean and Standard Deviations

	Male			*Female*		
Age	*Mean*	*SD*	*2SD*	*Mean*	*SD*	*2SD*
Less than 3 months	22.113	2.32	17.49	21.65	2.13	17.39
3 months +	24.68	1.58	21.52	23.98	2.40	21.80
6 months +	25.55	3.19	19.17	25.35	1.43	22.49
9 months +	27.36	1.77	23.82	26.26	1.52	23.22
1 year +	29.09	2.07	24.95	28.54	2.04	24.46
2 years +	32.13	2.10	27.93	31.53	2.28	26.97
3 years +	34.96	2.58	29.80	34.33	2.50	29.33
4 years +	37.80	2.65	32.50	37.20	2.50	32.20
5 years +	40.19	3.16	33.84	39.92	2.90	34.12
6 years +	42.71	2.81	37.09	42.28	3.41	35.46
7 years +	44.84	3.41	38.02	44.40	3.34	37.72
8 years +	46.96	2.89	41.18	46.53	3.03	40.47
9 years +	48.70	3.65	41.40	48.38	2.96	42.46
10 years +	48.97	3.93	41.11	50.55	3.15	44.25
11 years +	52.51	3.83	44.86	52.60	3.73	45.14
12 years +	54.45	3.99	46.47	54.80	4.03	46.74
13 years +	56.93	3.84	49.25	56.65	3.63	49.39
14 years +	59.10	3.95	51.20	58.07	3.82	50.43
15 years +	61.22	3.94	53.34	58.89	3.27	52.35

Contd...

Contd...

	Male			*Female*		
Age	*Mean*	*SD*	*2SD*	*Mean*	*SD*	*2SD*
16 years +	62.79	3.84	55.11	59.44	2.80	53.84
17 years +	63.54	4.11	55.32	59.64	2.95	53.74
18 years +	64.21	3.76	56.69	59.72	2.31	55.10
21 years	64.64	2.40	59.84	60.24	2.24	55.76

GUIDELINES FOR EVALUATION OF PPI IN AMPUTEES

Basic Guidelines

1. In case of multiple amputees if the total sum of permanent physical impairment is above 100%, it should be taken as 100% only.
2. If the stump is unfit for fitting the prosthesis, additional weightage of 5% should be added to the value.
3. In case of amputation in more than one limb percentage of each limb is added by combining formula and another 10% will be added but when only toes or fingers are involved only 5% will be added.
4. Any complication in form of stiffness of proximal joint, neuroma, infection, etc., should be given upto a total of 10% additional weightage.
5. Dominant upper extremity should be given 4% additional weightage.

Upper limb amputations				*PPI and loss of physical function each limb*
1. Forequarter amputation				100%
2. Shoulder disarticulation				90%
3. Above elbow upto upper 1/3 of arm				85%
4. Above elbow upto lower 1/3 of fore arm				80%
5. Elbow disarticulation				75%
6. Below elbow upto 1/3 of forearm				70%

Contd...

Contd...

7. Below elbow upto 1/3 of forearm				65%
8. Wrist disarticulation				60%
9. Hand through carpal bones				55%
10. Thumb through CM or 1st MC joint				30%
11. Thumb disarticulation through MC Joint or. phalanx				25%
12. Thumb disarticulation through IP joint or distal phalanx				15%
	Index finger (15%)	*Middle finger (5%)*	*Ring finger (3%)*	*Little finger (2%)*
13. Amputation through proximal phalanx or disarticulation through MP	15%	5%	3%	2%
14. Amputation through middle phalanx or disarticulation through PIP joint	10%	4%	2%	1%
15. Amputation through distal phalanx or through DIP joint	5%	2%	1%	1%

Lower limb amputations	*PPI and loss of physical function each limb*
1. Hind quarter	100%
2. Hip disarticulation	90%
3. Above knee upto upper 1/3 of thigh	85%
4. Above knee upto lower 1/3 of thigh	80%
5. Through knee	75%
6. BK upto 8 cm	70%
7. BK up to lower 1/3 of leg	60%

Contd...

Contd...

Lower limb amputations	*PPI and loss of physical function each limb*
8. Through ankle	55%
9. Syme's amputation	50%
10. Upto midfoot	40%
11. Upto forefoot	30%
12. All toes	20%
13. Loss of first toe	10%
14. Loss of second toe	5%
15. Loss of third toe	4%
16. Loss of fourth toe	3%
17. Loss of fifth toe	2%

EVALUATION OF PPI OF CONGENITAL DEFICIENCIES OF THE LIMBS

Transverse Deficiencies

1. Functionally congenital transverse limb deficiencies are comparable to acquired amputations and can be called synonymously as congenital amputation, however, in some cases revision of amputation is required to fit prosthesis.
2. The transverse limb deficiencies therefore should be assessed on basis of the guidelines applicable to the evaluation of PPI in cases of amputees as given in the preceding chapter.

For example:

Deficiency	*Equivalent to amputation*	*PPI*
1. Transverse deficiency right arm complete	(Shoulder disarticulation)	90%
2. Transverse deficiency at thigh complete	(Hip disarticulation)	90%
3. Transverse deficiency proximal upper arm	(Above elbow amputation)	85%
4. Transverse deficiency at lower thigh 1/3)	(Above knee amputation lower	80%

Contd...

Contd...

Deficiency	*Equivalent to amputation*	*PPI*
5. Transverse deficiency fore arm complete	(Elbow disarticulation)	75%
6. Transverse deficiency lower forearm	(Below elbow amputation)	65%
7. Transverse deficiency carpal complete	(Wrist disarticulation)	60%
8. Transverse deficiency	(Disarticulation through metacarpal complete carpal bones)	55%

Longitudinal Deficiencies

Basic Guidelines

1. In cases of longitudinal deficiencies of limbs, due consideration should be given to functional impairment.
2. In upper limb, loss of ROM, Muscle Strength and Hand functions like prehension, etc. should be tested while assessing the case for PPI.
3. In lower limb clinical method of assessing the stability component and shortening of lower limb should be given due weightage.
4. Apart from functional assessment the lost joint/part of body should also be valued as per distribution given in chapter. 'Guidelines for Evaluation of PPI in Upper and Lower Extremity'. The values so obtained should be added with the help of combining formula.

Example:
Congenital absence of humerus where forearm bones directly articulate with scapula. There will be mild reduction in ROM and strength of muscles in the existing joints apart from loss of body part. Loss of shoulder joint can be given 30%.

Loss of ROM of elbow/shoulder and wrist all the components should be added together by the combining formula of

- In case of loss of single bone in forearm the evaluation should be based on the principles of evaluation of arm component which include evaluation of ROM, muscle strength and coordinated activities. The values so obtained should be added together with the help of 'combining formula'.

- In case of loss of single bone in leg the evaluation should be based on the principles of evaluation of mobility component and stability components of the lower extremity. The values obtained should be added together with the help of 'combining formula.'

GUIDELINES FOR EVALUATION OF PHYSICAL IMPAIRMENT DUE TO CARDIOPULMONARY DISEASES

Basic Guidelines

1. Modified New York Heart Association subjective classification should be utilized to assess functional disability.
2. The assessing physician should be alert to the fact that patients who come for disability claims are likely to exaggerate their symptoms. In case of any doubt, patients should be referred for detailed physiological evaluation.
3. Disability evaluation of cardiopulmonary patients should be done after full medical, surgical and rehabilitative treatment available because most of these diseases are potentially treatable.
4. Assessment of cardiopulmonary impairment should also be done in diseases, which might have associated cardiopulmonary problems, e.g. Amputees, Myopathies, etc.
5. For respiratory assessment, routine respiratory functions test should be done. However, in cases of interstitial lung diseases, diffusion studies may be done.
6. In cases of Angina Pectoris (chest pain) baseline studies in resting ECG should be done. When there is persistence of symptoms, exercise or stress test should be done.

Proposed classification with loss of function is as follows:

Group 0: A patient with cardiopulmonary disease who is asymptomatic (i.e. has no symptoms of breathlessness, palpitation, fatigue or chest pain).

Group 1: A patient with cardiopulmonary disease who becomes symptomatic during his ordinary physical activity but has mild restriction (25%) of his physical activities.

Group 2: A patient with cardiopulmonary disease who becomes symptomatic during his ordinary physical activity and has 25–50% restriction of his ordinary physical activities.

Group 3: A patient with cardiopulmonary disease that becomes symptomatic during less than ordinary physical activity, so that his ordinary physical activities are 50–75% restricted.

Group 4: A patient with cardiopulmonary disease who is symptomatic even at rest or on mildest exertion so that his ordinary physical activity is severely or Completely restricted (75–100%).

Group 5: A patient with cardiopulmonary disease who gets intermittent symptoms at rest (i.e. patients with bronchial asthma, paroxysmal nocturnal dyspnea, etc.).

GUIDELINES FOR ASSESSMENT OF VISUAL DISABILITY

1. *Definition:* Blindness refers to a condition where a person suffers from any of the condition, namely,
   a. Total absence of sight; or
   b. Visual acuity not exceeding 6/60 or 20/200 (Snellen) in the better eye with best correcting lenses; or
   c. Limitation of field of vision subtending an angle of 20 degrees or worse;
2. *Low vision:* Persons with low vision means a person with impairment of vision of <6/18–6/60 with best correction in the better eye or impairment of field in any one of the following categories:
   a. Reduction of fields less than 50 degrees
   b. Hemianopia with macular involvement
   c. Altitudinal defect involving lower fields.
3. Process of certification

   A disability certificate shall be issued by a Medical Board duly constituted by the Central/State Government having, at least three members. Out of which, at least one members shall be a specialist in ophthalmology. It was also decided that whenever required the Chairman of the Board may co-opt other experts including that of the members constituted for the purpose by the Central and the State Government. On representation by the applicant, the Medical Board may review its decision having regard to all the facts and circumstances of the case and pass such order in the matter as it thinks fit. If visual disability is associated with one or more other disability (other than visual disability), the guidelines for multiple disability in disability assessment has to be followed.

4. Variables in assessing vision disability (PPI)
   In vision disability following variables need to be taken into consideration while assessing function loss resulting permanent physical impairment (disability).
   a. Vision
   b. Acuity of vision
   c. Field of vision (in degrees)
   d. Hemianopia
   e. Altitudinal defect (in lower field)
5. Categories of visual disability all with correction

Category	*Better eye*	*Worse eye*	*%age impairment*
Category 0	6/9–6/18	6/24–6/36	20%
Category I	6/18–6/36	6/60—Nil	40%
Category II	6/60–4/60 or Field of vision 10–20	3/60—Nil	75%
Category III	3/60–1/60 or Field of vision 10°	FC at1 ft—Nil	100%
Category IV	FC at 1 ft—Nil Or field of vision 10°	FC at 1 ft—Nil	100%
One eyed persons 6/6		FC at 1 ft—Nil or Field of vision 10°	30%

Abbreviation: FC, finger count.

MENTAL RETARDATION

Definition

Mental retardation is a condition of arrested or incomplete development of the mind, which is especially characterized by impairment of skills manifested during the development period which contributed to the overall level of intelligence, i.e. cognitive, language, motor and social abilities.

Categories of Mental Retardation

Mild Mental Retardation

The range of 50-69 (standardized IQ test) is indicative of mild retardation. Understanding and use of language tend to be delayed to a varying degree and executive speech problems that interfere with the development of independence may persist into adult life.

Moderate Mental Retardation

The IQ is of 35 to 49 discrepant profiles of abilities are common in this group with some individuals achieving higher levels in visuospatial skills than in tasks dependent on language while others are markedly clumsy, do not enjoy social interaction and simple conversation. The level of development of language is variable. Some of those affected can take part in simple conversations while others have only enough language to communicate their basic needs.

Severe Mental Retardation

The IQ is usually in the range of 20 to 34. In this category, most of the people suffer from a marked degree of motor impairment or other associated deficits indicating the presence of clinically significant damage to or maldevelopment of the central nervous system.

Profound Mental Retardation

The IQ in this category estimated to be under 20. The ability to understand or comply with requests or instructions are severely limited. Most of such individuals are immobile or severely restricted in mobility incontinent and capable at most of only very rudimentary forms of nonverbal communication. They posses little or no ability to care for their own basic needs and require constant help and supervision.

Process of Certifications

A disability certificate shall be issued by a Medical Board consisting of three members duly constituted by the Central/State Government. At least one shall be a specialist in the area of mental retardation, namely Psychiatrist, Pediatrician and Clinical Psychologist. Copy of the Certificate for Mental Retardation/Illness is enclosed.

It was also decided that whenever required the Chairman of the Board may co-opt other experts including that of the members constituted for the purpose by the Central and the State Government.

Variables in Assessing Disability (PPI)

Following variables need to be taken into consideration while assessing function loss resulting permanent physical impairment (disability) in mental retardation/mental illness.

a. Clinical assessment,
b. Assessment of adaptive behavior and
c. Intellectual functioning.

Assessment of Permanent Physical Impairment in Mental Illness based on Indian Disability Evaluation and Assessment Scale (IDEAs)

A scale for measuring and quantifying disability in mental disorders, developed by the Rehabilitation Committee of Indian Psychiatric Society, December 2000.

Items:

- *Self-care:* Includes taking care of body hygiene, grooming, health including bathing, toileting, dressing, eating, taking care of one's health.
- *Interpersonal activities (Social relationships):* Includes initiating and maintaining interactions with others in contextual and social appropriate manner.
- *Communication and understanding:* Includes communication and conversation with others by producing and comprehending spoken/written/nonverbal messages.
- *Work:* Three areas are Employment/Housework/Education measures on any aspect.
  1. *Performing in work/job:* Performing in work/employment (paid) employment/self-employment/family concern or otherwise. Measure ability to perform tasks at employment completely and efficiently and in proper time includes seeking employment.
  2. *Performing in housework:* Maintaining household including cooking, caring for other people at home, taking care of belongings, etc. Measures ability to take responsibility for and perform household tasks completely and efficiently and in proper time.
  3. *Performing in school/college:* Measures performance education-related tasks.

Scores for each item:

0 No disability (none, absent, negligible)
1 Mild disability (slight, low)
2 Moderate disability (medium, fair)

3. Severe disability (high, extreme)
4. Profound disability (total, cannot do).

TOTAL SCORE

Add scores of the 4 items and obtain a total score
Additional weightage for duration of illness (DOI):

<2 years:	score to be added is 1
2–5 years:	add 2
6–10 years:	add 3
>10 years:	add 4

GLOBAL DISABILITY

Total disability score + DOI score = Global disability score percentages:

0	No Disability = 0%
1-6	Mild Disability = <40%
7–13	Moderate Disability = 40–70%
14–19	Severe Disability = 71–99%
20	Profound Disability = 100%

Cut off for welfare measures.

MANUAL FOR "IDEAS"

In order to score this instrument, information from all possible sources should be obtained. This will include interview of patient, the care giver and case notes when available.

Self-care

This should be regarded as activity guided by social norms and conventions. The broad areas covered are:

a. Maintenance of personal hygiene and physical health
b. Eating
c. Maintenance of personal belongings and living space
d. Does he look after himself, wash his clothes regularly, and take a bath and brush his teeth?
e. Does he have regular meals?
f. Does he take food of right quality and quantity?
g. What about his table manners?

h. Does he take care of his personal belongings with reasonable standard of cleanliness and orderliness?

0 = No disability

Patient's level and pattern of self-care and normal, within the social cultural and economic context.

1 = Mild

Mild deterioration in self-care and appearance (not bathing, shaving, changing clothes for the occasion as expected). Does not have adverse consequences such as hazards to his health to his health. No embarrassment to family.

2 = Moderate

Lack of concern for self-care should be clearly established such as mild deterioration of physical health, obesity, tooth decay and body odors.

3 = Severe

Decline in self-care should be marked in all areas. Patient wearing torn clothes, would only wash if made to and would only eat if told. Evidence of serious hazards to physical health. (Malnutrition, infection, patient unacceptable in public).

4 = Profound

Total or near total lack of self-care (e.g. risk to physical survival, needs feeding, washing, putting on clothes, etc. constant supervision necessary).

Interpersonal Activities

Includes patient's response to questions, requests and demands of others. Activities of regulating emotions. Activities of initiating, maintaining and terminating interactions and activities of engaging in physical intimacy.

Guiding questions

a. What is his behavior with others?
b. Is he polite?
c. Does he respond to questions?
d. Is he able to regulate verbal and physical aggression ?
e. Is he able to act independently in social interactions?
f. How does he behave with strangers?
g. Is he able to maintain friendship?
h. Does he shows physical expression of affection and desire?

Scoring

0 = No

Patients gets along reasonably well with people personal relationships, no friction in interpersonal relationships.

1 - Mild

Some friction on isolated occasions. Patient known to be nervous or irritable but generally tolerated by others.

2 = Moderate

Factual evidence that pattern of response to people is unhealthy. May be seen on more than few occasion. Could isolate himself from others and avoid company.

3 = Severe

Behavior in social situations is undesirable and generalized. Causes serious problem in daily living/or work. Patient is socially ostracized.

4 = Profound

Patient in serious and lasting conflict, serious danger to problems or others, family afraid of potential consequences.

Communication and Understanding

Understanding spoken messages as well as written and nonverbal messages and ability to reduce messages in order to communicate with others.

1. Questions
   a. Does he avoid talking to people?
   b. When people come home what does he do?
   c. Does he ever visit others?
   d. Is he able to start, maintain and end a conversation?
   e. Does he understand body language and emotions of others such as, crying, screaming, etc.
   f. Does he indulge in reading and writing?
   g. Do you encourage him to be more sociable?

Scoring:

0 = No disability

Patient mixes, talks and generally interacts with people as much as can be expected in his sociocultural context. No evidence of avoiding people.

1 = Mild

Patient described as uncommunicative or solitary in social situations. Sings of social anxiety might be reported.

2 = Moderate

A very narrow range of social contact, evidence of active avoidance of people on some occasions and interference with performance of social rules causes concern to family.

3 = severe

Evidence of more generalized, active avoidance of contact with people (leave the room when visitors arrive and would not answer the door or phone).

4 = Profound

Hardly has contacts and actively avoids people nearly all the time, e.g. may lock himself inside the room. Verbal communication is nil or a bare minimum.

Work

This includes employment, housework and educational performance. Score only one category in case of an overlap.

Employment:

Guiding questions

a. Is he employed/unemployed?
b. If employed, does he go to work regularly?
c. Does he like his job and coping well with it?
d. Can you rely on him financially?
e. If unemployed, does he make any efforts to find a job?

Scoring:

0 = No disability—Patient goes to work regularly and his output and quality of work performance are within acceptable levels for the job.

1 = Mild—Noticeable decline patient's ability to work, to cope with it and meet the demands of work. May threaten to quit.

2 = Moderate—Declining work performance, frequent absences, lack of concern about all this. Financial difficulties foreseen.

3 = Severe—Marked decline in work performance, disruptive at work, unwilling to adhere to disciplines of work. Threat of losing his job.

4 = Profound—Has been largely absent from work, termination imminent. Unemployed and making no efforts to find jobs. In similar ways, housewives should be rated on the amount, regularity

and efficiency in which tasks in the following areas are completed. Consider the amount of help required completing these. Acquiring daily necessities, making, storing and serving of food, cleaning the house, working with those helping with domestic duties such as maids, cooks, etc. looking after possessions and valuable in the house.

Student: Assess an score on performance in school/college, regularity discipline, interest in future studies, behavior at educational institutions. Those who had to discontinue education on account of mental disability and unable to continue further should be given a score of 4.

IDEAS SCORING SHEET

Items	*0*	*1*	*2*	*3*	*4*
Self-care					
Interpersonal activities					
Communication and understanding					
Work					
A. Total score					
B. DOI score					
Global score (A + B)					

STANDARD FORMAT OF THE CERTIFICATE OF MENTAL RETARDATION FOR GOVERNMENT BENEFITS (NAME AND ADDRESS OF THE INSTITUTE/HOSPITAL ISSUING THE CERTIFICATE)

Certificate No. .... Date.......................

This is to certify that /Sh/Kum ....

Son/Daughter of .... of Town/City

....

.... with particulars given below:

a. Age

b. Sex

c. Signature/Thumb impression

CATEGORIZATION OF MENTAL RETARDATION

Mild/Moderate/Severe/Profound
Validity of the Certificate: Permanent

Signature of the Government
Doctor/Hospital with seal

Chairperson Mental Retardation
Certification Board

Recent Attested Photograph
Showing the disability affixed here

Dated:

Place:

SPEECH AND HEARING DISABILITY

1. *Definition of hearing:* A person with hearing impairment having difficulty of various degrees in hearing sounds is an impaired person.
2. *Points to be remembered in hearing disability assessment:*
   a. Hearing has been taken as 100% and percentage of disability in such cases should be calculated in relation to this and not thinking human body as 100%
   b. Disability percentage should be calculated following latest guidelines notified (2001) and not of personal opinion.
   c. Disability guidelines are based on loss in function (hearing) taking medical diagnosis into account and not mere based on medical diagnosis.
   d. The assessment has to be done after possible correction, mechanical cleaning of ear canal but without hearing aid.
   e. Hearing in both ear should be tested separately.
   f. In calculating disability percentage, hearing and speech discrimination have to be taken into account.
   g. While calculating disability, age, sex, education and nature of work being performed by individual have no role to play.

h. In multiple disability, if a person has disability other than hearing, it should be added as per guidelines and not mere summing percentage of two disability.
i. The board may review certificate issued by it, on the request/ representation of disabled.
j. The DGHs, Government of India is final authority (Appellate authority)

2. Variables in assessing hearing impairment (PPI)
   a. Hearing loss in units of dB level in each ear separately
   b. Speech discrimination
   c. Categories of hearing impairment.

Category	*Type of impairment*	*dB level*	*Speech discrimination*	*%age of impairment*
I	Mild hearing	dB 26 to 40 dB in better ear	80 to 100% in better ear	Less than 40%
II (a)	Moderate hearing	41 to 60 dB in better ear	50 to 80% in better ear	40 to 50%
II (b)	Severe hearing impairment	61 to 70 dB in better ear	40 to 50% in better ear	51 to 70%
III	a. Profound hearing Impairment b. Total deafness	71 to 90 dB 91 dB and above/in better ear/no hearing	Less than 40% in better ear/very poor discrimination	71 to 100%

- Pure tone average of hearing in 500 and 2000 HZ, 4000 HZ by conduction (AC and BC) should be taken as basis for consideration as per the test recommendations.
- When there is only an island of hearing present in one or two frequencies in better ear, it should be considered as total loss of hearing.
- Wherever there is no response (NR) at any of the 4 frequencies (500, 1000, 2000 and 4000 HZ), it should be considered as equivalent to 100 dB loss for the purpose of classification of disability and in arriving at the average.

4. Process of certification.
   A disability certificate shall be issued by a Medical Board duly constituted by the Central and State Government. Out of which at least one member shall be a specialist in the field of ENT.

CHAPTER 17

National District Level Rehabilitation Program

OBJECTIVES OF THE PROGRAM

To develop rehabilitation services and provide opportunities for all disabled people in all states in India.

Specific Objectives

- To make all basic rehabilitation services available at the community level.
- To increase participation of people with disabilities in community life including all the main stream development activities.
- To develop equal opportunities in all the existing health, education, social welfare, rural development and other programs.
- To develop appropriate technology to enhance participation of disabled people in all main stream program.
- To protect the human and civil rights of people with disabilities and to promote the representation and empowerment of such persons and their families.
- To remove physical and psychological barriers.
- To ensure full participation of the state and national government and that of the communities in CBR program.

ACTIVITY FRAME WORK

Activities

- Identification of disabled people and assessment of their needs.
- Functional training with the assistance of families and the community.
- Preparation for the inclusion of disabled children in to main stream education.
- Organization of self-help groups that will share the care of severely disabled persons and prepare them for main stream education and employment.
- Provision of aids and appliances by using existing welfare scheme.
- Setting up workshops for aids and appliances at district level, with decentralization of maintenance and supply of simple appliances to the Taluk level.
- Prevocational assessment and training using existing rural development programs.
- Vocational training using existing rural development programs.
- Creation of opportunities for self-employment and group employment through existing rural development and welfare schemes.

FRAMEWORK FOR SERVICE DELIVERY

When setting up a framework for service delivery, it is proposed to follow the recommendations and directives made by the Rehabilitation Council of India. The Council Act of 1992 requires that organizations that deliver services for persons with disabilities will employ only personnel that meet the requirements for competence. For a CBR program, the council has decided that it is appropriate to use a "Multipurpose Rehabilitation Worker (MRW)". At the community (Gram Panchayat) level, a community worker Local Facilitator (LF) should be chosen by the community and trained.

The principles of the service delivery system as shown above may be described as follows:

At the Gram Panchayat level, the local Panchayat committee or a special rehabilitation committee will micromanage the CBR program. It decides if and when the community will start a CBR program, what resources to provide (such as employing and training a community facilitator), and assists in providing access to schemes for functional training, inclusive education, rural development, health, social welfare benefits, care and economic support.

- At the Taluk level, the MRW will be responsible for the information to community leaders and to persons with disabilities and their families about disability and what the community can do to provide services and opportunities using already available resources. The MRW will cooperate with personnel at PHC, education, labor, social welfare NGOs and others, which will make services available and open opportunities for persons with disabilities.
- At the district level, a district technical rehabilitation coordinator will monitor and guide the work carried out at more peripheral levels. Liaisons will be established with specialists at referral levels in a two-way system. Not only will disabled persons living in the community get access to specialized care; also disabled persons in centers will be referred back to their homes and continue the rehabilitation process there. A report system will be set up to serve the state administration.
- At the state level, a cell will be created within the nodal department, the Department of Disabled Welfare. This CBR coordination cell will be involved in macromanagement, planning, monitoring, evaluation, guiding technical development and overseeing training programs for MRWs, LFs and other categories of personnel involved in the program. It should be remarked that there is also another option for a service delivery system, namely to add the responsibilities to an already existing category of personnel. The experience of this option is rather negative for four reasons:

The personnel chosen from one sector will most often neglect or even be ignorant of how other sectors engage to meet the needs of disabled people, The training costs are substantially higher, as often 8–10 times more personnel will have to be trained, There is most often a lack of clear responsibility for the whole rehabilitation program, which is avoided when MRWs are employed, and the personnel will most often lack sufficient experience.

Duties and Responsibilities of Implementing Agency Personnel

The LF is a Community Worker who

1. May work on full time or part-time basis,
2. Is chosen by the community and under the management of its leaders,
3. Is trained and subsequently supervised by the MRW

4. Undertakes tasks related to the identification of disabled people, followed by locating, motivating and preparing a trainer for each of them,
5. Undertakes the transfer of rehabilitation technology to the family and community members,
6. Assists in the functional training and in the production of simple rehabilitation appliances,
7. Contacts other community members or local authorities to arrange for disabled people's participation in all locally available development programs, such as those related to poverty alleviation, preschool activities, schooling and other special education, vocational training and other job-oriented program, legal protection, home care, etc.,
8. Contacts welfare or other activities which provide benefits or grants for disabled people;
9. Initiates social contacts and participation in all aspects of community life, with the aim of fully integrating disabled people, and
10. Keeps records and monitors and reports progress of the programs to all those concerned.

The Multipurpose Rehabilitation Worker (MRW)

The MRW will work at the Taluk level:

1. Initiating contacts with communities and providing the information requested on the CBR Program,
2. Visiting communities to advise them on the practical aspects of the CBR Program,
3. Designing, conducting and evaluating courses to train local facilitators (LFs),
4. Assisting in the development of multisectoral contact, so disabled people will be involved in mainstream rural development schemes, receive primary healthcare, education, and ability training, and be given opportunities for gainful employment,
5. Contacting referral services, public authorities, or private organizations, regarding disabled people in need of diagnostic, therapeutic or rehabilitation services and/or opportunities for assessment, guidance, counseling, schooling, and ability training such as vocational training,
6. Monitoring all aspects of the legal protection of disabled people to ensure observance of their human rights and adequate

representation of the disabled people and their families in all community affairs that are of special interest to them.

7. Ensuring appropriate monitoring of the CBR Programs of all communities in the district and taking steps to correct problems that become apparent on monitoring; reporting monitored information and data to higher levels, and responding to directives aimed at reprogramming or at other changes, and
8. Assisting, in co-operation with the local and district administrations, with the necessary administrative action to ensure smooth functioning of the program.

The District CBR Coordinator

The coordinator:

1. Plans for, monitors and guides all CBR programs, including the training of LFs, in the district,
2. Provides technical support and liaison with referral levels for the rehabilitation activities that cannot be carried out at community or Taluk levels,
3. Reports on the district activities to the district authorities and committees and to the state level, and
4. Provides orientation and awareness courses for all personnel at district level who are involved in CBR Programs.

The State CBR Coordinator

The state coordinator:

1. Undertakes all planning for resource requirements and provisions for the entire state, including the budgeting process,
2. Monitors and evaluates all reports, intervenes to correct managerial problems, and reports to the appropriate authorities on the outcomes of the program,
3. Supervises all training of personnel engaged in CBR, and
4. Liaisons with the State Commissioner and the Coordination Executive Committees and other bodies as required.

Duties and Responsibilities of the Committees

State Level Committees

The duties and responsibilities of the State Coordination and Executive Committees are defined in the 1995 Act. These committees, in addition to those mentioned in the Act, should also make room for representation of the disabled people, families with disabled people, NGOs implementing CBR and other departments concerning poverty alleviation, education and other development activities.

Interdepartmental Coordination

The active collaboration of the following departments is a prerequisite for an optimal functioning of the CBR Program:

- Department of Education,
- Department of Women and Child Welfare,
- Department of Health,
- Department of Rural Development,
- Department of Social Welfare, and
- Department of Labor.

Duties and Responsibilities of Nodal Agency

The Department for Welfare of Disabled is:

1. To select a nodal training agency and arrange for MRW training,
2. To recruit and employ,
3. To select districts with the target of covering 80% of disabled people of all districts in ten years time,
4. To ensure economic support to Panchayats from the existing development program and schemes for disabled people,
5. To establish linkages between Panchayats at district, Taluk and village levels with concerned government departments at all levels,
6. To set up District CBR Coordinating committees at Jilla Panchayat office,
7. To ensure that Taluk CBR Coordination committees are set up at the Taluk Panchayat office, and
8. To ensure that village level CBR coordinating committees are set up at the gram Panchayat office.

Duties and Responsibilities of Nodal Training Agency

1. To set up a training center for MRW training,
2. To implement the MRW training curriculum approved by the Rehabilitation Council of India,
3. To arrange accommodation for 60 MRW's per year,
4. To train 540 MRW's in 10 years,

5. To set up a CBR Training coordination committee with a Director for Disabled Welfare, Disabled persons, NGOs, experts on CBR, and representatives from Education, Health, Welfare, Rural Development, Labor and other concerned departments, and
6. To report to the State CBR Coordination Committee once a year.

Decentralized Levels

Duties and Responsibilities of District CBR Committee

1. To set up Taluk CBR Coordination Committees comprised of disabled persons, NGOs, families with disabled persons, and representatives from health, education, welfare, rural development and other concerned departments, with Taluk Panchayat president as the Chairperson of the committee. The person responsible for the execution of its decision is the District CBR Coordinator,
2. To ensure the establishment of appropriate monitoring systems,
3. To ensure that the resources for rehabilitation services are available in time for village Panchayat,
4. To motivate village Panchayats to take up CBR program (Flowchart 7.1).

Flowchart 17.1: Framework for CBR Program proposed managerial structure and linkages for CBR

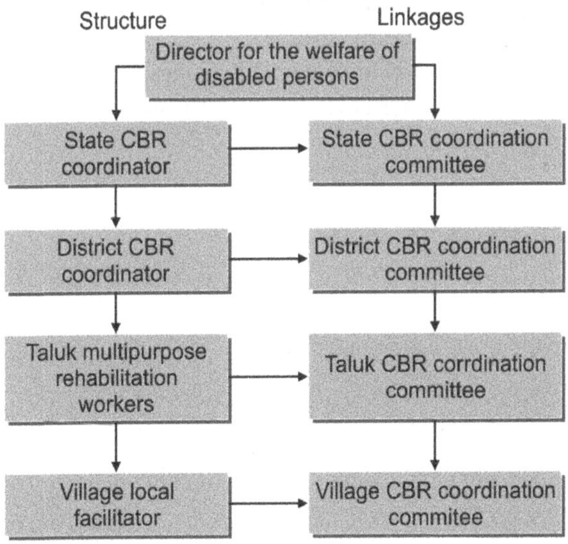

Note: At each district, there will be one MRW working at the Taluk level for one lakh people. At each village Panchayat, there will be one LF for about 5000 people.

5. To establish necessary linkages with various departments to assist the village Panchayats to avail the benefits from the existing schemes, and
6. To report to the state CBR coordinator every month.

Duties and Responsibilities of Taluk CBR committees

1. To ensure that village level CBR coordination is established,
2. To assist the village Panchayat to mobilize resources,
3. To establish linkages with various departments in order to assist the village Panchayat to avail the benefit from the existing scheme for people with disabilities,
4. To assist, guide, and monitor the function of MRWs, and
5. To report to Jilla Panchayat once in a month.

Duties and Responsibilities of the Village Panchayat

1. To select and arrange for training and appoint a local facilitator,
2. To pay honorarium for the local facilitator,
3. To monitor the CBR program,
4. To arrange for rehabilitation services by using existing schemes for disabled, rural development schemes, and education schemes, and by mobilizing local resources,
5. To ensure full participation of people with disabilities and their families in CBR program, and
6. To ensure the evaluation of the CBR program at the end of the 3rd year and revise the scheme based on the evaluation results.

CHAPTER

18

Screening and Prevention of Disability

DEFINITION

Screening is search for unrecognized disease or defect by means of rapidly applied test, examination or other procedures in apparently healthy individuals.

Screening simply differs from diagnosis in three aspects:

1. Capable of wide applications.
2. Relatively inexpensive.
3. Require little physician time.

TABLE 18.1: Differences between screening and diagnosis

Screening	*Diagnosis*
1. Done on apparently healthy	1. In whom sickness prevails or those indicated
2. Applied to group	2. Applied in a single patient
3. Test results are arbitrary and final	3. Not final but it is the evidence of
4. Based on first criterion or cut off point	4. Based on evaluation
5. Less accurate	5. More accurate
6. Less expensive	6. More expensive
7. Not basis for treatment	7. Basis for treatment
8. Initiation from agency or investigation	8. Initiation from patient with complaint

SCREENING TEST

1. Apparently normal
   a. Periodic rescreening done.

2. Apparently abnormal.
   a. Normal—periodic rescreening.
   b. Intermediate—for surveillance.
   c. Abnormal—for treatment.

USES OF SCREENING

Screening is used for following purposes:
1. Case detection.
2. Control of disease.
3. Research purpose.
4. Educational opportunities.

Case Detection

It is prescriptive screening.

For example—
- Neonatal screening (polio drops for all, BCG,)
- Bacterial infection during pregnancy
- Breast cancer
- Deaf children
- Diabetes mellitus
- Iron deficiency anemia
- Pulmonary tuberculosis.

Control of Disease

- It is prospective screening
- People examined for benefit of others.

Research Purpose

For example, hypertension, cancer.

Educational Opportunities

Creating awareness among people.

TYPES OF SCREENING

A. Mass screening
B. High risk/selective screening
C. Multiphasic screening.

Mass Screening

- Screening of large number of people, group or subgroup.
- Group must be a specific one.
  For example, all students for hepatitis B, pregnant woman, children under two year.

Effects: Suitable treatment in appropriate time with decrease duration of illness and results in good outcome.

High Risk/Selective Screening

- Screening of "specially and selectively adapted" high-risk group, e.g. drivers prove for low back ache, upper middle class for hypertension and coronary artery disease and diabetes mellitus, upper middle class woman—cancer cervix.

Effect: Help in eliminating and treatment diabetes mellitus, coronary artery disease, occupational hazards, etc.

Multiphasic Screening

Two or more screening in combination is used for a large group of people at a time than carrying out individual screening tests.

For example, chemical hematological test on blood, urine specimens,

Lung function assessment,audiometry and measurement of visual acuity.

Effect: Largely on decrease time and offering multiple benefits to the people undergoing screening.

EVALUATION OF SCREENING PROGRAM

1. Randomized control trial.
2. Uncontrolled trials.
3. Other method.

Randomized Control Trial

Here a group of people is randomly selected. The screening program will be implemented with a specific type of personnel's, equipment and procedures.
For example, cancer patients.

Uncontrolled Trials

These are the trial without controls (comparison group) because necessity is not felt due to peculiar nature of the outcome. This is used for group of people who were detected through screening and diagnosed and treatment still left over with the disease.

For example, in human rabies, the mortality is 100%. If a new drug for human rabies is invented, control group is not required. In other words, 'historical controls" (i.e. experience of earlier untreated patients) are used.

Other Method

Evaluations such as case control studies and comparison in trends between areas with different degrees of screening coverage.

Following screening tests cover

(i) Pregnancy, (ii) infancy, (iii) Middle-aged male and female, (iv) Elderly

- Pregnancy
  - Anemia
  - Hypertension
  - Toxemia
  - Rh status
  - Syphilis
  - Diabetes
  - Cardiovascular diseases
  - Neural tube defect
  - Down syndrome
  - HIV
- Infancy
  - Congenital diaphragmatic hernia (CDH)
  - Coronary heart disease (CHD)
  - Spina bifida
  - Cerebral palsy (CP)
  - Hg defect
  - Visual defect
  - Hypothyroidism
  - Developmental screening test
  - Sickle cell anemia
- Middle-aged male and female
  - Hypertension
  - Cancer
  - Diabetes mellitus

- Serum cholesterol
- Obesity
- Elderly
  - Nutritional deficiencies
  - Cancer
  - TB
  - Chronic bronchitis
  - Cataract
  - Glaucoma.

PREVENTION OF DISABILITIES

Prevention is usually defined at 4 levels:

1. Primary prevention.
2. Secondary prevention.
3. Tertiary prevention.
4. Primordial prevention.

Primary Prevention

Action taken prior to the onset of the disease/disability, which will remove the possibility that a disease/disability will occur.

This includes health promotional and specific protection measures.

Health Promotional Measures

- Health education of the community regarding prevention of disease and disabilities need, use, why, how, and what of immunization defluoridation of water, iodization of common salt, good nutrition, provision of perinatal care
- Improvement of housing, provision of potable drinking water, sanitation facilities, improved standard of living, etc.
- Avoiding certain drugs, unnecessary medication or exposure to X-ray during pregnancy
- Better care during delivery, antenatal/postnatal/perinatal periods
- Prevention of head injuries—using helmets and seat belts
- Improvement in vehicle design and provision of medical facilities, stronger, enforcement of regulations concerning the compulsory use of seat belts (four wheel vehicles) and helmet (two wheel vehicles) and restriction on alcohol consumption and other substance abuse combined with driving will mean greater changes of survival from road accidents and these should therefore be encouraged.

Specific Protection Measures

- Immunization against six killer diseases
- Defluoridation of water
- Use of iodized salt vitamin A prophylaxis.

Essentially primary prevention aims at aborting the onset of event like injury/disease which may lead to disease/disability—effort may take sometime to be obvious, but will reduce the burden of disability in a big way. Primary prevention programs are vital for both developed and developing countries. It is more so in developing countries where childhood disabilities are prevalent even today.

Secondary Prevention

Action, which halts the progress of the disease/disability at its incipient stage and prevents complications. The specific interventions are early diagnosis and adequate treatment.

Early diagnosis/early identification of disease and treatment/management of diseases/injury/event will help to reduce occurrence of disability. Examples of this are: early identification of patches due to leprosy and institution of prompt treatment will prevent occurrence of disabilities.

Early recognition of vitamin A deficiency and prompt treatment, nutritional supplementation will prevent occurrence of blindness due to vitamin A deficiency.

Screening for cataract and surgery will help people have better vision. Identification, needed surgery, therapeutic measures will prevent contractures and deformities in persons with paralysis due to poliomyelitis.

Tertiary Prevention

All measures available to reduce or limit impairments and disabilities, and minimize suffering caused by existing disability. This phase is also called rehabilitation, which includes physical, psychosocial and vocational measures taken to restore the patient back to normal or near normal condition.

It is extremely important that the women undertake adequate and effective preventive measures during their pregnancy and immediate postnatal period and also for their children especially during the early childhood period, in order to significantly reduce the incidence of impairment and disabilities in them. Therefore, in this chapter examples of easily understood primary preventive measures, for mother and child are summarized.

General Preventive Measures

1. Marriage between very close blood relations like uncle, niece, first cousin should be avoided for prevention of hereditary disorders.
2. Avoid pregnancies before the age of 18 years and after the age of 35 years.
3. Consult a doctor before planning the pregnancy;
   a. If there is incidence of birth defects in your family.
   b. If you have had difficulty in conceiving or have had a series of miscarriages, still births, twins, delivery by operation (Caesarean), obstructed labor/prolonged labor (more than 12 hours) and/or severe bleeding in previous pregnancy.
   c. If you have Rh-negative blood type.
   d. If you have diabetes.

Care during Pregnancy

1. Avoid hard physical work such as carrying heavy loads, especially in fields, and other accident-prone activities such as walking on slippery ground or climbing stools and chairs.
2. Avoid unnecessary drugs and medications. Even the normally considered safe drugs which are sold commonly can potentially cause serious defects in an unborn child.
3. Avoid smoking, chewing tobacco, consuming alcohol and narcotics.
4. Avoid X-rays, and exposure to any kind of radiation.
5. Avoid exposure to illnesses like measles, mumps, etc., especially during the first 3 months of pregnancy.
6. Avoid sexual contact with a person having venereal disease.
7. Take precautions against lead poisoning.
8. Avoid too much use of 'Surma' and 'Kohl.'
9. Eat a well-balanced and nourishing diet supplemented with green leafy vegetables, proteins and vitamins.
10. All women of the child-bearing age need 0.4 mg of folic acid daily. It is Also available in folic acid plus iron tablets which should be taken for at least 3 months during the third trimester when the risk of developing iron deficiency anemia is greatest.
11. Ensure weight gain of at last 10 kg. Have regular medical check- ups.
12. All pregnant women should be given tetanus injection.
13. Woman at 'high-risk,' whose weight is <38 kg, height is less than 152 cm, weight gain during pregnancy <6 kg or who is severely

anemic (Hb <8 mg), having frequent pregnancies, having a history of miscarriage/abortion/premature deliveries, must get expert prenatal care so as to have a normal baby.

14. Must consult a doctor, in case of edema (swelling) of feet, persistent headache, fever, difficulty or pain in passing urine, bleeding from the vagina, and yellowness of eyes (jaundice).

Care at the Time of Birth

1. Delivery must be conducted by trained personnel, preferably in a hospital where all facilities are available.
2. If a baby does not cry immediately after birth, resuscitation measures should be undertaken at once.
3. Babies born prematurely and with a low birth weight (<2.5 kg) may need neonatal intensive care.
4. If the baby's head appears to be abnormally small or large then a physician should be consulted, preferably a pediatrician. The approximate head size for a male child at birth is 35 cm and for female child is 34.5 cm.
5. To protect a child from infections, breastfeeding must be started immediately after birth. First milk (colostrums) must be fed to the baby and should not be thrown away, as it has antibodies which are protective.

Early Childhood Care

1. Do not allow a child's temperature to rise above 101°F because of any reason. It can cause febrile seizures.
2. If a child gets a fit take him to doctor immediately.
3. Every child should be immunized against infectious diseases as per the recommended schedule of immunization.
4. Do not allow a child to have too much contact with paint, newsprint ink, lead, etc. as they are toxic.
5. Take precautions against head injury, and other accidents.
6. Ensure that the child gets a well-balanced diet and clean drinking water.
7. Introduce additional foods of good quality and in sufficient quantity when the child is 4–6 months old.
8. Vitamin A deficiency and its consequences including night blindness can be easily prevented through the use of vitamin A supplementation.

9. Protect a child from meningitis and encephalitis by providing a hygienic environment which is free of overcrowding.
10. Common salt must be iodized as a precaution against goiter and cretinism.
11. Do not allow a child to use hairpins, matchsticks and pencils, to remove wax from the ears.
12. Use ear protectors to reduce the exposure to high levels of noise, if children are living or working in a noisy environment.
13. Do not slap a child over the face as this may lead to injury of the eardrum and consequent hearing loss.

Primordial Prevention

Primordial prevention is an important level of prevention. this especially helps us to prevent occurrence of diseases like hypertension, diabetes, coronary artery disease, stroke, obesity, etc. if intervene in early child hood, childhood and adolescence, prevents occurrence, suffering and disabilities due to noncommunicable diseases, especially if we change our lifestyle. Health education and counseling on diet, physical activity and tobacco use at high school level may help in attempting primordial prevention. Basically, primordial prevention aims at risk factor prevention.

APPROACHES FOR THE PRIMORDIAL PREVENTION

1. Population strategy.
2. High-risk strategy.

Population Strategy

This is directed at the whole population, for example, a small reduction in the average blood pressure or serum cholesterol in the population, goes a long way in reducing the prevalence of coronary artery disease in the community. This approach is directed towards changes in lifestyle of the population by health education from the childhood itself.

High-risk Strategy

This is directed to those individuals, who are at high risk of getting the disease. These high-risk group can be detected by screening procedures.

CHAPTER

19

Assessment of Different Types of Disabilities

Despite all the best efforts at prevention, children may be born with or develop the following disabilities in early childhood, from the causes which are not yet fully understood or could be prevented.

TYPES OF DISABILITIES

- Visual impairment
- Hearing impairment
- Locomotor impairment; Cerebral palsy
- Mental retardation and mental illness
- Children with learning disabilities
  - Dyslexia
  - Dysgraphia
  - Dyscalculia
  - Attention deficit and hyperactivity disorder (ADHD).

DEFINITIONS

Disability as defined by the Act (Persons with Disability Act, 1995) covers blindness, low vision, leprosy-cured, hearing impairment, locomotor disability, mental retardation and mental illness as well as multiple disability. The Act does not cover disabilities like autism, or learning disabilities. However, definitions/concepts of all relevant disabilities are given below:

- *Blindness:* A condition where a person suffers from any of the following conditions namely:
  - Total absence of sight or
  - Visual acuity not exceeding 6/60 or 20/200 (snellen) in the better eye with correcting lenses; or
  - Limitation of the field vision subtending an angle of 20° or worse.
- *Person with low vision:* A person with impairment of visual functioning even after treatment or standard refractive correction but who uses or is potentially capable of using vision for the planning or execution of a task with appropriate assistive device.
- *Cerebral palsy:* A group of non-progressive conditions characterized by abnormal motor control posture resulting from brain insult or injuries occurring in the perinatal, neonatal or infant period of development.
- *Hearing impairment:* Loss of sixty decibels or more in the better ear in the conversational range of frequencies.
- *Leprosy-cured person:* Any person who has been cured of leprosy but is suffering from loss of sensation in hands or feet as well as loss of sensation and paresis in the eyelid but with no manifest deformity; manifest deformity and paresis but having sufficient mobility in their hands and feet to enable them to engage in normal economic activity; extreme physical deformity as well as advanced age which prevents him from undertaking any gainful occupation.
- *Locomotor disability:* Disability of the bones, joint or muscles leading to substantial restriction of the movement of the limbs or a usual form of cerebral palsy. Some common conditions giving raise to locomotor disability could be poliomyelitis, cerebral palsy, amputation, injuries of spine, head, soft tissues, fractures, muscular dystrophies, etc.
- *Mental illness:* Any mental disorder other than mental retardation
- *Mental retardation:* A condition of arrested or incomplete development of mind of a person which is especially characterized by sub-normality of intelligence, i.e. cognitive, language, motor and social abilities.
- *Autism:* A condition of uneven skill development primarily affecting the communication and social abilities of a person, marked by repetitive and ritualistic behavior.

- *Multiple disability:* A combination of two or more disabilities as defined in clause (i) of section 2 of the Person with Disabilities (Equal Opportunities, Protection of Rights and Full Participation) Act 1995 namely Blindness/low vision Speech and Hearing impairment Locomotor disability including leprosy cured Mental retardation and Mental illness.
- *Learning disabilities (Dyslexia):* Affect person's ability to acquire, process, and/or use either, spoken, read, written or nonverbal information (organization/planning, functional literacy skills, memory, reasoning, problem solving, perceptual skills) or in other words in short—difficulty with language in its various uses (not always reading).
  - *Dyspraxia:* The inability to motor plan, to make an appropriate body response.
  - *Dysgraphia:* Difficulty with the act of writing both in the technical as well as the expressive sense. There may also be difficulty with spelling.
  - *Dyscalculia:* Difficulty with calculations.
  - *Attention deficit* and hyperactivity, distractibility and impulsivity hyperactivity disorder (ADHD).
- *Impairment:* Missing or defective body part, an amputated limb, paralysis after polio, restricted pulmonary capacity, diabetes, nearsightedness, mental retardation, limited hearing capacity, facial disfigurement or other abnormal condition.
- *Disabilities:* As a result of an impairment may involve difficulties in walking, seeing, speaking, hearing, reading, writing, counting, lifting, or taking interest in and making one's surrounding.

  Temporary total disability: Period in which the affected person is totally unable to work. During this period, he may receive orthopedic, ophthalmological, auditory or speech any other medical treatment.

  Temporary partial disability: Period when recovery has reached the stage of improvement, so that person may began some kind of gainful occupation.

  Permanent disability: Permanent damage or loss of use of some part/parts of the body after the stage of maximum improvement (from any medical treatment) has been reached and the condition is stationary.
- *Handicap:* A disability becomes a handicap when it interferes with doing what is expected at a particular time in one's life.

- *Rehabilitation:* Refers to a process aimed at enabling persons with disabilities to reach and maintain their optimal physical, sensory, intellectual, psychiatric or social functional levels;
- *'Person with Disability':* A person suffering from not less than 40% of any disability as certified by a medical authority.
- *Institution for persons:* An institution for the reception, care, protection, with disabilities education, training, rehabilitation or any other service of persons with disabilities.

Note: Various State Governments have also adopted different sets of definitions for example, Government of Tamil Nadu declared one-eyed persons in the same category as blind persons and have extended various concessions.

IDENTIFICATION AND ASSESSMENT OF THE DISABILITIES

Timely identification of impairments, a secondary prevention, can reduce the impact of the impairment on the functional level of the individual and also in checking the impairments from becoming a disabling condition. Initially they need to be identified as soon as possible at home by the parents and outside (in the Anganwadi centers/schools/subhealth centers/through camps), and then they need to be assessed through a team of specialists to plan necessary interventions.

AT HOME

Parents can observe and identify the children with disabilities by using the following checklist for early identification of disabilities:

Hearing Impairment

Screening Newborn

1. Is there anyone in the family with deafness since childhood?
2. Did the mother take an abortifacient drug or any other medicine in large doses during the first three months of pregnancy?
3. Is the birth weight below 1500 g.
4. Did the child had a delayed cry after birth?
5. Did the child have significant jaundice (yellowness of eyes) during the first 10 days after birth?

6. Does the child have a cleft in the lip or palate, or a malformed pinna?

Screening Children in the Age Group of 6 Months to 2 Years

1. Does a child turn towards the source of sound which is located either at the back or towards one side of the body?
2. Does he/she have discharge from the ear?

Screening Children above 2 Years Age

1. Does he/she turn when called from behind?
2. Uses gestures excessively.
3. The child does not speak or has a defective speech.
4. The child does not understand the spoken language.
5. The child has an ear discharge.

Visual Impairment

1. The child does not follow an object moving before his eyes by 1 month's age.
2. The child does not reach for toys and things held in front of him by 3 months age.
3. One eye moves differently from the other; including squint.
4. Eyes are either red or have a yellow discharge or the tears flow continuously.
5. The child has tendency to bring pictures or books very near the eyes.

Mental Retardation

1. Does the child respond to name/voice by 4th month?
2. Does the child smiles at others by 6th month?
3. Does the child hold the head steadily by 6th month?
4. Does the child sit without support by 12th month?
5. Can the child stand without support by 18th month?
6. Can the child walk well by 20th month?
7. Can the child talk 2-3 word sentences by 3rd year?
8. Can a child eat/drink by himself by 4th year?
9. Can he tell his name by 4th year?
10. Does he have toilet control by 4th year?
11. Does he avoid simple hazards?
12. Does he get fits?

Locomotor Disability

1. The child is not able to raise both the arms fully without any difficulties.
2. The child is not able to grasp objects without any difficulty.
3. The child has absence of any part of the limb.
4. The child has a difficulty in walking.

OUTSIDE

In the rural and tribal areas as well as in the urban-slums, early identification is done through door-to-door surveys, screening children at the Anganwadis, schools, health centers, subhealth centers, rehabilitation centers or through camps usually organized by the voluntary workers, or else.

1. *Anganwadi Center—ICDS:* The Department of Women and Child Development under the Ministry of Human Resource Development, has been implementing the program of Integrated Child Development Scheme (ICDS) since 1975. An Angandwadi center under the program is located in each village and is run by an Anganwadi worker. Some of the important objectives of the scheme include improvement of the nutritional status of the children in the age group of 0–6 years, providing nutrition and health education for every woman in the age group of 15–44 years and improving the capability of the mothers to look after the normal health and nutritional needs of their children. An Anganwadi worker is required to do early detection of the disabilities in children present at their Anganwadi centers.
2. *Subhealth Centers—Primary Health Centers:* India has a well-established network of Primary Health Centers, each catering to a population of 30,000 to 40,000. These have subhealth centers at the field level. Each subhealth center caters to a population of around 3000 persons and is managed by one female health worker. Under the program of MCH (Mother and Child Health), the worker takes care of the children by providing immunization, and vitamin A supplementation to children below 6 years of age. She also identifies the health problems which may lead to disability and takes further preventive action.
3. *Rehabilitation Services are provided to all the eligible persons by the Ministry of Social Justice and Empowerment through its various Programs:*

a. *Camps under District Rehabilitation Centers (DRCs) in 11 districts:* Comprehensive Rehabilitation Services are provided to the rural disabled at their door steps mainly through camps organized by voluntary organizations. Grass-root functionaries like Anganwadi workers, health workers, are also involved. These Centers provide services for the prevention and early detection, medical intervention and surgical correction, fitting of artificial aids and appliances, therapeutic services such as physiotherapy, occupational and speech therapy, provision of training for acquisition of skills through vocational training, job placement in local industries, etc.

b. *Composite Rehabilitation Services (District Center):* Rehabilitation services in more than 107 districts in the country are being provided at the door steps of persons with disabilities. These services include promotion of early detection and prevention of disability, fitting, follow-up and repair of assistive devices, provide vocational training and help in finding gainful-employment. At the field level, grass-root level functionaries—Anganwadi workers, health workers and PRIs are helping in implementation of the program (List of District Centers may be seen at annexure-III C).

c. *National Program for Rehabilitation of Persons with Disabilities (NPRPD):* The program of NPRPD has recently been launched as a State Sector Scheme. Under the scheme, there is a provision of 2 Community-based Rehabilitation Workers at each Gram Panchayat and 2 Multi-purpose Rehabilitation Workers at Block level. The focus at grass-root level would be prevention, early detection and information dissemination. Services at district level would be provided through various professionals like physiotherapists, occupational therapists, orthotic and prosthetic engineers, etc. At the State Referral Center, higher services would be provided.

4. *School:* Teachers in all the primary, upper primary and secondary government schools have a responsibility to identify children with disabilities.

Check list for identification of children with special needs:
(School teachers and parents should use this check list).

Visual

- Watering of eyes
- Recurrent redness
- Often irritation
- Frequent blinking
- Squint
- Inappropriate stumbling over objects or bump into other people
- Tilting of the head or closure of one eye
- Headache while doing fine work
- Difficulty in counting the fingers of an outstretched hand at a distance of one meter
- Moving head side-to-side while reading
- Difficulty in recognizing distant objects
- Difficulty in counting the fingers of an outstretched hand at a distance of one meter
- Moving head side-to-side while reading
- Difficulty in recognizing distant objects
- Difficulty in doing other fine work requiring perfect vision
- Holding books too close or too far from the eyes
- Frequently ask other children when taking down notes from the blackboard
- Exhibit difficulty in reading from the blackboard
- Hitting against the objects on the side.

Note: If any of the above 4 responses are yes, then the child should be properly examined by a qualified ophthalmologist to see if the existing condition can be improved by medical treatment or by using spectacles.

Hearing

- Malformation of the ear
- Discharge from ear
- Pain in ear
- Irritation in ear
- Trying to listen from a closer distance
- Ask for the instructions repeatedly
- Not able to write properly
- Trying to listen to the echo reflection rather than from the speaker
- Make errors while copying from black board

- Frequently ask a colleague to show his workbook
- Problems in paying attention in the class
- Favor one ear for listening purposes
- Problems when anyone speaks from behind
- Child speaks loudly or too softly
- Exhibit voice problem and mispronunciation
- Tune the TV/Radio too loud
- Irrelevant answers
- The child keeps away from his age mates
- The child is unable to respond when you call from the other room
- The child understands only after few repetitions.

Note: If any of the above 3–4 questions elicits response that indicates some kind of hearing/speech loss, then the child should be carefully examined by a qualified ENT specialist, an audiologist, and also by a speech therapist for complete evaluation. In case the child is below 4–5 years, a psychologist should also be consulted to address and identify any associated psychological problems which may not be overtly evident.

Speech

- Inappropriate sound in speech
- Stammering
- Baby speech
- Inability to learn correct sound and use incorrect speech
- Incomprehensible speech.

Physical Disabilities

- Deformity in neck, hand, finger, waist, legs
- Difficulty in sitting, standing, walking
- Difficulty in lifting, holding, keeping things on floor
- Difficulty in moving or using any part of the body
- Difficulty in holding pen
- Using a stick to walk
- Jerks in walking
- Lack bodily coordination
- Epileptic behavior/have tremors
- Joint pains
- Any part of the body is amputated.

Note: If answer to any of the above written statements is positive, the child should be carefully examined by a qualified orthopedic surgeon and referred to a physiotherapist and/or prosthetic/orthotic technician as needed.

Mental Retardation

- If the child does not sit unassisted even much after 12–15 months
- Or starts to walkeven much after 2 ½ years
- Or starts to talk even much after 2 ½ years
- If a child has undue problems in doing independently any of the following:
  Activities by the age of 6 years:
  - Eating
  - Dressing or
  - Toilet activity
- Problems in holding a pencil/or using a scissors
- Unable to play with a ball; or play 'gilli-danda' with his peers
- Frequent tantrums, while playing with the peers
- Usual inattentiveness to the spoken speech or addressal
- Requires too many repetitions to remember simple things
- Problems in naming even 5 fruits, vegetables or plants
- Problems in naming the days of the week
- Exhibit problems in expressing the needs in a clear language unlike the other peers
- Unable to concentrate on tasks even for a short period of time
- Inappropriate oral responses
- Difficulty in performing daily routine work
- Poor comprehension of lessons taught in the school class
- Difficulty in learning new things
- Difficulty in conceptualization
- Does not get well along with the children of same age group
- More efforts are required in learning or practicing as compared to the peers
- Takes an unreasonable amount of time in perfecting any work
- Poor academic achievements
- Show an undue dependency on visual clues or material for learning.

Note: If the responses to any of the above 4 indicators is positive when compared to the average school going peers of same age group and class then the child should be properly assessed by a qualified psychologist or a teacher who is especially trained to take care of the mentally challenged children.

Learning Disabilities

- Difficulty in counting
- Lack of concentration or easily distraction by the surroundings, either at home or school
- Difficulty in sitting quietly in the classroom
- Does not write down the spoken words correctly
- In appropriate additions to the right word; e.g. 'ischool' in place of school
- Always confused between right and left
- Unreasonable difficulty in remembering the verbal instructions
- General difficulty in memorizing the things
- Extreme restlessness in a child which significantly interferes with the timely completion of various tasks
- Reverses letters or symbols too frequently while reading for example b as d, saw as was, etc.
- Reverses numbers too frequently while reading or writing for example 31 as 13, as 9, etc.
- Excessive errors during reading like loose place or repeat/insert/substitute/omit words
- Poor in mathematical calculations
- Problems in accurate copying from the common sources like a book or a blackboard, even though the vision is normal
- Write letters or words either too close or too far (spacing problems)
- The child appears to comprehend satisfactorily but is not able to answer the questions.

Note:

i. If the answer to any of the above 3–5 statements is positive, the child should be carefully examined by a qualified psychologist/pediatrician/or a special educator for initial screening and further consultations.

ii. One of the main characteristics children with learning disabilities is that their verbal skills are often much better than the writing skills. Therefore, they should be formally tested in order to elucidate their disability in detail.

ASSESMENT OF IMPAIRMENT

Impairment is assessed through a team of specialists in order to plan the necessary interventions. Each category of disability has been divided into four groups viz., mild, moderate, severe and profound; the latter can extend up to total deafness.

HEARING IMPAIRMENT CATEGORIES

Sl. No.	*Type of impairment*	*DB level and/or*	*Speech discrimination*	*Percentage of impairment*
1.	Mild	26 to 40 dB in better ear	80 to 100% in better ear	Less than 40%
2	Moderate	41 to 60 dB in better ear	50 to 80% in better ear	40 to 50%
3.	Severe	61 to 70 dB hearing impairment in better ear	40 to 50% in better ear	50 to 75%
4.	a. Total deafness b. Near total c. Profound	No hearing 91 dB and above in better ear 71 to 90 dB	No discrimination. Very poor discrimination Less than 40% in better ear	100% 100% 100% 71 to 100%

a. Pure tone average of hearing in 500, and 2000 HZ, 4000 Hz by conduction (AC and BC) should be taken as the basis for consideration as per test recommendations.
b. When there is only an island of hearing present in one or two frequencies in the better ear, it should be considered as total loss of hearing.
c. When there is no response (NR) at any of the 4 frequencies (500, 1000, 2000 and 4000 HZ) it should be considered as equivalent to 100 dB loss for the purpose of classification of disability and in arriving at the average.

Note: As per the latest guidelines for evaluation of disabilities (2001), definition of hearing disability is : 'A person with hearing impairment having difficulty of various degrees in sounds is an impaired person.'

- *Contact ENT specialist:* Available at block, district, state hospital for assessment
- *Assessment process:* Audiological assessment through battery of tests
- *Organizations for education:* Formal schools, open school, special school
- *Organizations for providing:* Field: Subhealth Center, Primary Health Center
- *Aids and appliances:* Gram Panchayat, Rehabilitation center if available

  NGOs working in the field of disability
- *Block:* Block Welfare Officer
- *District:* District Welfare Officer
  Students get aids and appliances in schools.

VISUAL IMPAIRMENT CATEGORIES

		Better eye	*Worse eye*	*Percentage impairment*
Category O Category I	Mild	6/9 to 6/18 6/18 to 6/36	6/24 to 6/36 6/60 to nil	20% 40%
Category II	Moderate	6/60 to 4/60 or Field of vision 10-20	3/60 to nil	75%
Category III	Severe	3/60 to 1/60 or Field of vision 10 degree	FC at 1 ft to nil	100%
Category IV or one eyed persons	Profound	FC at 1 ft to Nil Field of vision 10 6/6	FC at 1 ft to nil Field of vision 100 FC at 1 ft to nil	100% 30%

Low vision: Impairment of vision less than 6/18 to 6/60 with best correction in better eyes or impairment of field in any one of the following categories:

a. Reducation of fields less than 50 degrees
b. Hemianopia with macular involvement
c. Altitudinal defect involving lower fields.

IF THE CHILD IS BLIND OR HAS A LOW VISION, CONTACT

- *Ophthalmologist:* Available at block, district, state hospital for assessment, assessment can be done at eye camps, etc. also.
- *Organizations for education:* Formal schools, open school
  - Special school for blind children,
  - Non-governmental organizations working in the field of blindness.
- *Organizations for providing:* Field: Subhealth center, primary health center, *aids and appliances* Gram Panchayat, rehabilitation center if available,
  - NGOs working in the field of disability.
  - *Block:* Block Welfare Officer
  - *District:* District Welfare Officer
  - *Students:* in schools.

Note: Impairment of 20 to 40% or less may only be entitled to aids and appliances.

DEGREE OF MENTAL RETARDATION

Clinical classification	*Educational classification*	*IQ range*	*Adult mental age*	*Focus of training*	*Education achievement as adults*	*Level of adaptive behavior*
Profound	Life support	<20	<3.08 years	–	–	Dependant for self-care
Severe	Trainable	20–34	3:09–6 years	Self-care skills	Academic training not effective	Self-care under supervision
Moderate	Trainable	35–49	6:01 8:05 years	Self-care skills Practical skills - equivalent of IInd or	-equivalent of IInd or IIIrd grade children	Independent in self-care

Contd...

Contd...

Clinical classification	*Educational classification*	*IQ range*	*Adult mental age*	*Focus of training*	*Education achievement as adults*	*Level of adaptive behavior*
Mild	Educable	50–69	8:06 year 10: 10 years	Vocational training Personal social skills Functional education	IV–V grade level Cannot handle money without supervision	Independent in self-care - engage in semi-skilled or simple skilled jobs
Borderline	Slow learner	70–80	10–11 years 13:03 years	Academic skill Vocational training	Some pass 10th standard through open school	Achieve adequate social and vocational adjustment—capable of skilled and semi-skilled jobs

Source: Centers for Assessment of IQ
Child Guidance Clinics:
Clinical Psychologist/Psychiatrist/Paediatrician in Clinics/Hospitals
Note: All categories of mental retardation, i.e. mild/moderate/severe/profound are eligible for government benefits.

LEARNING DISABILITIES WHAT TO LOOK FOR: SOME FIRST SIGNS OF TROUBLE KEEPING UP WITH THE FLOW OF EXPECTATIONS

	Language	*Memory*	*Attention*	*Fine motor skill*	*Other functions*
Preschool	Pronunciation problems, slow vocabulary growth. Lack of interest in story telling	Trouble learning numbers, alphabet, days of week, etc. Poor memory for routines	Trouble sitting still. Extreme restlessness. Impersistence at tasks	Trouble learning self help skills (e.g. tying shoe laces). Clumsiness. Reluctance to draw or trace	Trouble learning left from right (Possible visual spatial confusion). Trouble interacting (Poor social skills)

Contd...

Contd...

	Language	*Memory*	*Attention*	*Fine motor skill*	*Other functions*
Lower grades	Delayed decoding abilities for reading. Trouble following directions. Poor spelling	Slow recall of facts. Organizational problems. Slow acquisition of new skills. Poor spelling	Impassivity, lack of planning, careless errors, Insatiability, distractibility	Unstable pencil grip. Trouble with letter formation	Trouble learning about time (Temporal sequential disorganization. Poor grasp of math concepts)
Middle grades	Poor reading comprehension. Lack of verbal participation in class. Trouble with word problems	Poor intelligible writing. Slow or poor recall of math facts. Failure of automatic recall	Inconsistency. Poor self-monitoring, Great knowledge of Trivia. Distaste for fine detail	First-like or tight pencil illegible, slow or inconsistent writing. Reluctance to write	Poor learning strategies. Disorganization in time or space, peer rejection
Upper grades	Weak grasp of explanations. Foreign language problems. Poor written expression. Trouble summarizing	Trouble studying for tests. Weak cumulative memory. Slow work place	Memory problems due to weak attention. Mental fatigue	(lessening relevance of fine motor skills)	Poor grasp of abstract concepts. Failure to elaborate. Trouble taking tests. Multiple choice (e.g. SAT's)

Note: These are guideposts for parents, teachers and other involved. They should not be used in isolation, but may lead you to seek further assessment. Many children will, from time-to-time, have difficulty with one or more of these items. They should always be reviewed in a broader content of understanding about a child.

CATEGORIES OF LOCOMOTOR DISABILITIES

- Permanent physical impairment of upper limb
- Permanent physical impairment of lower limb
- Permanent physical impairment of trunk (spine)
- Permanent physical impairment in case short stature/dwarfism
- Permanent physical impairment in amputees
- Longitudinal deficiencies
- Permanent physical impairment in neurological conditions
- Permanent physical impairment due to cardiopulmonary diseases
- The estimation of permanent impairment depends upon the measurement of functional impairment.
- *Impairment:* An impairment in any loss or abnormality of psychological, physiological or anatomical structure or function in a human being.
- *Functional limitations:* Impairment may cause functional limitations which are partial or total inability to perform these activities necessary for motor, sensory or mental function within the range or manner of which a human being is normally capable.

If the child has locomotor disability contact:

- *Orthopedic surgeon or specialist in physical medicine and rehabilitation:* Available at block, district, state hospital for assessment,
- *Organizations for education:* Formal schools, open school non-governmental organizations working in the field of locomotor disabilities.
- *Organizations for providing:* Field: Subhealth center, primary health center, aids and appliances Gram Panchayat, rehabilitation center if available, NGOs working in the field of disability.
- *Block:* Block Welfare Officer
- *District:* District Welfare Officer.

EDUCATION PROGRAMS FOR CHILDREN WITH SPECIAL NEEDS

The community at large is often unaware of the potential of children with special needs. In the popular mind, special needs are usually identified with very low expectations. Parent should believe in the value of educating children with special needs. The higher the expectations, the higher will be their acceptance in the family.

All the children with special needs must be enrolled in primary schools. After the assessment of their disabilities by a team of a doctor, a psychologist, and a special educator, in schools, the child will be placed in appropriate educational settings.

Children with mild and moderate disabilities of any kind may be integrated in normal schools, severe in special schools/remedial schools, dropouts who have problems in availing benefits of normal schools can join open schools. All the children with learning disabilities alone are first managed in the normal schools. Open and special schools also offer vocational courses also for children with disabilities.

Formal Schools

The Ministry of Human Resource Development (Department of Secondary and Higher Education) has been implementing a scheme of 'Integrated Education for the Disabled Children' (IEDC) in formal schools since 1982. The main objective of the scheme is to provide educational opportunities for the disabled children in normal schools so as to facilitate their retention in the school system. The disabled children who are placed in special schools should be considered for integration into common schools once they acquire the communication and daily living skills at a functional level.

The following types of children with disabilities must be integrated in the normal school system—formal as well as in non-formal schools.

- Children with locomotor handicaps (OH)
- Mildly and moderately hearing impaired
- Partially sighted children
- Mentally handicapped educable group (IQ 50–70)
- Children with multiple handicaps (blind and orthopedic, hearing impaired and orthopedic, educable mentally retarded and orthopedic, visual impaired and mild hearing impaired) A three-member assessment team comprising of a doctor, a psychologist and a special educator is formed and their assessment report recommends whether a child can be enrolled directly into a normal school or should receive preparation in a special school/ or a special preparatory class in Early Childhood Education Center (ECCE) specially equipped for this purpose. Under the IEDC scheme, resources and itinerant teachers are provided. Children are also given certain incentives like book allowance, equipment allowance, transport allowance, etc.

Integrated Education for Disabled Children (IEDC) in District Primary Education Program (DPEP)

The DPEP which was launched in 1994, aims at Universalization of Primary Education (UPE) and is operational in 271 districts in the country. Its aim cannot be achieved until and unless 10% of children with special needs are integrated in the education system. With this aim, since 1998, IEDC program has been receiving special emphasis under DPEP and endeavoring to integrate children with disabilities in DPEP primary schools. DPEP supports for the activities like community mobilization and early detection, in service teacher training, resource support, educational aids and appliances, architectural designs in schools, etc.

Children with learning disabilities also get special care in primary schools under DPEP. In the other non-DPEP districts, the same IEDC activities will be supported by the program of Sarva Shiksha Abhiyan (SSA) which has recently been approved. Earlier, there were no activities for children with learning disabilities under the program of IEDC. Estimates of prevalence rate of children with learning disabilities seem to be very high, ranging from 1–30% in the 'school population' depending on the criteria used to determine the disability. Some studies estimate the prevalence of learning disabilities to be 7–8% whereas others indicate a prevalence rate of 15% in the general population. Now under SSA and DPEP such children are being especially taken care of. Strategies of teaching such children have been developed.

Special Schools

This is a program of the Ministry of Social Justice and Empowerment. Children with severe multiple disabilities who have difficulty in coping with regular schools are referred to such special schools. Most of these special schools are located in urban areas and run by voluntary organizations. A majority of them are residential schools, and boarding-lodging and other services are provided free of cost. At present, more than 3000 special schools for the disabled children are functioning across the country. Out of them approximately 900 institutions are specialized for the hearing impaired, 400 for the visually impaired, 1000 for the mentally retarded and the remaining 700 are for the children with physical disabilities. About 40% disability of any such particular types is a benchmark for identification and certification for admission in these special schools.

National Open School (NOS)

The NOS was established as an Autonomous Registered Society in 1989 with the mission to provide education through an open learning system at the school stage as an alternative to the formal system. It is especially suited to the needs of certain categories such as school dropouts, girls, mentally or physically disabled, etc. It has also developed educational materials for teaching children with special needs in their own homes. At present, there are 1459 NOS study centers in the country. It offers courses like the foundation course, notionally equivalent to class VIII level, secondary education and higher secondary courses and vocational courses. The NOS also provides the program of Open Basic Education for Universal Elementary Education (UEE), which includes program for the disabled children. It offers Open Basic Education courses through the following:

a. *Open Basic Education (OBE):* This project is for out of school children in the age group 6–14 and also for adult learners. It has 3 levels: Preparatory, i.e. (A), Primary, i.e. (B) and elementary, i.e. (C), which are equivalent to a formal school standard of class III, V and VIII respectively.
b. *Special Accredited Institutions for Education of the Disadvantaged (SAIED):* To cater to the needs of the people with physical or mental disabilities the NOS has accredited institutions for education of the disadvantaged. Academic courses like open basic education (OBE), secondary and senior secondary courses and vocational courses are offered either independently or in combination with an academic subject(s) through SAIED.

SPECIAL FEATURES OF NOS

- It allows total freedom to learn at one's own speed. One gets a period of 5 years and 9 chances to complete the course
- Flexibility in choice of subjects
- There is no age limitation for admission in NOS programmers
- For admission, a person is required to submit the following supporting documents:
  - Attested copy of birth certificate, obtained in one of the following ways:

  - From the Admission Register of the last school attended or
  - Birth certificate from Registrar of Births and Death or
  - From a recognized Hospital or
  - Affidavit from parents countersigned by first class/ subdivision magistrate.
- Minimum education qualifications:
  - Self-certificate or certificate of class V/Matriculation/ Higher secondary pass.
- About 5% passport size (3 cm × 2 cm) photographs are also required
- Handicapped are exempted from payment of registration and cost of course material.
  - Candidates with disabilities are required to produce a certificate from a government hospital and not from a private nursing home.

TEACHING STRATEGIES FOR CHILDREN WITH LEARNING DISABILITIES

Children with learning disabilities show greater learning when techniques like task analysis, peer teaching, cooperative learning, learning corners and multisensory approach are used. The following strategies would be helpful to both the parents and teachers when trying to teach such children.

STRATEGIES FOR READING SKILLS

- Prepare the student by presenting new concepts and vocabulary
- Guide the student in to reading a story by asking questions which bring up the purpose or goal of the reading
- Develop or strengthen skills relating to the material through drills or worksheet activities
- Assign work in order to apply the skills acquired during a lesson
- Read aloud to students regularly
- Devote a few minutes every day to sustained silent reading
- Use writing activities that provide opportunities for the teacher to model writing strategies and skills
- Include journal writing as part of the student's individualized educational program

- Provide meaningful printed materials in the instructional setting (e.g. dictionaries, categorized lists of words)
- Establish a network of communication with other teachers, and thus using holistic techniques in working with such students
- Let the child read aloud (oral reading). If the child makes mistakes, they can be easily identified by the teacher and corrected
- Reading can be done with peers or with parents (paired reading). This will enhance the confidence of the child
- Reading in a group (choral reading). Here they get both auditory and visual stimulus to correct themselves
- Use color-coded textbooks (e.g. green equals start, red equals stop)
- Have a small group of class read aloud simultaneously.

STRATEGIES FOR WRITING SKILLS

- A sufficient amount of time should be allocated for writing. (e.g. four times per week) because students can learn and develop as writer only by writing
- Expose students to a broad range of writing tasks. Students should participate in writing activities that present highly structured problem-solving situations as well as activities that involve self-selected and expressive writing
- Create a social climate conducive to writing development. Teachers need to be encouraging in as non-threatening environment and should try to develop a sense of community by promoting student sharing and collaboration
- Integrate writing with subjects such as language and arts so as to stimulate the writing skills
- Help students develop the processes central to effective writing. The composition process of writing can be divided into a series of discrete stages (e.g. prewrite, write and rewrite), and students can be taught appropriate task-specific and metacognitive strategies (e.g. self-instructional strategy training)
- Help students develop explicit knowledge about the characteristics of good writing. Students should be given exposure to the characteristics of various literary compositions either through reading or teacher presentation of writing or live models that incorporate a specific skill or style
- Help students develop the skills and abilities to carry out more sophisticated composing processes

- Assist students in the development of goals for improving their written products
- Goal setting and having students evaluate their own writing according to specific criteria can help students accurately monitor and evaluate progress
- Tape alphabets forms to the floor. Have students walk or hop around the form.

Have them reproduce the form with colored yarn.

- Have students use a stick (broom handle) and their bodies to form the letters
- Spray shaving cream can be used to form large letters. Paper provides a suitable surface
- Have students use a torch light beam to trace letters on a chalkboard
- Have students form letters in wet fingerprint/paint/sand
- Use colored directional cues such as green arrows and red dots
- Help students to form an association for a letter they have difficulty remembering
- Have students orally describe their movements as the letter is being written. This provides auditory reinforcement.

STRATEGIES FOR MATHEMATICS

- Use manipulatives such as buttons and beads. Let the students drop beads into a clear plastic cup and count while seeing how many beads represent the number. The child also gets auditory input to support this concept
- Use visuals. Materials for younger students usually have a generous display of visual illustrations. Materials for older pupils tend to rely more on abstract presentations. A teacher may need to supplement teaching by drawing and constructing visual representations
- Try providing verbal reinforcement with visual material. Describing the computation process while working problems alongwith clapping activities are other examples of verbal reinforcement
- Try using tactile presentations. These can be materials such as sandpaper number or paper strips of various lengths used to demonstrate concepts such as more or less. Another type of tactile presentation is to trace a number or problem on the back of the student's hand

- Use color cues. Colored chalk and marking pens can be used to indicate these steps and direction of the process. Highlighters can be used to call attention to process signs (+, ×) and clue words ("more than", "times")
- Provide a sample problem for each assignment. The referent problem can be particularly helpful for students with memory difficulties
- Relate class activities to increase temporal awareness to time. Using phrases such as 'in five minutes' "earlier today" and "yesterday" will provide some basis for understanding time. Calendar work is useful, particularly in regard to special events and holidays
- Reduce the number of examples in the assignment. Some work pages are overwhelming to the pupil because of the sheer numbers of examples. They may also lose their place because of figure-ground deficits. These pupils are also slower in their rate of production
- Use display charts
- Play tallying games. Develop word problems based on game scores
- Have students use playing cards to develop games that require arithmetic computation
- Apply measurement in the classroom. Chart the growth of class members (a long-term project for certain ages), the growth of plants, and other measurements. Have students estimate distances, weights and possible answers
- Have students use an abacus to facilitate their calculations
- Reinforce high rates of correct responses
- Set a rate goal
- Chart performances and terminate daily practice once the goal is achieved
- Tell students to work faster
- Challenge students to beat their last rate score
- Teach students to use rules. (e.g. any number times 2 is double that number)
- Drill difficult problems with flash cards
- Play instructional math games
- Teach students the relationship between addition and subtraction or multiplication and division when they are learning the respective facts
- Use color-coded textbooks (e.g. green equals start, red equals stop)
- Use concrete manipulations

- Use meaningful examples and materials
- Have students use graph paper to help organize numbers and columns on mathematical assignments
- Teach key vocabulary in mathematics.

STRATEGIES FOR ATTENTION DEFICIT AND HYPERACTIVE DISORDER

- Reward the student for being prepared by allowing him/her to participate in favorite activities, conferring classroom privileges (like making the child monitor of the class)
- Establish routines for placing objects—especially routinely used objects such as books or assignments
- Point out to the salient features of the assignments (topic sentences, headings or table of contents)
- Provide the student with a list of materials needed for each task. Limit the list to only those materials necessary to complete the task
- Enhance the clarity of instructions. Repeat as often in a clear, clam tone.

Shorten the task by breaking one task into smaller parts to be completed

- Make tasks more interesting
- Increase the novelty of the task by using a game format
- Use high interest curriculum materials.

GENERAL INTERVENTIONS

- Show, demonstrate and model
- Utilize multisensory learning
- Break information down into smaller units
- Utilize peer tutoring and cooperative learning
- Use a developmentally appropriate approach
- Make information as concrete as possible
- Provide a small group of instructions
- Read test materials to the student
- Find out how the student learns best, and utilize this learning channel
- Provide opportunity for continuous success
- Use consistent vocabulary when teaching a new skill
- All students should be encouraged and given time to work collaboratively and

- Solve problems up to whatever levels they can attain
- Give students a chance to share and justify their thinking in different ways
- Make greater use of problem driven tasks and open-ended questions
- Increase expectations for student's reasoning, and encourage multiple solution strategies
- Lay greater emphasis on inter student dialogue and collaboration
- Make less use of teacher directed instruction.

ROLE OF THE PARENTS

No one is prepared to be the parent of a handicapped child. The parent(s) primarily learn about their child through an experience of family living, and the professionals working with these parents must focus on their experiences which are unique in every individual case. Although, parents may share common problems and reactions; the combinations of possible reactions, the intensity of the reactions, and the duration of the reactions are some factors that necessitate that each family be considered individually.

Parental adjustment may consist of any or all the following stages:

- Awareness of the problem
- Recognition of the problem
- Search for a cause
- Search for a cure, and
- Acceptance of the child.

The parents should bear the following in mind:

- Foster feelings of self-esteem in your child
- Do not compare the performance of their child with other siblings
- All children have strengths and competencies, and these strengths must be identified and reinforced
- Parents who convey hope provide a major force in helping children overcome adversity and become resilient
- Parents can help children develop a sense of responsibility and contribution to their family, and the ward in general
- Parents can provide opportunities for their child to make choices and decisions, and promote self-discipline
- Parents can help the children deal effectively with their mistakes and failures
- If possible, parents should attend training programmers along with the community.

CHAPTER

20

Developmental Disorders

INTRODUCTION

Developmental disabilities are a group of conditions due to an impairment in physical, learning, language, or behavior areas. These conditions begin during the developmental period, may impact day-to-day functioning, and usually last throughout a person's lifetime.

DEVELOPMENTAL MILESTONES

Skills such as taking a first step, smiling for the first time, and waving "bye-bye" are called developmental milestones. Children reach milestones in how they play, learn, speak, behave, and move (for example, crawling and walking).

Children develop at their own pace, so it is impossible to tell exactly when a child will learn a given skill. However, the developmental milestones give a general idea of the changes to expect as a child gets older.

As a parent, you know your child best. If your child is not meeting the milestones for his/her age, or if you think there could be a problem with your child's development, talk with your child's doctor or health care provider and share your concerns. Do not wait.

DEVELOPMENTAL MONITORING AND SCREENING

Developmental Monitoring

Your child's growth and development are kept track of through a partnership between you and your health professional. At each well-child visit the doctor looks for developmental delays or problems and talks with you about any concerns you might have. This is called developmental monitoring (or surveillance). Any problems noticed during developmental monitoring should be followed-up with developmental screening.

Children with special health care needs should have developmental monitoring and screening just like those without special needs. Monitoring healthy development means paying attention not only to symptoms related to the child's condition, but also to the child's physical, mental, social, and emotional well-being.

Developmental Screening

Well-child visits allow doctors and nurses to have regular contact with children to keep track of—or monitor— your child's health and development through periodic developmental screening. Developmental screening is a short test to tell if a child is learning basic skills when he/she should, or if there are delays. Developmental screening can also be done by other professionals in health care, community, or school settings.

The doctor might ask you some questions or talk and play with the child during an examination to see how he/she plays, learns, speaks, behaves, and moves. A delay in any of these areas could be a sign of a problem.

The American Academy of Pediatrics recommends that all children be screened for developmental delays and disabilities during regular well-child doctor visits at:

- 9 months
- 18 months
- 24 or 30 months.

Additional screening might be needed if a child is at high-risk for developmental problems due to preterm birth, low birth weight, or other reasons.

If your child's doctor does not routinely check your child with this type of developmental screening test, you can ask that it be done.

IMPORTANCE OF DEVELOPMENTAL SCREENING

Many children with developmental delays are not being identified as early as possible. As a result, these children must wait to get the help they need to do well in social and educational settings (for example, in school).

In the United States, about 13% of children 3 to 17 years of age have a developmental or behavioral disability such as autism, intellectual disability (also known as mental retardation), and attention-deficit/hyperactivity disorder. In addition, many children have delays in language or other areas that can affect school readiness. However, fewer than half of children with developmental delays are identified before starting school, by which time significant delays already might have occurred and opportunities for treatment might have been missed.

EARLY INTERVENTION SERVICES

Research shows that early intervention treatment services can greatly improve a child's development. Early intervention services help children from birth through 3 years of age (36 months) learn important skills. Services include therapy to help the child talk, walk, and interact with others.

The Individuals with Disabilities Education Act (IDEA) says that children younger than 3 years of age (36 months) who are at risk of having developmental delays might be eligible for early intervention treatment services even if the child has not received a formal diagnosis. These services are provided through an early intervention system in each state.

In addition, treatment for particular symptoms, such as speech therapy for language delays, often does not require a formal diagnosis. Although early intervention is extremely important, intervention at any age can be helpful.

IMPORTANT MILESTONES: YOUR BABY AT TWO MONTHS

Milestone Checklist

How your child plays, learns, speaks, and acts offers important clues about your child's development. Developmental milestones are things most children can do by a certain age.

Check the milestones your child has reached by the end of 2 months.

Take this with you and talk with your child's doctor at every visit about the milestones your child has reached and what to expect next.

What most babies do at this age:

- Social and Emotional
  - Begins to smile at people
  - Can briefly calm himself (may bring hands to mouth and suck on hand)
  - Tries to look at parent
- Language/Communication
  - Coos, makes gurgling sounds
  - Turns head toward sounds.

Cognitive (Learning, Thinking, Problem-solving)

- Pays attention to faces
- Begins to follow things with eyes and recognize people at a distance
- Begins to act bored (cries, fussy) if activity does not change.

Movement/Physical Development

- Can hold head up and begins to push up when lying on tummy
- Makes smoother movements with arms and legs.

Act early by talking to your child's doctor if your child:

- Does not respond to loud sounds
- Does not watch things as they move
- Does not smile at people
- Does not bring hands to mouth
- Cannot hold head up when pushing up when on tummy.

  The American Academy of Pediatrics recommends that children be screened for general development using standardized, validated tools at 9, 18, and 24 or 30 months and for autism at 18 and 24 months or whenever a parent or provider has a concern. Ask your child's doctor about your child's developmental screening.

IMPORTANT MILESTONES: YOUR BABY AT FOUR MONTH

Milestone Checklist

How your child plays, learns, speaks, and acts offers important clues about your child's development. Developmental milestones are things most children can do by a certain age.

Check the milestones your child has reached by the end of 4 months.

Take this with you and talk with your child's doctor at every visit about the milestones your child has reached and what to expect next.

What most babies do at this age:

- Social and emotional
  - Smiles spontaneously, especially at people
  - Likes to play with people and might cry when playing stops
  - Copies some movements and facial expressions, like smiling or frowning
- Language/Communication
  - Begins to babble
  - Babbles with expression and copies sounds he hears
  - Cries in different ways to show hunger, pain, or being tired.

Cognitive (Learning, Thinking, Problem-solving)

- Lets you know if she is happy or sad
- Responds to affection
- Reaches for toy with one hand
- Uses hands and eyes together, such as seeing a toy and reaching for it
- Follows moving things with eyes from side-to-side
- Watches faces closely
- Recognizes familiar people and things at a distance.

Movement/Physical Development

- Holds head steady, unsupported
- Pushes down on legs when feet are on a hard surface
- May be able to roll over from tummy to back

- Can hold a toy and shake it and swing at dangling toys
- Brings hands to mouth
- When lying on stomach, pushes up to elbows.

Act early by talking to your child's doctor if your child:
- Does not watch things as they move
- Does not smile at people
- Cannot hold head steady
- Does not coo or make sounds
- Does not bring things to mouth
- Does not push down with legs when feet are placed on a hard surface
- Has trouble moving one or both eyes in all directions.

IMPORTANT MILESTONES: YOUR BABY AT SIX MONTHS

Milestone Checklist

How your child plays, learns, speaks, and acts offers important clues about your child's development. Developmental milestones are things most children can do by a certain age.

Check the milestones your child has reached by the end of 6 months. Take this with you and talk with your child's doctor at every visit about the milestones your child has reached and what to expect next.

What most babies do at this age:
- Social and emotional
  - Knows familiar faces and begins to know if someone is a stranger
  - Likes to play with others, especially parents
  - Responds to other people's emotions and often seems happy
  - Likes to look at self in a mirror
- Language/Communication
  - Responds to sounds by making sounds
  - Strings vowels together when babbling ("ah," "eh," "oh") and likes taking turns with parent while making sounds
  - Responds to own name
  - Makes sounds to show joy and displeasure
  - Begins to say consonant sounds (jabbering with "m," "b")

Cognitive (Learning, Thinking, Problem-solving)

- Looks around at things nearby
- Brings things to mouth
- Shows curiosity about things and tries to get things that are out of reach
- Begins to pass things from one hand to the other.

Movement/Physical Development

- Rolls over in both directions (front to back, back to front)
- Begins to sit without support
- When standing, supports weight on legs and might bounce
- Rocks back and forth, sometimes crawling backward before moving forward.

Act early by talking to your child's doctor if your child:

- Does not try to get things that are in reach
- Shows no affection for caregivers
- Does not respond to sounds around him
- Has difficulty getting things to mouth
- Does not make vowel sounds ("ah", "eh", "oh")
- Does not roll over in either direction
- Does not laugh or make squealing sounds
- Seems very stiff, with tight muscles
- Seems very floppy, like a rag doll
- What most babies do at this age?
- Social and emotional
- May be afraid of strangers
- May be clingy with familiar adults
- Has favorite toys.

Language/Communication

- Understands "no"
- Makes a lot of different sounds like "mama mama" and "bababababa"
- Copies sounds and gestures of others
- Uses fingers to point at things.

Cognitive (Learning, Thinking, Problem-solving)

- Watches the path of something as it falls
- Looks for things he/she sees you hide
- Plays peek-a-boo
- Puts things in her mouth
- Moves things smoothly from one hand to the other
- Picks up things like cereal o's between thumb and index finger.

Movement/Physical Development

- Stands, holding on
- Can get into sitting position
- Sits without support
- Pulls to stand
- Crawls.

Act early by talking to your child's doctor if your child:

- Does not bear weight on legs with support
- Does not sit with help
- Does not babble ("mama", "baba", "dada")
- Does not play any games involving back-and-forth play
- Does not respond to own name
- Does not seem to recognize familiar people
- Does not look where you point
- Does not transfer toys from one hand to the other.

IMPORTANT MILESTONES: YOUR CHILD AT ONE YEAR

Milestone Checklist

How your child plays, learns, speaks, and acts offers important clues about your child's development? Developmental milestones are things most children can do by a certain age.

Check the milestones your child has reached by his/her first birthday. Take this with you and talk with your child's doctor at every visit about the milestones your child has reached and what to expect next.

What most children do at this age:

- Social and emotional
  - Is shy or nervous with strangers?
  - Cries when mom or dad leaves?

  - Has favorite things and people?
  - Shows fear in some situations?
  - Hands you a book when he wants to hear a story
  - Repeats sounds or actions to get attention
  - Puts out arm or leg to help with dressing
  - Plays games such as "peek-a-boo" and "pat-a-cake".
- Language/Communication
  - Responds to simple spoken requests
  - Uses simple gestures, like shaking head "no" or waving "bye-bye"
  - Makes sounds with changes in tone (sounds more like speech)
  - Says "mama" and "dada" and exclamations like "uh-oh!"
  - Tries to say words you say.

Cognitive (Learning, Thinking, Problem-solving)

- Explores things in different ways, like shaking, banging, throwing
- Finds hidden things easily
- Looks at the right picture or thing when it's named
- Copies gestures
- Starts to use things correctly; for example, drinks from a cup, brushes hair
- Bangs two things together
- Puts things in a container, takes things out of a container
- Lets things go without help
- Pokes with index (pointer) finger
- Follows simple directions like "pick up the toy".

Movement/Physical Development

- Gets to a sitting position without help
- Pulls up to stand, walks holding on to furniture ("cruising")
- May take a few steps without holding on
- May stand alone.

Act early by talking to your child's doctor if your child:

- Doesn't crawl
- Can't stand when supported
- Doesn't search for things that she sees you hide
- Doesn't say single words like "mama" or "dada"
- Doesn't learn gestures like waving or shaking head.

IMPORTANT MILESTONES: YOUR CHILD AT EIGHTEEN MONTHS

Milestone Checklist

How your child plays, learns, speaks, and acts offers important clues about your child's development. Developmental milestones are things most children can do by a certain age.

Check the milestones your child has reached by the end of 18 months. Take this with you and talk with your child's doctor at every visit about the milestones your child has reached and what to expect next.

What most babies do at this age:

- Social and emotional
  - Likes to hand things to others as play
  - May have temper tantrums
  - May be afraid of strangers
  - Shows affection to familiar people
  - Plays simple pretend, such as feeding a doll
  - May cling to caregivers in new situations
  - Points to show others something interesting
  - Explores alone but with parent close by.
- Language/Communication
  - Says several single words
  - Says and shakes head "no"
  - Points to show someone what he wants.

Cognitive (Learning, Thinking, Problem-solving)

- Knows what ordinary things are for; for example, telephone, brush, spoon
- Points to get the attention of others
- Shows interest in a doll or stuffed animal by pretending to feed
- Points to one body part
- Scribbles on his own
- Can follow one-step verbal commands without any gestures; for example, sits when you say "sit down"

Movement/Physical Development

- Walks alone
- May walk up steps and run
- Pulls toys while walking
- Can help undress herself
- Drinks from a cup
- Eats with a spoon.

Act early by talking to your child's doctor if your child:

- Does not point to show things to others
- Cannot walk
- Does not know what familiar things are for
- Does not copy others
- Does not gain new words
- Does not have at least 6 words
- Does not notice or mind when a caregiver leaves or returns
- Loses skills he once had.

IMPORTANT MILESTONES: YOUR CHILD AT THREE YEARS

Milestone Checklist

How your child plays, learns, speaks, and acts offers important clues about your child's development. Developmental milestones are things most children can do by a certain age.

Check the milestones your child has reached by his or her third birthday. Take this with you and talk with your child's doctor at every visit about the milestones your child has reached and what to expect next.

What most babies do at this age:

- Social and emotional
  - Copies adults and friends
  - Shows affection for friends without prompting
  - Takes turns in games
  - Shows concern for crying friend
  - Understands the idea of "mine" and "his" or "hers"
  - Shows a wide range of emotions

  - Separates easily from mom and dad
  - May get upset with major changes in routine
  - Dresses and undresses self.
- Language/Communication
  - Follows instructions with 2 or 3 steps
  - Can name most familiar things
  - Understands words like "in," "on," and "under"
  - Says first name, age, and sex
  - Names a friend
  - Says words like "I," "me," "we," and "you" and some plurals (cars, dogs, cats)
  - Talks well enough for strangers to understand most of the time
  - Carries on a conversation using 2 to 3 sentences.

Cognitive (learning, Thinking, Problem-solving)

- Can work toys with buttons, levers, and moving parts
- Plays make-believe with dolls, animals, and people
- Does puzzles with 3 or 4 pieces
- Understands what "two" means
- Copies a circle with pencil or crayon
- Turns book pages one at a time
- Builds towers of more than 6 blocks
- Screws and unscrews jar lids or turns door handle.

Movement/Physical Development

- Climbs well
- Runs easily
- Pedals a tricycle (3-wheel bike)
- Walks up and downstairs, one foot on each step.

Act early by talking to your child's doctor if your child:

- Falls down a lot or has trouble with stairs
- Drools or has very unclear speech
- Cannot work simple toys (such as peg boards, simple puzzles, turning handle)
- Does not speak in sentences
- Does not understand simple instructions.

- Does not play pretend or make-believe
- Does not want to play with other children or with toys
- Does not make eye contact
- Loses skills he once had
- How your child plays, learns, speaks, and acts offers important clues about your child's development. Developmental milestones are things most children can do by a certain age.
- Check the milestones your child has reached by his or her second birthday. Take this with you and talk with your child's doctor at every visit about the milestones your child has reached and what to expect next.

What most babies do at this age:

- Social and emotional
  - Copies others, especially adults and older children
  - Gets excited when with other children
  - Shows more and more independence
  - Shows defiant behavior (doing what he has been told not to)
  - Plays mainly beside other children, but is beginning to include other children, such as in chase games.
- Language/Communication
  - Points to things or pictures when they are named
  - Knows names of familiar people and body parts
  - Says sentences with 2 to 4 words
  - Follows simple instructions
  - Repeats words overheard in conversation
  - Points to things in a book.

Cognitive (Learning, Thinking, Problem-solving)

- Finds things even when hidden under two or three covers
- Begins to sort shapes and colors
- Completes sentences and rhymes in familiar books
- Plays simple make-believe games
- Builds towers of 4 or more blocks
- Might use one hand more than the other
- Follows two-step instructions such as "Pick up your shoes and put them in the closet"
- Names items in a picture book such as a cat, bird, or dog.

Movement/Physical Development

- Stands on tiptoe
- Kicks a ball
- Begins to run
- Climbs onto and down from furniture without help
- Walks up and downstairs holding on
- Throws ball overhand
- Makes or copies straight lines and circles.

Act early by talking to your child's doctor if your child:

- Does not use 2-word phrases (for example, "drink milk")
- Does not know what to do with common things, like a brush, phone, fork, spoon
- Does not copy actions and words
- Does not follow simple instructions
- Does not walk steadily
- Loses skills he/she once had.

IMPORTANT MILESTONES: YOUR CHILD AT FOUR YEARS

Milestone Checklist

How your child plays, learns, speaks, and acts offers important clues about your child's development. Developmental milestones are things most children can do by a certain age.

Check the milestones your child has reached by his or her fourth birthday. Take this with you and talk with your child's doctor at every visit about the milestones your child has reached and what to expect next.

What most babies do at this age:

- Social and emotional
  - Enjoys doing new things
  - Plays "Mom" and "Dad"
  - Is more and more creative with make-believe play
  - Would rather play with other children than by himself
  - Cooperates with other children
  - Often cannot tell what's real and what's make-believe
  - Talks about what she likes and what she is interested in.
- Language/Communication
  - Knows some basic rules of grammar, such as correctly using "he" and "she"

- Sings a song or says a poem from memory such as the "Itsy Bitsy Spider" or the "Wheels on the Bus"
- Tells stories
- Can say first and last name.

Cognitive (Learning, Thinking, Problem-solving)

- Names some colors and some numbers
- Understands the idea of counting
- Starts to understand time
- Remembers parts of a story
- Understands the idea of "same" and "different"
- Draws a person with 2 to 4 body parts
- Uses scissors
- Starts to copy some capital letters
- Plays board or card games
- Tells you what he thinks is going to happen next in a book.

Movement/Physical Development

- Hops and stands on one foot up to 2 seconds
- Catches a bounced ball most of the time
- Pours, cuts with supervision, and mashes own food.

Act early by talking to your child's doctor if your child:

- Cannot jump in place
- Has trouble scribbling
- Shows no interest in interactive games or make-believe
- Ignores other children or doesn't respond to people outside the family
- Resists dressing, sleeping, and using the toilet
- Cannot retell a favorite story
- Does not follow 3-part commands
- Does not understand "same" and "different"
- Does not use "me" and "you" correctly
- Speaks unclearly
- Loses skills he once had.

UNDER FIVE CLINICS

Under five clinic is center, where preventive, promotive, curative, referral and educational, services are provided in a package manner to under

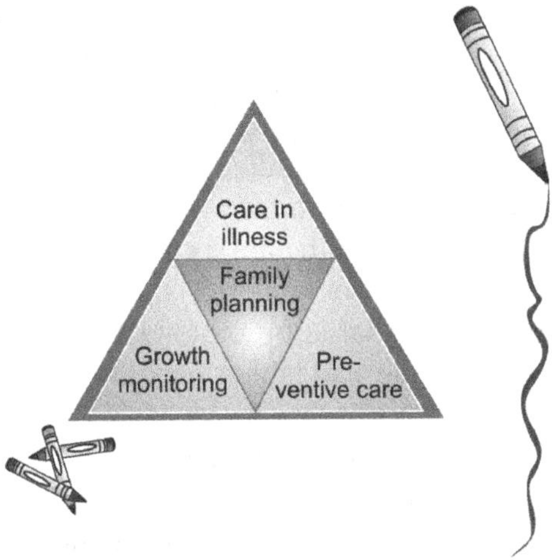

Fig. 20.1: Symbol of under-five clinic

five children under one roof. The services are made available through trained nurses, so that not only the services become economical but also available to larger population of children population in the community. Since, the services are provided by anon medical person, it constitute an example of primary health center. The sub center, The PHC function as under five clinics one afternoon every week. The pediatric outpatient department in the hospitals function as under five clinic every day. In recent time "well baby clinics" are giving way to concept of the under-five clinics.

Importance

The services are concentrated to under five clinics because of the following reasons:

- They constitute nearly 15% of total population
- They are nutritionally vulnerable
- They constitute human resource of country in future
- They are responsible for the progress of the country.

AIMS

The aim of the clinic is to provide comprehensive health care to under-fives through non-medical person, in an economical way.

Functions of Under Five Clinics

1. Registration of all infants and toddlers and preparation of a specific card.
2. Medical check-up on scheduled visit, at least on by medical officer and on other occasions by the MCH staff.
3. Regular recording of health data such as height, weight to verify normal growth and development.
4. Distribution of natural supplements (supplementary food, vitamin and iron folic acid tablets or solution).
5. Routine immunization.
6. Reporting of all registered children to health assistant so that he may check and update his vital statistic records.
7. Early detection of any communicable and non-communicable disease or congenital defect.
8. Prompt treatment of disease and defect.
9. Referral to specialist.
10. Training to mothers regarding child feeding and other aspects of mother craft.
11. Advice about family planning.
12. Health education by arranging health exhibitions and well body competitions.

Other Welfare Services Required for Children

Crèches (Day Care Centers)

They are compulsory for factories under Factories Act 1948, if more than 50 woman are employed. It is worthwhile having such crèches or nurseries in towns and big Gram Panchayats. A woman worker, qualified as a health visitor, nurse, midwife or public health nurse is required to look after the children. A doctor should be available on call.

Care for the Handicapped

- For the mentally handicapped, there should be child guidance clinics, as also schools, and home for the mentally retarded
- For the physically handicapped children, such as the deaf, dumb, blind, spastic and paralyzed, there are special institutions, such as the All India Institute of Physical Medicine and Rehabilitation, Mumbai, Spastics Society of India, Mumbai and Delhi, Occupational Therapy School, Nagpur, etc. the Ali Yavar Jung National Institute for the hearing handicapped.

CHAPTER

21

Important Definitions in Community-based Rehabilitation

CAPACITY

The ability, power or strength of a community or an organization.

Capacity Building; Capacity Development

Increasing the "capacity" (ability) of a community or an organization. Capacity building, also referred to as capacity development, is a conceptual approach to social or personal development that focuses on understanding the obstacles that inhibit people, governments, international organizations and non-governmental organizations from realizing their development goals.

CATALYST

In chemistry, a catalyst is a chemical that affects the rate of a chemical process, without becoming part of that process. It usually speeds up the process. The word, therefore, is a good one to describe a mobilizer or social animator. The mobilizer does not develop or change a community.

The community develops or changes itself. The mobilizer stimulates that change, without becoming part of the social organization of the community. Most importantly, the mobilizer provides temporary leadership, without becoming a community leader.

CELEBRATION

A celebration is a happy recognition of an event, usually one that changes the status of a person or thing. A celebration is a public party. For a mobilizer, celebration of completion of a community project is an important element of community empowerment, where the community is publicly recognized for successfully engaging in self-help. It is also an opportunity to start a new beginning, another mobilization cycle.

CHARITY

The helping of poor or needy people is a universal value, and found in all the major world religions. But there is giving and giving. If your gift makes the receiver dependent upon you, then you are not helping to strengthen the receiver, or helping him or her become more self-reliant.

When you give some coins to a beggar on the street, then you are training that person to be more of a beggar. If your assistance is well-thought out, and helps to strengthen the receiver then it is a much more useful gift.

CITY

A human settlement (habitat) that is characterized by (1) a large population, (2) population density and (3) social complexity (e.g. division of labor, heterogeneity).

There are no universally agreed measurements for these three variables, so hamlets and villages lay near one end of the spectrum and cities and mega-cities lay near the other end, with towns and semi-urban settlements in between. These three variables affect methods of community strengthening.

CIVIC ENGAGEMENT

For some mobilizers, the authorities are seen as the "enemy" or "opposition" and see their task as organizing the poor communities to oppose those "oppressors."

That may be an appropriate approach in some situations, and is often seen as "civic engagement" rather than as "community participation".

The methodology in these modules (developed mainly in Africa) sees the bringing of those authorities on side is more likely to lead to sustainability and a consistent national policy and program of poverty elimination.

COMMON VALUES

Common values belong to one of the sixteen elements of strength, power or capacity of a community or organization. These are the degree to which members of the community share values, especially the idea that they belong to a common entity that supersedes the interest of members within it.

The more that community member share, or at least understand and tolerate, each other's values and attitudes, the stronger their community will be. (Racism, prejudice and bigotry weaken a community or organization). When simulating a community to organize and act, the mobilizer needs to be aware of the role of common values in empowering that community or organization.

COMMUNAL FACILITIES AND SERVICES

In a human settlement, some facilities are owned by individuals or families, usually housing. Other facilities, like roads, water supply or schools, are owned by the group as a whole. These are communal.

Communal services and facilities are one of the sixteen elements of strength, power or capacity of a community or organization. Human settlements facilities and services (such as roads, markets, potable water, access to education, health services), their upkeep (dependable maintenance and repair), sustainability, and the degree to which all community members have access to them.

The more members have access to needed communal facilities, the greater their empowerment. (In measuring capacity of organizations, this includes office equipment, tools, supplies, access to toilets and other personal staff facilities, working facilities, physical plant). When simulating a community to organize and act, the mobilizer needs to be aware of the role of communal services and facilities in empowering that community or organization.

COMMUNICATION

Communication is one of the sixteen elements of strength, power or capacity of a community or organization. Within a community, and between itself and outside, communication includes roads, electronic methods (e.g. telephone, radio, TV, Internet), printed media (newspapers, magazines, books), networks, mutually understandable languages, literacy and the willingness and ability to communicate (which implies tact, diplomacy, willingness to listen as well as to talk) in general.

As a community gets better communication, it gets stronger. (For an organization, this is the communication equipment, methods and practices available to staff). Poor communication means a weak organization or community. When simulating a community to organize and act, the mobilizer needs to be aware of the role of communication in empowering that community or organization.

COMMUNITY

The word "community" has been used in several different contexts. Biologists talk of community as meaning several individuals in a single species, or several different species, living, competing, cooperating, to make a larger whole.

Since, the advent of the Internet and information technology, various collections of persons, often those sharing a single interest have grown-up, without geographical boundaries, and who communicate electronically.

The focus on this website in this training series, is on a more orthodox meaning of community, a community of living human beings, one which usually has geographic boundaries (except those may be stretched, as in nomadic communities), associated, for example in communities that range from local neighborhoods in large urban areas, to remote rural villages.

A community is not just a collection of individual human beings. It is a super-organism that belongs to and is part of culture, composed of interactions between people, everything that is learned. Its six dimensions include technology, economy, political power, social patterns, shared values, beliefs and ideas. It is not transmitted by biological means, but by learning. Like a tree or other life form that transcends the very atoms, which compose it, its human members can come of go, through death, birth or migration, and it still continues to live and grow. It is never homogeneous, having many factions, schisms, competition and conflicts within it. A community is a whole that is greater than the sum of its parts.

COMMUNITY-BASED

For a project or organization to be community based, it must originate in a community, must have community members responsible, and have its decisions (policy and executive) made by community members.

An outside agency or project that is merely located in a community cannot rightly claim to be community based. Also, consulting with community leaders does not make it community-based.

There is a big difference between community-based and community-located. If an agency sets up a service in a community (e.g. a clinic, an IG program), then that is community-located. To be called community-based correctly, an activity, construction, service, or organization, must be chosen, selected and controlled by the community as a whole (not just some factions). The important thing is for decision-making to be community-based; the decisions must be made inside and by the community.

COMMUNITY-BASED ORGANIZATION

A community-based organization (CBO) is an organization that has been formed and developed within a community, where the decision-making (management and planning) is from the community as a whole. An agency that is formed from outside, and has decisions made for it from outside, may be community located, but is not community-based.

COMMUNITY-BASED REHABILITATION

Rehabilitation in this context means physical (biological), emotional or mental rehabilitation (or habilitation) of persons who are disabled by some physical, emotional or mental incapacity. Where rehabilitation is community-based, then the decision-making and responsibility for the habilitation of those disabled individuals are in the community, and do not originate outside the community.

COMMUNITY CONTRIBUTION

When we point out that community participation is not the same thing as community contribution (though many mistakenly assume it is), we also note that both are necessary. While community participation means the decision-making that makes any activity community-based or community centered, community contribution is necessary to ensure that the community members feel that they own the project, i.e. that they have invested in it, not just received it.

We recommend that at least 50% of the inputs of any community project that we support must come from the community itself. At first this is often viewed with anxiety and despair from many community members. Then we point out that the donated communal labor alone has to be fairly calculated, and that if they did so, they would be pleasantly surprised at how much value that would add to the community input.

We point out that the time spent by community members, especially those that sit on the executive committee, deciding and planning the project, are donations of executive and management skills, time and labor. The donated labour should be fairly accounted. Furthermore, we point out that the value of donations of sand and dirt, too, are often underestimated, and should be recognized, with fair cost estimates, as community inputs.

COMMUNITY DEVELOPMENT

When a community develops, it grows. It does not necessarily mean getting bigger or getting richer. It means getting more complex and stronger. A community does not get developed by a mobilizer and more than a flower grows taller by someone pulling it up. A community (as a social institution) develops itself. A mobilizer can only stimulate, encourage and guide members of the community.

Some people assume that community development simply means getting richer—an increase in per capita wealth or income. It can be, but is more. It is social change, where a community becomes more complex, adding institutions, increasing its collective power, changing qualitatively in its organization. Development means growing in complexity and strength in all six dimensions of culture.

COMMUNITY EMPOWERMENT

To increase capacity of a community is to increase its ability to do things for itself. It is more than just adding some communal services or facilities like roads, sanitation, water, access to education and health care. It means increased ability and strength. It means more skills, more confidence, and more effective organization. It cannot come about by charity or donation of resources from outside. It can be facilitated through action such as community projects, but only when all community members become involved from the beginning, to decide upon a community action, to identify hidden resources from within the community, and by developing a sense of ownership and responsibility of communal facilities from the start to the finish. While increased democratisation may be helped by Government devolving some law making power to the community, its capacity to make use of its legal decision-making depends upon it having practical capacity, i.e. the ability to make decisions about its own development, to determine its own future. Power, strength, capacity, ability, empowerment.

COMMUNITY IMPLEMENTATION COMMITTEE

The community implementation comittee (CIC) is the Executive, Development Committee or Project Committee of the community, chosen by the community as a whole, responsible for carrying out the wishes of the whole community. Community Project Executive. Community Project Committee. Community Implementation Executive. Development Committee. This is the executive organization at village level that carries out construction or maintenance of a communal facility or service.

COMMUNITY MANAGEMENT TRAINING

Community management training is aimed at poverty reduction, the strengthening of low-income communities in the planning and management of human settlements communal facilities and services, their construction, operation and maintenance. This is training for action, not just for skill transfer or for giving information to individuals. Training, as a method for strengthening low-income communities, for poverty reduction, for promoting community participation, for practical support to democratisation and decentralization, is far from being only the transfer of information and skills to the trainees. It also includes mobilizing and organizing. This is non-orthodox training. Formalization and institutionalization of this kind of training brings with it the danger of emasculating the training, of emphasizing the skill transfer over the encouragement, mobilization and organizing aspects of the training.

Management training in this sense was developed for strengthening the effectiveness of top and middle management in profit making corporations. It has been modified here, and integrated with techniques of trade union organizing, for the purposes of mobilizing and strengthening the capacity of low-income communities to come together, help themselves, for developmental social change.

COMMUNITY PARTICIPATION

Community participation is far more than the contribution of labor or supplies; it is participating in decision-making, to chose a community project, plan it, implement it, manage it, monitor it, control it. It differs from community contribution. Social animation promotes the activities of a target community, with a view to the community taking more responsibility for its own development, starting with decisions about what projects to undertake, and stimulation to mobilize resources and organize activities. Community participation promotion aims at ensuring that decisions affecting the community are taken by all (not only a few) community members (not by an outside agency).

In the community empowerment methodology, community contribution is encouraged, for it helps the community to become more responsible for the activity if they invest their own resources in it. We also encourage Government, and outside donors to discuss their activities with the whole community; this is community consultation. Community participation here should not be used as the equivalent of community contribution or community consultation (as is misleadingly done by many assistance agencies); participation here means participation in decision-making, in control and in coordination.

CONCEPTUAL-BELIEF DIMENSION OF COMMUNITY

The belief-conceptual dimension of community is another structure of ideas, also sometimes contradictory, that people have about the nature of the universe, the world around them, their role in it, cause and effect, and the nature of time, matter, and behavior. Beliefs, like all cultural elements, are transmitted by communicating symbols, not by genetic (biological) inheritance. The beliefs and perceptions of reality shared by members of a community are affected by your mobilizing activities, and should be a major consideration in your planning of mobilizing activities.

CONFIDENCE

Confidence is one of the sixteen elements of strength, power or capacity of a community or organization. While expressed in individuals, how much confidence is shared among the community as a whole? For example, an understanding that the community can achieve whatever it wishes to do. Positive attitudes, willingness, self-motivation, enthusiasm, optimism, self-reliant rather than dependency attitudes, willingness to fight for its rights, avoidance of apathy and fatalism, a vision of what is possible. Increased strength includes increased confidence. When simulating a community to organize and act, the mobilizer needs to be aware of the role of confidence in empowering that community or organization.

CONSTRAINT

A constraint is any hindrance or barrier to reaching desired objectives. A good project design courageously identifies constraints, and then generates strategies to use available resources to overcome them.

CONSULT

When an aid agency or donor organization consults with community leaders or representatives, they often ask if the community wants a project. That answer is likely to be, "Yes". The agency may then report to its board or donors that there was community participation. That is incorrect. What has taken place is a consultation, not genuine community participation in decision-making, choosing and planning a project from among the community priorities (in contrast to the agency's priorities).

CONTEXT (POLITICAL AND ADMINISTRATIVE ENVIRONMENT)

Context is one of the sixteen elements of strength, power or capacity of a community or organization. A community will be stronger, more able to get stronger and sustain its strength more, the more it exists in an environment that supports that strengthening. An environment that supports strengthening includes political (including the values and attitudes of the national leaders, laws and legislation) and administrative elements (attitudes of civil servants and technicians, as well as Governmental regulations and procedures), and the legal environment. When politicians, leaders, technocrats and civil servants, as well as their laws and regulations, take a provision approach, the community is weak, while if they take an enabling approach to the community acting on a self-help basis, the community will be stronger. Communities can be stronger when they exist within a more enabling context. When simulating a community to organize and act, the mobilizer needs to be aware of the role of context in empowering that community or organization.

CONTRIBUTION

Some people will confuse participation with contribution. Many people, when they hear the phrase, community participation. Assume it only means community contribution. They think only of the communal labor that members will put into the project. Unfortunately, there have been many cases in the past where community members were treated as serfs or slaves and forced to contribute their labor (or other resources, e.g. land, food). The methodology promoted in this handbook is quite the opposite. Participation here means participation in decision-making, not merely the contribution of resources.

CORRUPTION

Dishonesty, one of the major factors of poverty.

COURAGE

Courage roughly means "bravery," and is often referred to as the bravery necessary to do the difficult but right thing, such as being honest and transparent with group or public funds. It is also the core of the word "encourage," which is what the mobilizer tries to do to community members to stimulate them to drop their apathy and fatalism and engage in self-help activity, and what a good manager does as a leader of staff.

CRITICISM

One of the most important bits of wisdom to learn is that when we see something wrong, to criticize it usually does not make it right, or correct the problem. Instead, it usually makes the problem worse. Why? Because human beings feel threatened and under attack when someone is criticizing them. Criticism lowers our/their self-confidence and self-esteem. We become defensive when criticized, and instead of correcting the mistake, we tend to defend it.

When we are mobilizing communities, coordinating volunteers, or managing staff, we must learn to expect that they will make mistakes and be prepared to deal with those mistakes in ways that further our aims. Showing our anger, criticizing the person who makes the mistake, may serve a purpose of "venting," but we pay a huge price for that personal relief.

CROSS TALK

In regular group discussions you allow, indeed you encourage, participants to speak their opinions and respond to others. In the Brainstorm Session, in contrast, cross talk is forbidden. Participants must direct their responses only to the facilitator, and not respond to the contribution of other participants. This ground rule is necessary for successful participatory group decision-making in the brainstorm session. It is not a feature of your work outside the brainstorm session.

CULTURE

More than merely songs and dances, culture, in social science, means the overall social system, the total of all learned attitudes and behavior, consisting of sociocultural systems belonging to six dimensions: technological, economic, political, interactive, ideological and world view. The basic unit of culture is the "symbol". Culture is not genetic; it is transmitted by communicating symbols. Sometimes called the "super-organic," because it is composed of systems that transcend the biological entities, humans, that compose and bear culture.

CURRICULUM

A "curriculum" is a plan of action applied to a training program. This website contains many modules, each of which includes half dozen or so training documents. Together they represent the content of a curriculum for training mobilizers and related professionals working to empower low-income communities. A summary and description of this curriculum material is in the document, which can be used for planning a program for strengthening low-income communities.

CHAPTER

22

Prosthesis and Orthosis

PROSTHESIS

A prosthesis (plural: prostheses; from Ancient Greek prosthesis, "addition, application, attachment") is an artificial device that replaces a missing body part, which may be lost through trauma, disease, or congenital conditions. Prosthetic amputee rehabilitation is primarily coordinated by a prosthetist and an inter-disciplinary team of health care professionals including psychiatrists, surgeons, physical therapists, and occupational therapists.

GENERAL PRINCIPLES

In surgeons try to save as much length of the limb as possible while providing a residual limb that is able to tolerate the stress of the prosthesis and return to mobility. Sometime compromises are necessary between retaining maximum bone length and avoiding scars and other deformities that may interfere with prosthetic fitting.

TYPE OF PROSTHESIS

In theory, any part of the body—from your ear or nose to your finger or toe—could be replaced by prosthesis. In practice, there are four common types of prosthetic limb, which replace either a partial or complete loss of an arm or leg:

- Below the knee (BK, transtibial): An prosthetic lower leg attached to an intact upper leg (Fig. 22.1)
- Above the knee (AK, transfemoral): A prosthetic lower and upper leg, including a prosthetic knee
- Below the elbow (BE, transradial): A prosthetic forearm
- Above the elbow (AE, transhumeral): A prosthetic lower and upper arm, including a prosthetic elbow

Surgery attention is paid not only to the bones but also to the muscles and nerves.

PART OF THE PROSTHESIS

Prosthesis consists of a number of different parts includes:

1. The prosthetic limb
2. The socket (the connection or "interface" between the prosthetic limb and the patient's body)
3. The attachment mechanism and
4. The control system.

Prosthetic Limb

The construction of prosthesis depends largely on the job it will have to do. While cosmetic hands are concerned purely with appearance, prosthetic legs are substitutes for a major structural part of someone's body and have to bear their entire weight. Typically, a prosthetic arm or leg is made from a strong and durable but lightweight material such as carbon fiber, covered with foam padding (for comfort) or flesh-colored plastic. The weight of prosthetic limbs is a very important factor.

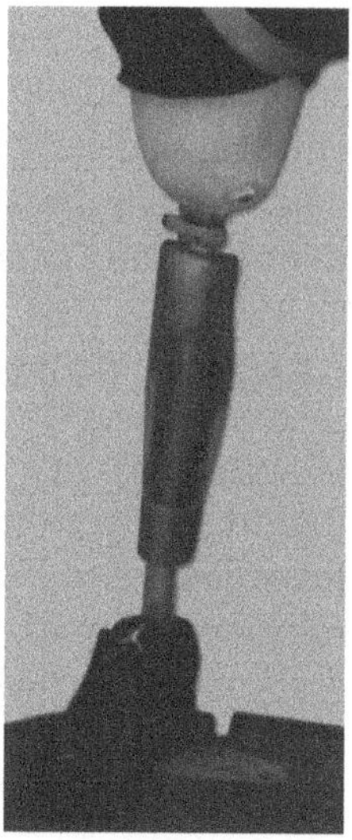

Fig. 22.1: Below knee prosthesis *(For color version see Plate 2)*

Socket

The comfort and effectiveness of a prosthesis is largely governed by how well it fits onto the remaining part of the patient's own limb, which is called their residual limb (or sometimes, informally, the "stump"—a term some people understandably find offensive, though it is, nevertheless, widely used in the medical world). The connecting part of prosthesis is called the socket and it is carefully molded around a plaster cast taken from the residual limb. The fit of a socket has to be precise or the new limb may damage the residual one, causing discomfort or tissue damage and perhaps even making it impossible to wear the prosthesis for a time. A patient's residual limb is likely to change shape and size over months and years so new sockets will be needed from time to time. More precisely fitting sockets can now be made by scanning a patient's residual limb with lasers and cutting-edge techniques such as 3D printing are also now being used. However, sockets are produced, it is important for them be custom-made and expertly fitted by an experienced prosthetist.

Attachment Mechanism

A well-fitting prosthesis is usually secured to a residual limb by what is called a suspension system (which might be an elastic sleeve, a suction socket, or old-fashioned straps and harnesses). A snug, secure fitting is vital for comfort—and ensures the limb can be properly controlled. Often the socket is itself a part of the attachment; for example, a prosthetic leg socket may consist of a large hollow plastic casing into which the residual limb is inserted.

Control System

Natural limbs are pulled back and forth by muscles stimulated by our brains; in much the same way, the simplest functional prostheses are operated by systems of cables that run through them, doing the job of the muscles. One common type of prosthetic hand is a pincer, sometimes worn inside a glove (for cosmetic reasons) that can be opened or closed by pulling cables attached to the opposite shoulder. Simple artificial legs work largely through gravity: the wearer learns to walk in them, through practice, by alternately swinging them into position and then balancing on them while they move their unimpaired leg in its turn. More sophisticated prostheses are electrically controlled and powered by rechargeable battery packs.

The most sophisticated (and expensive) prostheses are myoelectric. They use electrodes to sense muscular impulses in the residual limb (or elsewhere on the patient's body); electronic control systems detect those signals and amplify them to power electric motors that operate the prosthetic limb as though it were real. In other words, the patient thinks "I want to move my arm," their brain stimulates muscles in the residual arm, the electronic system commands the electric motors to move and the prosthetic limb shifts accordingly.

CLASSIFICATION OF PROSTHESIS

On the basis of prosthetic construction design prostheses are classified into:

1. Exoskeletal
2. Endoskeletal

Exoskeletal Prostheses

Exoskeletal is defined as structurally supported by an external frame. Exoskeletal prostheses are usually nonflexible foam or wood with an external plastic lamination. Exoskeletal structures may be laminated and then hollowed out to make them ultra-lightweight (Fig. 22.2).

Exoskeletal structures are non-adjustable/non-alignable. An exoskeletal prostheses gains its structural integrity from the outer

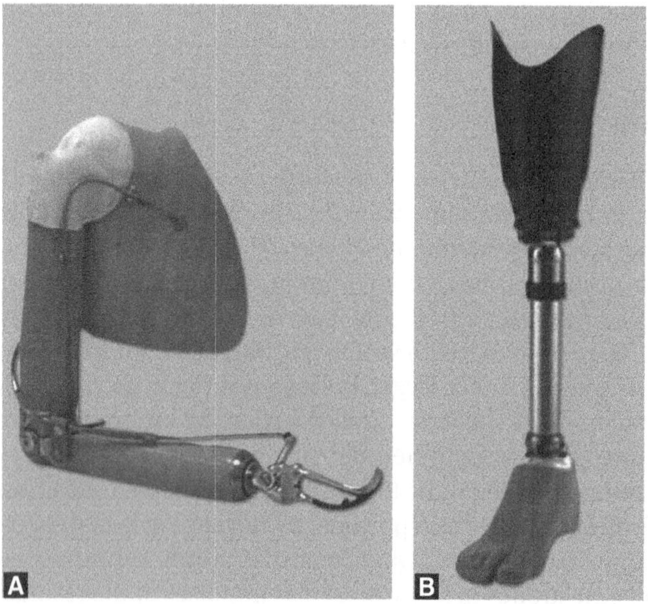

Figs 22.2A and B: Exoskeletal prostheses *(For color version see Plate 3)*

laminated shell, usually made up of resin, which is quite durable, over a filler material of wood or foam, which has been shaped to provide the cosmetic appearance of the prosthesis. However, prosthetic fitting should be very perfect, because otherwise lack of alignment and adjustability would pose great problems.

The development of prosthetic limbs did not progress much from the era of World War II through the era of the Vietnam War. Prior to the Vietnam War, prosthetic limbs were exoskeletal. These limbs were constructed with a laminate that formed the outside dimensions. The laminate was constructed to be strong enough to support the body weight of the patient and the forces that were placed on it by normal ambulation. These exoskeletal prostheses tended to be very heavy and fairly inflexible. This was especially a problem for those with above-knee amputations. Once constructed, there was very little adaptability. Materials could be added or shaved, but there was relatively little one could do to alter the limb once it was constructed. This lack of adaptability created a special problem for growing children. As body dimensions and the mechanics of ambulation changed, exoskeletal prostheses would have to be replaced in their entirety. The cost and inconveniences associated with obtaining the new limbs often led to children using these prosthetic limbs longer than they should have.

Endoskeletal Prostheses

Endoskeletal or modular is defined as structurally supported by an internal pipe/pylon that are constructed of aluminum, carbon composites, titanium and steel with a flexible foam cover that is cosmetically topped with a nylon hose.

Endoskeletal structures, however, are generally lighter in weight than exoskeletal, particularly when carbon composites and titanium are used. Generally, it is the adjustability and light-weight that makes the endoskeletal prosthesis indicated for most cases. As the user acquires mobility skills, the alignability of endoskeletal prosthesis allows moving of the foot in lateral, medial, anterior, posterior, inversion, eversion, dorsiflexion and plantar flexion. In an exoskeletal system, the lamination must be cut and reshaped with the desired change, while the endoskeletal usually has Allen screws at each connection that allow changing of the angle at that attachment. Replacing the required components in endoskeletal prostheses usually only requires a few minutes and an Allen wrench.

A socket change-out can usually be conducted in a few minutes and the prosthesis can then be aligned with the new component. The biggest advantage of the endoskeletal prosthesis is the component interchangeability and alignment adjustability. Besides being easier for the prosthetist or therapist to adjust, in the long run the interchangeability of components keeps the costs lower. One of the few possible disadvantages of the endoskeletal design is that variability may allow the patient to make unnecessary changes.

Limb Prostheses

Limb prostheses include both upper- and lower-extremity prostheses.

Upper-extremity Prostheses

Upper-extremity prostheses are used at varying levels of amputation: forequarter, shoulder disarticulation, transhumeral prosthesis, elbow disarticulation, transradial prosthesis, wrist disarticulation, full hand, partial hand, finger, partial finger.

Transradial prosthesis is an artificial limb that replaces an arm missing below the elbow. Two main types of prosthetics are available. Cable operated limbs work by attaching a harness and cable around the opposite shoulder of the damaged arm. The other form of prosthetics available is myoelectric arms. This work by sensing, via electrodes, when the muscles in the upper arm move, causing an artificial hand to open or close. In the prosthetic industry, a transradial prosthetic arm is often referred to as a "BE" or below elbow prosthesis.

Lower-extremity Prostheses

Lower-extremity prostheses provide replacements at varying levels of amputation. These include hip disarticulation, transfemoral prosthesis, knee disarticulation, transtibial prosthesis, Syme's amputation, foot, partial foot, and toe. The two main subcategories of lower-extremity prosthetic devices are transtibial (any amputation transecting the tibia bone or a congenital anomaly resulting in a tibial deficiency) and transfemoral (any amputation transecting the femur bone or a congenital anomaly resulting in a femoral deficiency).

Transfemoral prosthesis is an artificial limb that replaces a leg missing above the knee. Transfemoral amputees can have a very difficult time regaining normal movement. In general, a transfemoral amputee must use approximately 80% more energy to walk than a person with two whole legs. This is due to the complexities in movement associated with the knee. In newer and more improved designs, hydraulics, carbon fiber, mechanical linkages, motors, computer microprocessors, and innovative combinations of these technologies are employed to give more control to the user. In the prosthetic industry a transfemoral prosthetic leg is often referred to as an "AK" or above the knee prosthesis.

Transtibial prosthesis is an artificial limb that replaces a leg missing below the knee. A transtibial amputee is usually able to regain normal movement more readily than someone with a transfemoral amputation, due in large part to retaining the knee, which allows for easier movement. Lower, extremity prosthetics describes artificially replaced limbs located at the hip level or lower. In the prosthetic industry a transtibial prosthetic leg is often referred to as a "BK" or below the knee prosthesis.

AMBULATORY AIDS

Ambulatory aids are devices used to assist in functional independent ambulation (walking). These devices range from very basic items like a cane to a four-wheeled walker. Walkers and ambulatory aids are height adjustable and can be fitted to your body. Most walkers and ambulatory aids are made from lightweight materials to reduce user fatigue.

- Capable of walking; not bedridden: an ambulatory patient.
- Designed for or available to patients who are not bedridden: ambulatory care; ambulatory pediatrics.

Assistive devices for mobility/ambulation can be referred to as ambulatory aids. Ambulatory aids (e.g. canes, crutches, walkers) are used to provide an extension of the upper extremities to help transmit bodyweight and provide support for the patient.

A mobility aid is a device designed to assist walking or otherwise improve the mobility of people with mobility impairment.

There are various walking aids which can help people with impaired ability to walk and wheelchairs or mobility scooters for more severe disability or longer journeys which would otherwise be undertaken on foot. For people who are blind or visually impaired the white cane and guide dog have a long history of use. Other aids can help with mobility or transfer within a building or where there are changes of level.

Traditionally, the phrase "mobility aid" has applied mainly to low technology mechanical devices. The term also appears in government documents, for example, dealing with tax concessions of various kinds. It refers to those devices whose use enables a freedom of movement similar to that of unassisted walking or standing up from a chair.

Selection Criteria

Selection of walking aids for a particular person depends on:

- Degree of relief from weight bearing required
- Strength of the person's upper and lower limb
- Coordination of the limb
- Stability of patient
- Extent of improvement of the patient
- Other factor like motivation, age and acceptance
- Prognosis of the condition.

As the condition of the patient improves he may progress through different types of walking aids. Each aid gives a varying amount of stability and accordingly, a varying extent of mobility.

Benefits of Walking Aids or Appliances

Walking aids or appliances are useful:

- To improve balance
- To give proprioception
- To decrease pain
- To reduce weight bearing on injured or inflamed structures
- To compensate weak muscle
- To scan the immediate environment (for the visually impaired)
- To indicate to the bystanders of the disability of the individual (e.g. the white with a red tip indicates the user is visually impaired).

Walking Aids

Forearm Crutch

Walking aids include assistive canes (commonly referred to as walking sticks), crutches, and walkers. As appropriate to the needs of the individual user, these devices help to maintain upright ambulation by providing any or all of: improved stability, reduced lower-limb loading and generating movement.

Improved Stability

By providing additional points of contact the walking aid provides both additional support and a wider range of stable center of gravity positioning.

Reduced Lower-limb Loading

By directing load through the arms and the walking aid, lower impact and static forces are transmitted through the affected limbs.

Generating Movement

The walking aid and arms can substitute for the muscles and joints of the spine, pelvis and/or legs in the generation of dynamic forces during walking.

Cane

The cane or walking stick is the simplest form of walking aid. It is held in the hand and transmits loads to the floor through a shaft (Fig. 22.3).

The load which can be applied through a cane is transmitted through the user's hands and wrists and limited by these.

Crutches

A crutch also transmits loads to the ground through a shaft, but has two points of contact with the arm, at the hand and either below the

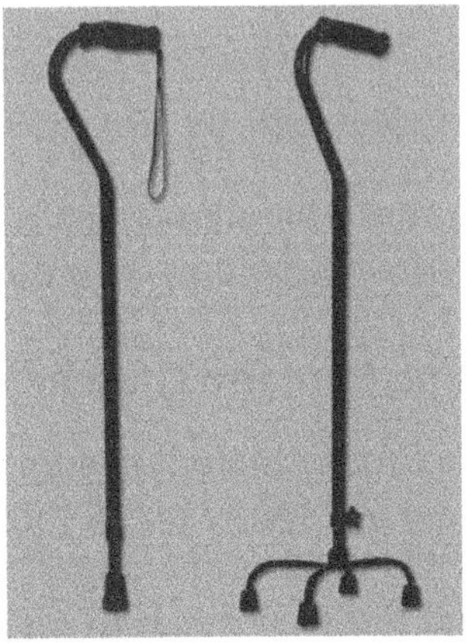

Fig. 22.3: Cane or walking stick

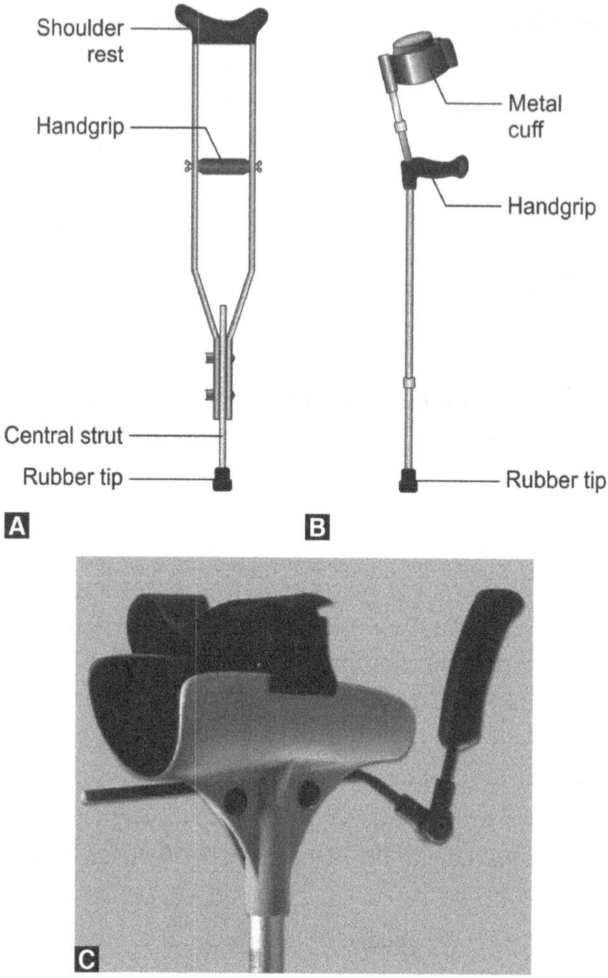

Figs 22.4A to C: (A) Axillary crutch; (B) Forearm crutch; (C) Gutter crutch

elbow or below the armpit. This allows significantly greater loads to be exerted through a crutch in comparison with a cane.

Canes, Crutches, and Forearm Crutch Combinations

Devices on the market today include a number of combinations for canes, crutches, and forearm crutches (Figs 22.4A to C). These crutches have bands that encircle the upper arms and handles for the patient to hold and rest their hands to support the bodyweight. The forearm crutch typically gives a user the support of the cane but with additional forearm support to assist in mobility. The forearm portion helps increase balance, lateral stability and also reduces the load on the wrist.

Walkers

A walker (also known as a Zimmer frame) is the most stable walking aid and consists of a freestanding metal framework with three or more points of contact which the user places in front of them and then grips during movement. The points of contact may be either fixed rubber ferrules as with crutches and canes, or wheels, or a combination of both. Wheeled walkers are also known as rollators (Figs 22.5A and B).

Walker Cane Hybrid

A walker cane hybrid adjusted to four configurations (Fig. 22.6).

A walker cane hybrid was introduced in 2012 designed to bridge the gap between a cane and a walker. The hybrid has two legs which provide lateral (side-to-side) support which a cane does not. It can be used with two hands in front of the user, similar to a walker, and provides an increased level of support compared with a cane. It can be adjusted for use with either one or two hands, at the front and at the side, as well as a stair climbing assistant. The hybrid is not designed to replace a walker which normally has four legs and provides 4-way support using both hands.

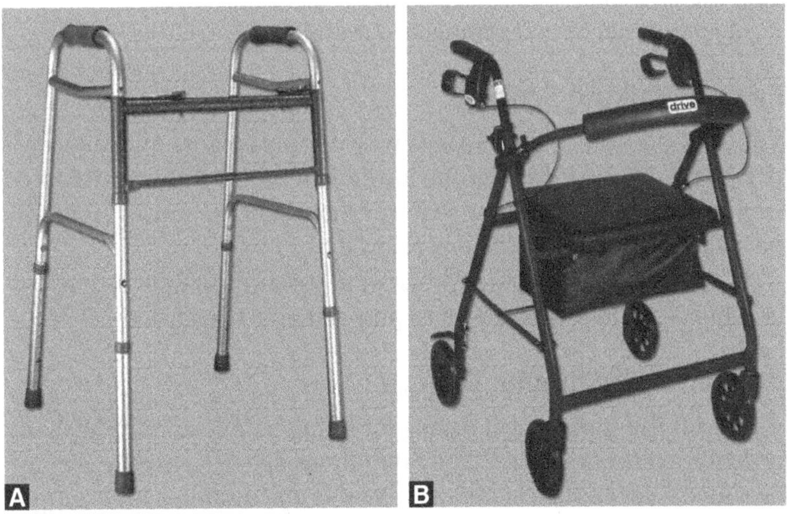

Figs 22.5A and B: (A) Walker; (B) Wheeled walker

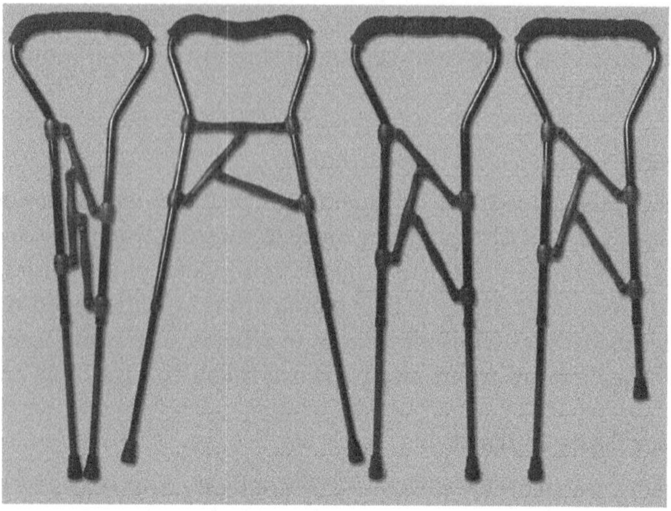

Fig. 22.6: Walker cane hybrid adjusted to four configurations

Gait Trainers

Another device to assist walking that has entered the market in recent years is the gait trainer. This is a mobility aid that is more supportive than the standard walker. It typically offers support that assists weight-bearing and balance. The accessories or product parts that attach to the product frame provide unweighting support and postural alignment to enable walking practice (Fig. 22.7).

A gait trainer as an example of a mobility aid.

Seated Walking Scooter

The walk aid scooter allows a user with normal balance and foot, knee or hip conditions to unload the lower extremities. The two-wheeled scooter has a bicycle-type seat and handlebars, and is manually propelled with one or both feet (Fig. 22.8).

This walking aid scooter provides more support than a cane and is lighter, less bulky and easier to propel than a wheelchair.

Stair Lifts and Similar Devices

A stair lift is a mechanical device for lifting people and wheelchairs up and downstairs (Fig. 22.9). Sometimes special purpose lifts are provided elsewhere to facilitate access for the disabled, for example, at entrances to raised bus stops in Curitiba, Brazil.

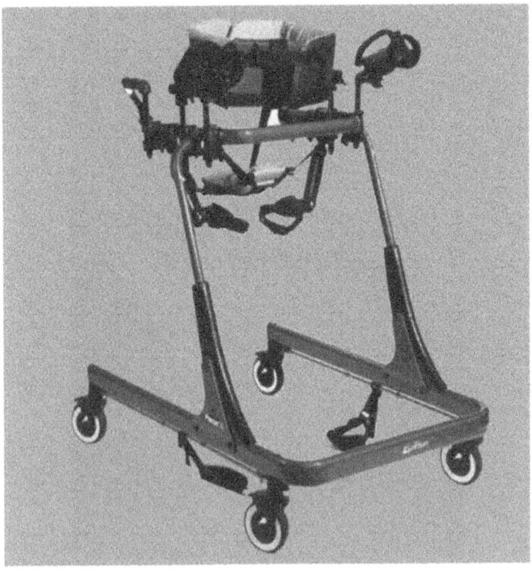

Fig. 22.7: Gait trainer

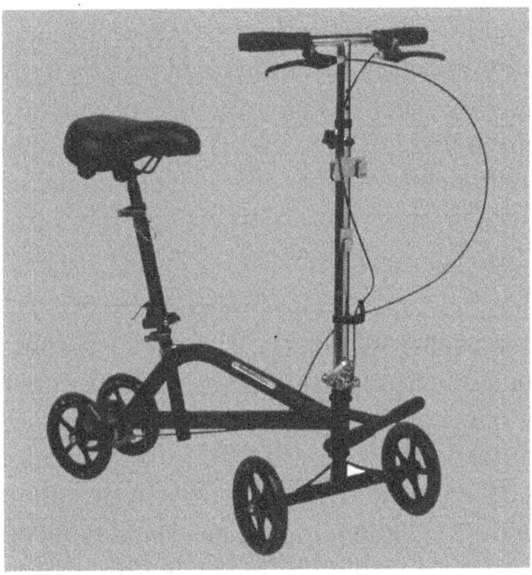

Fig. 22.8: Walking scooter

Wheelchairs and Scooters

Wheelchairs and mobility scooters substitute for walking by providing a wheeled device on which the user sits. Wheelchairs may be either manually propelled (by the user or by an aid) or electrically powered (commonly known as a "power chair"). Mobility scooters

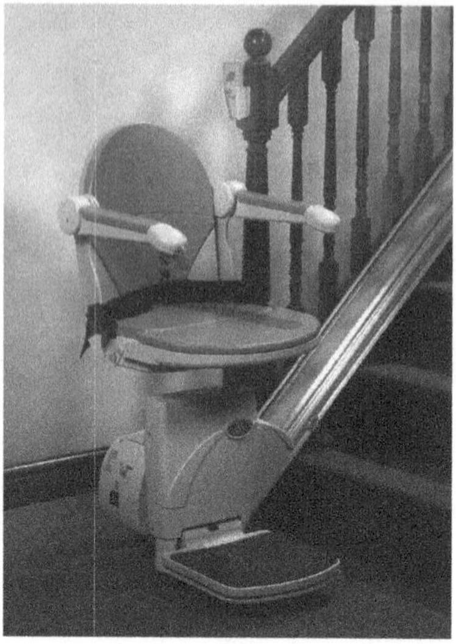

Fig. 22.9: Stairs lift

are electrically powered, as are motorized wheelchairs. Wheelchairs and scooters are normally recommended for any individual due to significant mobility/balance impairment. A registered occupational therapist or physiotherapist (few cases) are able to provide object and clinical testing to ensure proper and safe device recommendations (Figs 22.10 and 22.11).

Wheelchair

Wheelchair is a chair with wheels. The device comes in variations allowing either manual propulsion by the seated occupant turning the rear wheels by hand, or electric propulsion by motors. There are often handles behind the seat to allow it to be pushed by another person.

Wheelchairs are used by people for whom walking is difficult or impossible due to illness, injury, or disability. People who have difficulty sitting and walking often make use of a wheel bench (Fig. 22.10).

Types of Wheelchair

A basic manual wheelchair incorporates a seat, foot rests and four wheels: two caster wheels at the front and two large wheels at the back. The two larger wheels in the back usually have hand rims; two metal or plastic circles approximately 3/4" thick. The hand rims have

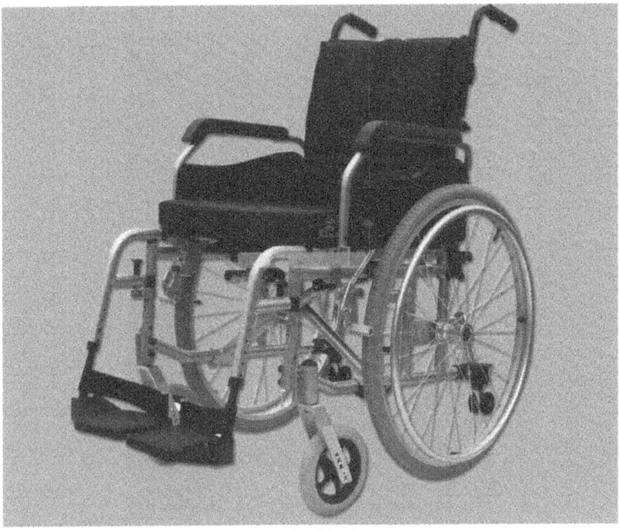

Fig. 22.10: Wheel chair

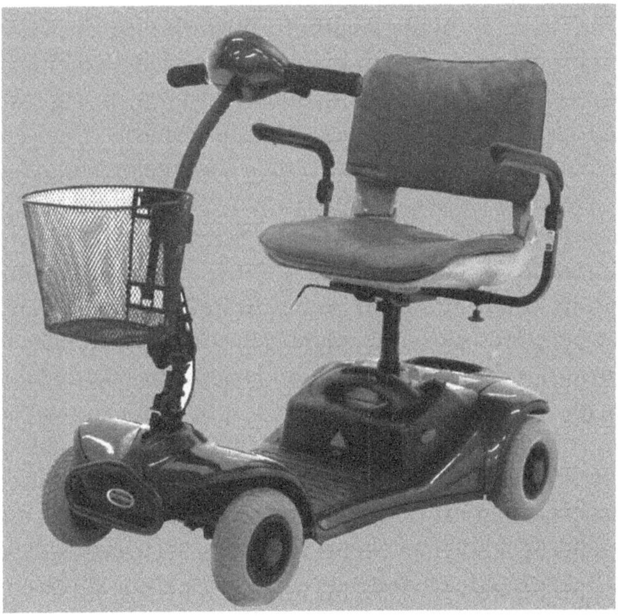

Fig. 22.11: Electric scooter

a diameter normally only slightly smaller than the wheels they are attached to. Most wheelchairs have two push handles at the top of the back to allow for manual propulsion by a second person.

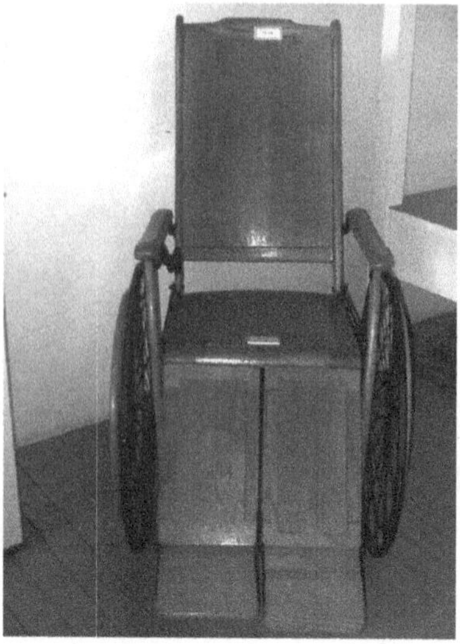

Fig. 22.12: Wooden wheelchair dating to the early part of the 20th century

Other varieties of wheelchair are often variations on this basic design, but can be highly customized for the user's needs. Such customizations may encompass the seat dimensions, height, seat angle (also called seat dump or squeeze), foot rests, leg rests, front caster outriggers, adjustable back rests and controls (Fig. 22.12).

Everyday manual wheelchairs come in two major designs—folding or rigid. The rigid chairs, which are increasingly preferred by active users, have permanently welded joints and many fewer moving parts. This reduces the energy required to push the chair by eliminating many points where the chair would flex as it moves. Welding the joints also reduces the overall weight of the chair. Rigid chairs typically feature instant-release rear wheels and back rests that fold down flat, allowing the user to dismantle the chair quickly for storage in a car.

Many rigid models are now made with ultralight materials such as aircraft aluminum and titanium. One major manufacturer, Tilite, builds only ultralights. Another innovation in rigid chair design is the installation of polymer shock absorbers, such as frog legs, which cushion the bumps over which the chair rolls. These shock absorbers may be added to the front wheels or to the rear wheels, or both. Rigid chairs also have the option for their rear wheels to have a camber. Wheels can have a camber, or tilt, which angles the tops of the wheels in toward the chair. This allows for better propulsion by the user which is desired by long-term users. Sport wheelchairs have large camber angles to improve stability.

Various optional accessories are available, such as anti-tip bars or wheels, safety belts, adjustable back rests, tilt and/or recline features, extra support for limbs or neck, mounts or carrying devices for crutches, walkers or oxygen tanks, drink holders, and clothing protectors.

Transport wheelchairs are usually light, folding chairs with four small wheels. These chairs are designed to be pushed by a caregiver to provide mobility for patients outside the home or more common medical settings.

Experiments have also been made with unusual variant wheels, like the omni wheel or the mecanum wheel. These allow for a broader spectrum of movement.

The electric wheelchair shown Figure 22.13 is fitted with Mecanum wheels (sometimes known as Ilon wheels) which give it complete freedom of movement. It can be driven forwards, backwards, sideways, and diagonally, and also turned round on the spot or turned around while moving, all operated from a simple joystick.

Transport Wheelchairs

Attendant-propelled chairs (or transport wheelchairs) are designed to be propelled by an attendant using the handles, and thus the

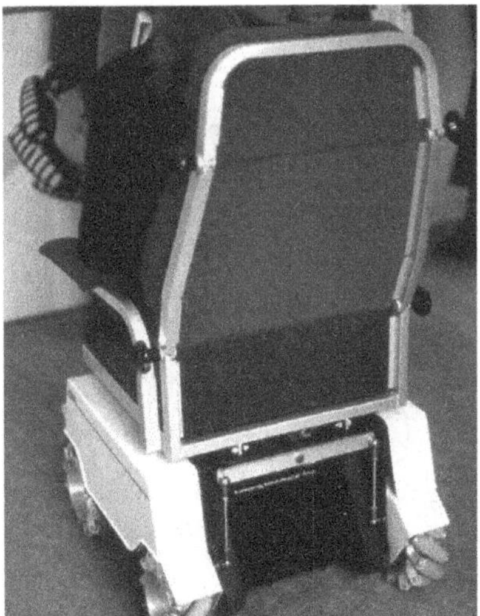

Fig. 22.13: Wheelchair fitted with Mecanum wheels, taken at an exhibition in the early 1980s

back wheels are rimless and often smaller. These chairs are often used as 'transfer chairs' to move a patient when a better alternative is unavailable, possibly within a hospital, as a temporary option, or in areas where a user's standard chair is unavailable. These chairs are commonly seen in airports. Special airplane transfer chairs are available on most airlines, designed to fit narrow airplane aisles and transfer wheelchair-using passengers to and from their seats on the plane.

Electric-powered

An electric-powered wheelchair is a wheelchair that is moved via the means of an electric motor and navigational controls which is usually a small joystick mounted on the armrest, rather than manual power. For users who cannot manage a manual joystick, head switches, chin-operated joysticks, sip-and-puff or other specialist controls may allow independent operation of the wheelchair (Fig. 22.14).

Wheelbase chairs are wheeled platforms with specially molded seating systems interfaced with them for users with a more complicated posture. A molded seating system involves taking a cast of a person's best achievable seated position and then either carving the shape from memory foam or forming a plastic mesh around it. This seat is then covered, framed, and attached to a wheelbase.

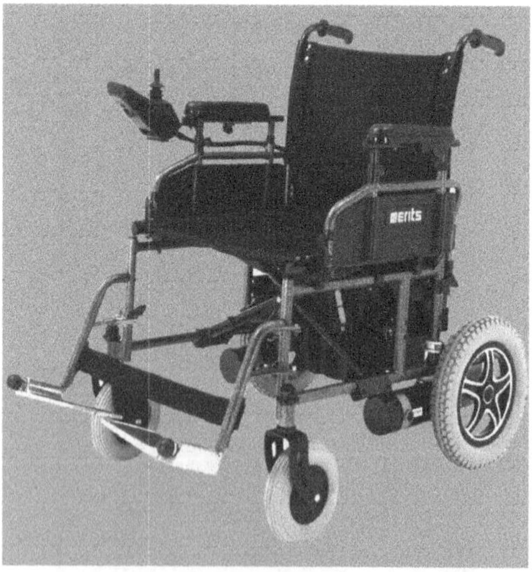

Fig. 22.14: Electric powered wheelchair

Other Variants

A dynamic tilt wheelchair has seating surfaces which can be tilted to various angles. It was developed by an orthotist, Hugh Barclay, who worked with disabled children and observed that postural deformities such as scoliosis could be supported or partially corrected by allowing the wheelchair user to relax in a tilted position. Invented in Kingston, Ontario, Canada, in the early 1980s, the dynamic tilt wheelchair type is now manufactured by a number of companies and used all around the world. This revolutionary adaptation of wheelchair design provides individuals with very complex health needs the opportunity for increased mobility.

A standing wheelchair is one that supports the user in a nearly standing position. They can be used as both a wheelchair and a standing frame, allowing the user to sit or stand in the wheelchair as they wish. They often go from sitting to standing with a hydraulic pump or electric-powered assist. Some options are provided with a manual propel model and power stand, while others have full power, tilt, recline and variations of power stand functions available as a rehabilitative medical device. The benefits of such a device include, but are not limited to: aiding independence and productivity, raising self-esteem and psychological well-being, heightening social status, extending access, relief of pressure, reduction of pressure sores, improved functional reach, improved respiration, reduced occurrence of urinary tract infection (UTI), improved flexibility, help in maintaining bone mineral density, improved passive range motion, reduction in abnormal muscle tone and spasticity, and skeletal deformities.

A bariatric wheelchair is one designed to support larger weights; most standard chairs are designed to support no more than 250 lb (113 kg) on average.

Pediatric wheelchairs are another available subset of wheelchairs. Hemi wheelchairs have lower seats which are designed for easy foot propulsion. The decreased seat height also allows them to be used by children and shorter individuals.

A knee scooter is a related device which may be substituted for a wheelchair when an injury has occurred to only one leg, below the knee. The patient rests the injured leg on the scooter, grasps the handlebars, and pushes with the uninjured leg.

A power-assisted wheelchair is a recent development that uses the frame and seating of a typical manual chair while replacing the standard rear wheels with wheels that have small battery-powered motors in the hubs. A floating rim design senses the pressure applied by the users push and activates the motors proportionately. This results in the convenience, small size and light-weight of a manual chair while providing motorized assistance for rough/uneven terrain and steep slopes that would otherwise be difficult or impossible to navigate, especially by those with limited upper-body function.

Orthosis

An orthosis is the correct term for an externally applied device that is designed and fitted to the body to achieve one or more of the following goals: Control biomechanical alignment. Correct or accommodate deformity. Protect and support an injury. The term orthosis refers to an exoskeletal appliance applied to a body part, and has replaced the traditional term, "bracing". A brace is considered to be an appliance that allows movement at the joint, whereas a splint does not allow movement at a joint.

Through the years, the term "splint" has been used, especially in the area of hand therapy, to mean a short-term orthosis and splints have been described as both static and dynamic. As a result, the terms orthosis, brace, and splint have become interchangeable across many allied health professions.

An orthosis (plural: orthoses) is an externally applied device used to modify the structural and functional characteristics of the neuromuscular and skeletal system.

The orthotist is the person who designs, fabricates, and repairs the orthotic appliance, however, physical and occupational therapists, as will as physicians, may fabricate low temperature thermoplastic.

An orthotist is the primary medical clinician responsible for the prescription, manufacture and management of orthoses. An orthosis may be used to control, guide, limit and/or immobilize an extremity, joint or body segment for a particular reason

- To restrict movement in a given direction
- To assist movement generally
- To reduce weight bearing forces for a particular purpose
- To aid rehabilitation from fractures after the removal of a cast
- To otherwise correct the shape and/or function of the body, to provide easier movement capability or reduce pain.

Orthotics combines knowledge of anatomy and physiology, pathophysiology, biomechanics and engineering. Patients who benefit from an orthosis may have a condition such as spina bifida or cerebral palsy, or have experienced a spinal cord injury or stroke. Equally, orthosis are sometimes used prophylactically or to optimize performance in sport.

The American Academy of Orthopaedic Surgeons and the American Orthotic and Prosthetic Association developed a standard of nomenclature devices. The acronyms used for the generic are listed in Table 22.1. Orthotics are named by the joints they encompass. Thus, foot orthoses (FO) are appliances applied to the foot and are placed inside or outside the shoe.

Biomechanical Principles of Orthotic Design

- The biomechanical principles of orthotic design assist in promoting control, correction, stabilization, or dynamic movement
- All orthotic designs are based on three relatively simple principles
  - Pressure
  - Equilibrium
  - The lever arm principle.

TABLE 22.1: Orthotic acronyms

LL orthoses			
FO	Foot orthosis	AFO	Ankle-foot orthosis
KO	Knee orthosis	KAFO	Knee-ankle-foot orthosis
HO	Hip orthosis	HKAFO	Hip-knee-ankle-foot orthosis
		RGO	Reciprocal gait orthosis
Spinal orthoses			
CO	Cervical orthosis	CTO	Cervical-thoracic orthosis
TO	Thoracic orthosis	CTLSO	Cervicothoraciclumbosacral orthosis
SO	Sacral orthosis	TLSO	Thoraciclumbosacral orthosis
SIO	Sacroiliac orthosis	LSO	Lumbosacral orthosis
UL orthoses			
HdO	Hand orthosis	WHO	Wrist-hand orthosis
WO	Wrist orthosis	EWHO	Elbow-wrist-Hand orthosis
EO	Elbow orthosis	SEO	Shoulder-elbow orthosis
SO	Shoulder orthosis	SEWHO	Shoulder-elbow-wrist-hand orthosis

These considerations include and are not limited to:

- The forces at the interface between the orthotic materials and the skin
- The degrees-of-freedom of each joint
- The number of joint segments
- The neuromuscular control of a segment, including strength and tone
- The material selected for orthotic fabrication
- The activity level of the client.

The following principles provide the foundation for all orthotic design keeping in mind that the more complicated the orthotic application, the more confounded the various principles become.

The Pressure Principle

It states that:

Pressure is equal to the total force per unit area

Clinically, what this means is that the greater the area of a pad or the plastic shell of an orthosis, the less force will be placed on the skin. Therefore, any material that creates a force against the skin should be of a dimension to minimize the forces on the tissues.

$$P = \frac{\text{Force}}{\text{Area of application}}$$

The Equilibrium Principle

It states that:

The sum of the forces and the bending moments created must be equal to zero.

The practical application is best explained by the most commonly used loading system in orthotics, the three-point pressure system (Fig. 22.15). The three-point pressure or loading system occurs when three forces are applied to a segment in such a way that a single primary force is applied between two additional counterforce's with the sum of all three forces equaling zero. The primary force is of a magnitude and located at a point where movement is either inhibited or facilitated, depending on the functional design of the orthosis.

The Lever Arm Principle

It states that:

The farther the point of force from the joint, the greater the moment arm and the smaller the magnitude of force required to produce a given torque at the joint.

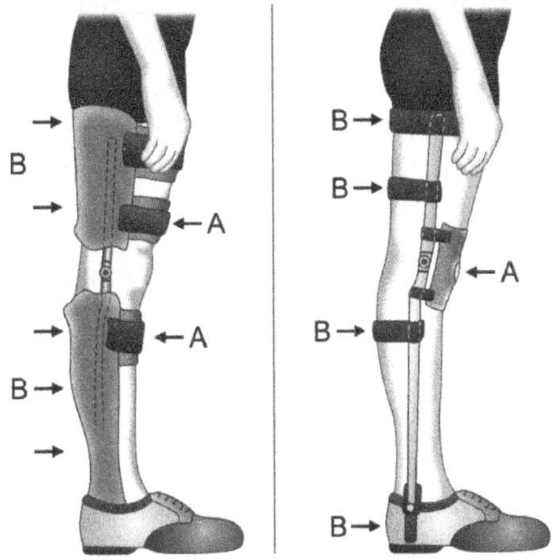

Fig. 22.15: Three point pressure system (A) Primary force; (B) The counterforce application. The sum of all forces will be equal to zero

This is why most orthoses are designed with long metal bars or plastic shells that are the length of an adjacent segment.

The greater the length of the supporting orthotic structure, the greater the moment or torque that can be placed on the joint or unstable segment.

Collectively, these three principles rarely, if ever, act independently of each other. Ideally, when designing or evaluating an orthotic appliance, the clinician should check that:

1. There is adequate padding covering the greatest area possible for comfort;
2. The total forces acting on the involved segment is equal to zero or there is equal pressure throughout the orthosis and no areas of irritation to the skin;
3. The length of the orthosis is suitable to provide an adequate force to create the desired effect and to avoid increased transmission of shear forces against the anatomic tissues.

Orthotic Considerations

- The goal of orthotic fitting is to meet the functional requirements of the client with minimal restriction
- To meet this goal, the rehabilitation team must evaluate each client individually without preconceived ideas of routine orthotic prescription based purely on the diagnosis

- It must be determined whether the appliance will be:
  - A temporary device to protect or assist the client until further restorative therapies have been progressed, or
  - A permanent orthosis fabricated for long-term use.

The functional considerations for an orthoses typically include one or more of the following.

1. *Alignment:* The correction of a deformity or maintenance of a body segment.

Clinical examples:

- Musculoskeletal considerations
  - Milwaukee brace for scoliosis
  - Dynamic splint to prevent scar shortening in clients with burns
- Neurologic considerations
  - Tone reducing AFOs in patient with cerebral palsy
  - CTLSO to prevent motion of the cervical region.

2. *Movement:* A joint requires assistance with motion or resistance to excessive motion.

Clinical examples:

- Assistance with joint motion
  - Musculoskeletal considerations
    - AFO with dorsiflexion assist for dorsiflexor weakness
    - Neurologic considerations
    - RGO assist clients with spinal cord injury with ambulation.
- Resistance of joint motion
  - Musculoskeletal considerations
    - Shoe insert for a patient with foot deformity.
    - Finger splints for arthritic hands
  - Neurologic considerations
    - Swedish knee cage for unstable knee
    - Arm sling for neurologic shoulder.

3. *Weight-bearing:* To reduce axial loading and reduce the forces placed on a joint.

Clinical examples:

- Musculoskeletal considerations
  - Shoe insert with metatarsal pad for a diabetic patient with foot deformity.
- Neurologic considerations
  - Heel wedge for the pronated foot of a child with cerebral palsy

4. ***Protection:*** Support or protect a segment against further injury or pain.

Clinical samples:

- Musculoskeletal considerations
  - Functional knee brace
- Neurologic considerations
  - Cock-up splints postspinal cord injury.

Contraindications for Orthotic Application

- The orthosis cannot provide the required amount of motion
- When greater stabilization is required than can be provided
- The orthosis actually limits function, and the client is more functional without the appliance, and
- Abnormal pressures from the orthosis would result in injury to the skin and other tissues.

Materials

The client is fitted with an orthotic appliance that is both functional and, in most cases, cosmetically acceptable. Selecting the appropriate material characteristics for the fabrication of an orthotic device requires careful consideration of a number of factors:

1. ***Strength:*** The maximum external load that can be sustained by a material.
2. ***Stiffness:*** The amount of bending or compression that occurs under stress. Clinically, when greater support is required, a stiffer material is used; when a more dynamic orthosis is desired, a more flexible material is used.
3. ***Durability (fatigue resistance):*** The ability of a material to withstand repeated cycles of loading and unloading. Selection of a material for orthotic appliances is frequently based on the ability of the material to withstand the day-to-day stresses of each individual client.
4. ***Density:*** The material's weight per unit volume. Generally, the greater the volume or thicker a material the more rigid and more durable it will be, however, this usually increases the overall weight of the finished orthosis.
5. ***Corrosion resistance:*** The vulnerability of the material to chemical degradation. Most materials will exhibit corrosion over time,

metals will rust and plastics will become brittle. Contact with human perspiration and environmental elements such as dirt, temperatures, and water accelerate the wearing effect on materials. Knowing the client's daily environment can assist in material selection.

6. ***Ease of fabrication:*** The equipments needed for fabrication of orthoses.

Manufacture and Materials

Orthoses were traditionally made by following a tracing of the extremity with measurements to assist in creating a well-fitted device. Subsequently, the advent of plastics as a material of choice for construction necessitated the idea of creating a plaster of Paris mold of the body part in question. This method is still extensively used throughout the industry. Currently, CAD/CAM, CNC machines and 3D printing are involved in orthotic manufacture.

Orthoses are made from various types of materials including thermoplastics, carbon fiber, metals, elastic, EVA, fabric or a combination of similar materials. Some designs may be purchased at a local retailer; others are more specific and require a prescription from a physician, who will fit the orthosis according to the patient's requirements. Over-the-counter braces are basic and available in multiple sizes. They are generally slid on or strapped on with Velcro, and are held tightly in place. One of the purposes of these braces is injury protection.

Classification

Under the International Standard terminology, orthoses are classified by an acronym describing the anatomical joints which they contain. For example, an ankle foot orthosis (AFO) is applied to the foot and ankle, a thoracolumbosacral orthosis (TLSO) affects the thoracic, lumbar and sacral regions of the spine. It is also useful to describe the function of the orthosis. Use of the International Standard is promoted to reduce the widespread variation in description of orthoses, which is often a barrier to interpretation of research studies.

Upper-limb Orthoses

Upper-limb (or upper extremity) orthoses are mechanical or electromechanical devices applied externally to the arm or segments thereof in order to restore or improve function, or structural characteristics of the arm segments encumbered by the device. In general, musculoskeletal problems that may be alleviated by the use of upper limb orthoses include those resulting from trauma or disease (arthritis for example). They may also be beneficial in aiding individuals who have suffered a neurological impairment such as stroke, spinal cord injury, or peripheral neuropathy.

Types of Upper-limb Orthoses

Upper-limb orthoses:
- Clavicular and shoulder orthoses
- Arm orthoses
- Functional arm orthoses
- Elbow orthoses
- Forearm-wrist orthoses
- Forearm-wrist-thumb orthoses
- Forearm-wrist-hand orthoses
- Hand orthoses
- Upper-extremity orthoses (with special functions).

Lower-limb Orthoses

A lower-limb orthosis is an external device applied to a lower-body segment to improve function by controlling motion, providing support through stabilizing gait, reducing pain through transferring load to another area, correcting flexible deformities, and preventing progression of fixed deformities. The term caliper or calipers remains in widespread use for lower-limb orthoses in the United Kingdom.

Foot Orthoses

Foot orthoses comprise a custom made insert or foot bed fitted into a shoe. Commonly referred to as "orthotics" these orthoses provide support for the foot by redistributing ground reaction forces as well as realigning foot joints while standing, walking or running. A great body of information exists within the orthotic literature describing the sciences that might be used to aid people with foot problems as well as the impact "orthotics" can have on foot, knee, hip, and spine deformities. They are used by everyone from athletes to the elderly to accommodate biomechanical deformities and a variety of soft tissue

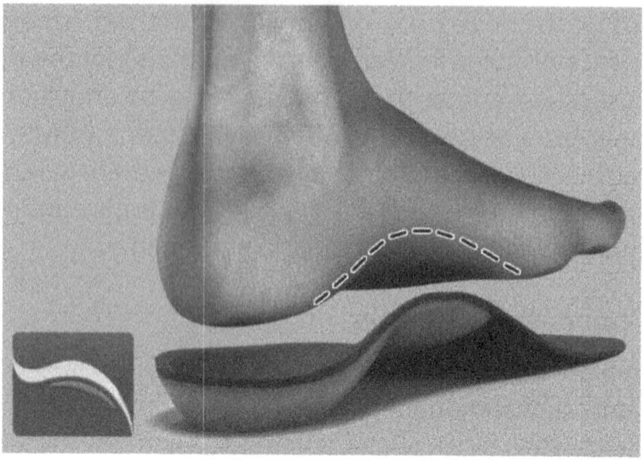

Fig. 22.16: Foot bed

inflammatory conditions such as plantar fasciitis. They may also be used in conjunction with properly fitted orthopedic footwear in the prevention of foot ulcers in the at-risk diabetic foot (Fig. 22.16).

Ankle-foot Orthosis

An AFO worn on the left foot with ankle hinge.

Schematic Ankle-foot Orthosis

An ankle-foot orthosis (AFO) is an orthosis or brace that encumbers the ankle and foot. AFOs are externally applied and intended to control position and motion of the ankle, compensate for weakness, or correct deformities. AFOs can be used to support weak limbs, or to position a limb with contracted muscles into a more normal position. They are also used to immobilize the ankle and lower leg in the presence of arthritis or fracture, and to correct foot drop; an AFO is also known as a foot-drop brace. Ankle-foot orthoses are the most commonly used orthoses, making up about 26% of all orthoses provided in the United States. An AFO is generally constructed of lightweight polypropylene-based plastic in the shape of an "L", with the upright portion behind the calf and the lower portion running under the foot. They are attached to the calf with a strap, and are made to fit inside accommodative shoes. The unbroken "L" shape of some designs provides rigidity, while other designs (with a jointed ankle) provide different types of control.

Obtaining a good fit with an AFO involves one of two approaches:

- Provision of an off-the-shelf or prefabricated AFO matched in size to the end user
- Custom manufacture of an individualized AFO from a positive model, obtained from a negative cast or the use of computer-aided imaging, design, and milling. The plastic used to create a durable AFO must be heated to 400 °F, making direct molding of the material on the end user impossible.

The International Red Cross recognizes four major types of AFOs:

Flexible AFOs	*Anti-Talus AFOs*	*Rigid AFOs*	*Tamarack Flexure Joint*
May provide dorsiflexion assistance, but give poor stabilization of the subtalar joint	Block ankle motion, especially dorsiflexion; do not provide good stabilization for the subtalar joint	Block ankle movements and stabilize the subtalar joint; may also help control adduction and abduction of the forefoot	Provide sub talar stabilization while allowing free ankle dorsiflexion and free or restricted plantar flexion. Depending upon the design; may provide dorsiflexion assistance to correct foot drop

The International Committee of the Red Cross published its manufacturing guidelines for ankle-foot orthosis in 2006. Its intent is to provide standardized procedures for the manufacture of high-quality modern, durable and economical devices to people with disabilities throughout the world.

Knee-ankle-foot Orthosis

A knee-ankle-foot orthosis (KAFO) is an orthosis that encumbers the knee, ankle and foot (Fig. 22.17). Motion at all three of these lower limb areas is affected by a KAFO and can include stopping motion, limiting motion, or assisting motion in any or all of the three planes of motion in a human joint: *saggital, coronal, and axial. Mechanical* hinges, as well as electrically controlled hinges have been used. Various materials for fabrication of a KAFO include but are not limited to metals, plastics, fabrics, and leather. Conditions that might benefit from the use of a

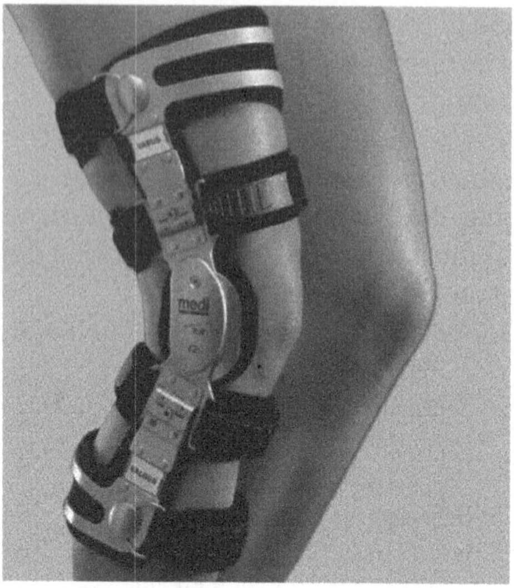

Fig. 22.17: Knee-ankle-foot orthosis

KAFO include paralysis, joint laxity or arthritis, fracture, and others. Although not as widely used as knee orthosis, KAFOs can make a real difference in the life of a paralyzed person, helping them to walk therapeutically or, in the case of polio patients, on a community level. These devices are expensive and require maintenance. Some research is being done to enhance the design; even NASA helped spearhead the development of a special knee joint for KAFOs.

Knee Orthosis

A knee orthosis (KO) or knee brace is a brace that extends above and below the knee joint and is generally worn to support or align the knee. In the case of diseases causing neurological or muscular impairment of muscles surrounding the knee, a KO can prevent flexion or extension instability of the knee. In the case of conditions affecting the ligaments or cartilage of the knee, a KO can provide stabilization to the knee by replacing the function of these injured or damaged parts. For instance, knee braces can be used to relieve pressure from the part of the knee joint affected by diseases such as arthritis or osteoarthritis by realigning the knee joint into valgus or varus. In this way a KO may help reduce osteoarthritis pain. However, a knee brace is not meant to treat an injury or disease on its own, but is used as a component of treatment along with drugs, physical therapy and possibly surgery.

When used properly, a knee brace may help an individual to stay active by enhancing the position and movement of the knee or reducing pain. Also used for elephants when traumatic amputation has occurred.

Prophylactic, Functional and Rehabilitation Braces

Prophylactic braces are used primarily by athletes participating in contact sports. Evidence about prophylactic knee braces, the ones football lineman wear are often rigid with a knee hinge, indicate they are ineffective in reducing anterior cruciate ligament tears, but may be helpful in resisting medial and lateral collateral ligament tears.

Functional braces are designed for use by people who have already experienced a knee injury and need support to recover from it. They are also indicated to help people who are suffering from pain associated with arthritis. They are intended to reduce the rotation of the knee and support stability. They reduce the chance of hyperextension, and increase the agility and strength of the knee. The majority of these are made of elastic. They are the least expensive of all braces and are easily found in a variety of sizes.

Rehabilitation braces are used to limit the movement of the knee in both medial and lateral directions—these braces often have an adjustable range of motion stop potential for limiting flexion and extension following ACL reconstruction. They are primarily used after injury or surgery to immobilize the leg. They are larger in size than other braces, due to their function.

Spinal Orthosis

Two different spinal orthosis used to treat scoliosis.

Scoliosis, a condition describing an abnormal curvature of the spine, may in certain cases be treated with spinal orthosis, such as the Milwaukee brace, the Boston brace, and Charleston bending brace. As this condition develops most commonly in adolescent females who are undergoing their pubertal growth spurt, compliance with wearing is these orthosis is hampered by the concern these individuals have about changes in appearance and restriction caused by wearing these orthosis. Spinal orthosis may also be used in the treatment of spinal fractures. A Jewett brace, for instance, may be used to facilitate healing of an anterior wedge fracture involving the T10 to L3 vertebrae. A body jacket may be used to stabilize more involved fractures of the

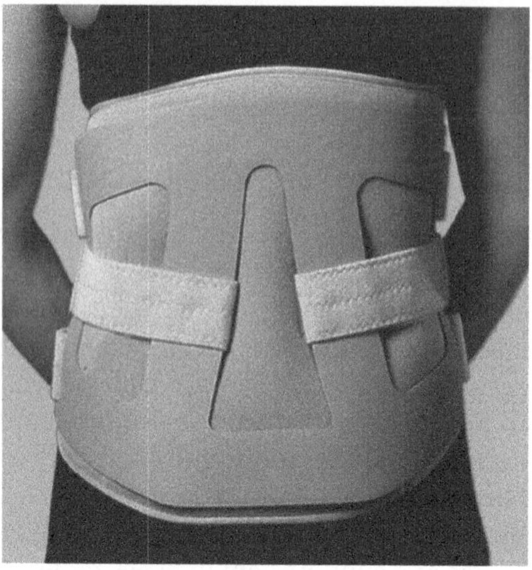

Fig. 22.18: Spinal orthosis

spine (Fig. 22.18). The halo brace is a cervical thoracic orthosis used to immobilize the cervical spine, usually following fracture. The halo brace allows the least cervical motion of all cervical orthosis currently in use; it was first developed by Vernon L Nickel at Rancho Los Amigos National Rehabilitation Center in 1955.

MEASUREMENT OF POP CAST TECHNIQUES

Cast Application

According to World Health Organization to prepare plaster of Paris bandage, use dry cotton gauze bandage 500 cm long and 15 cm wide unroll a portion of the bandage on a dry table with a smooth top. And apply plaster powder (anhydrous calcium sulfate or gypsum) evenly to the surface (Figs 22.19 to 22.21).

1. Clean the skin and apply dressings to any wound. If available, apply stockinet to the extremity, avoiding wrinkles. Next apply a uniform thickness of cotton padding over the stockinet and put extra padding over any bony prominence such as the patella, the elbow or the ankle.
2. Soak the plaster roll in a pail containing water at room temperature. Do not use warm water as the heat given off by the plaster as it

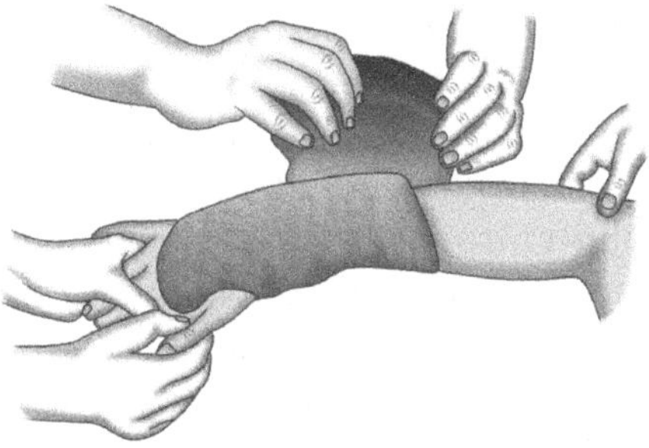

Fig. 22.19: Dressing

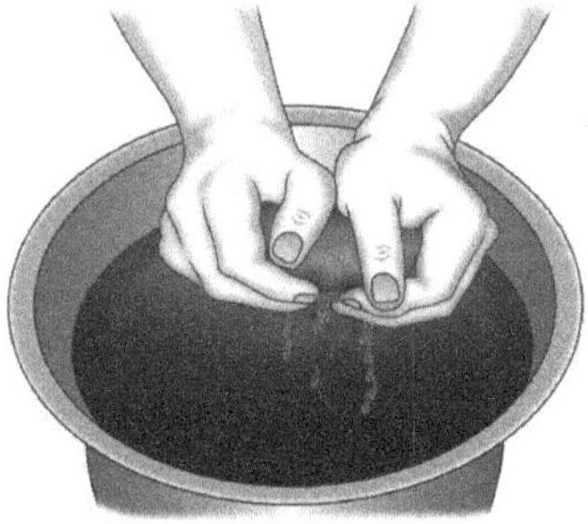

Fig. 22.20: Squeezing the bandage

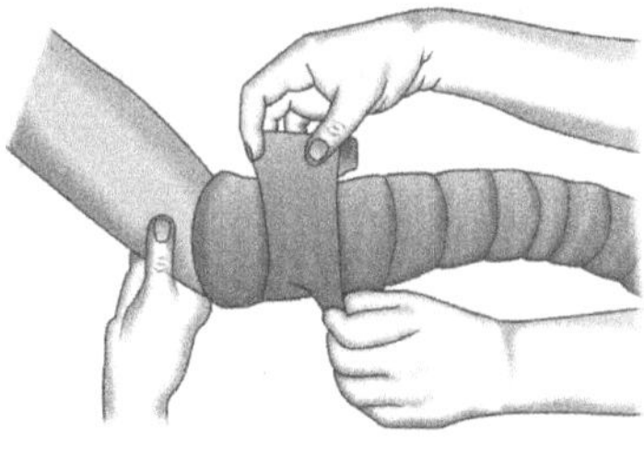

Fig. 22.21: Plaster application

sets may burn the patient. Leave the plaster in the water until it is completely soaked and the air bubbles cease to rise.

3. Gently pick up the ends of the bandage with both hands and lightly squeeze it, pushing the ends together without twisting or wringing.
4. While applying the plaster, hold the relevant part of the body steady in the correct position. Movement will cause ridges to form on the inside of the plaster. Work rapidly and without interruption,

rubbing each layer firmly with the palm so that the plaster forms a homogeneous mass rather than a discrete layer.

5. Apply the plaster by unrolling the bandage as it rests on the limb. Do not lift it up from the patient or apply tension to the roll. Overlap the previous layer of plaster by about half the width of the roll.
6. Mould the plaster evenly around the bony prominences and contours. Leave 3 cm of padding at the upper and lower margins of the cast to protect the skin from irritation by the edge of the cast. This can be folded back over the edge and incorporated in the last layer of plaster to provide a smooth edge.
7. Mould the cast until the plaster sets and becomes firm. Complete drying takes 24 hours, so advise the patient to take care not to dent the cast or apply weight to it during this time. The technique for application of a fiberglass cast is similar, but the fiberglass is slightly elastic and will contour to the body more easily. It sets firmly in about 30 minutes and will not be affected by water after that time.

SPLINT APPLICATION

Measure the length of material needed to secure the limb. Place 3–5 layers of the measured padding on a flat surface and unroll 5–10 layers of plaster on to the padding (Fig. 22.22).

Grasp the plaster layer at each end, dip into the water and gently squeeze together without twisting. Place the wet plaster on the padding and smooth with the palm into a homogeneous layer.

And alternative method is to split a circular cast lengthwise, remove the anterior half and secure it similarly with an elastic bandage (Fig. 22.23).

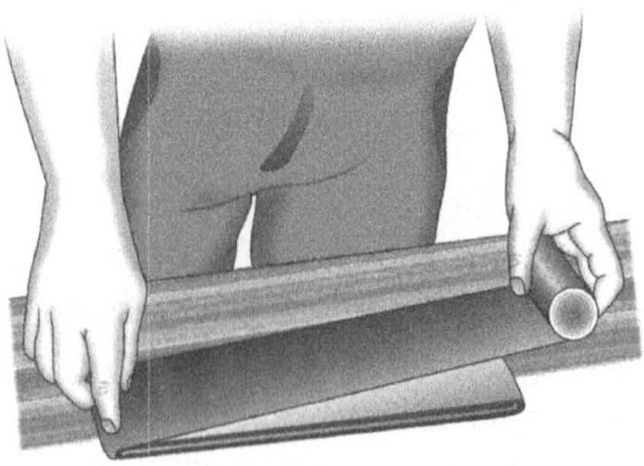

Fig. 22.22: Measurement of length of material

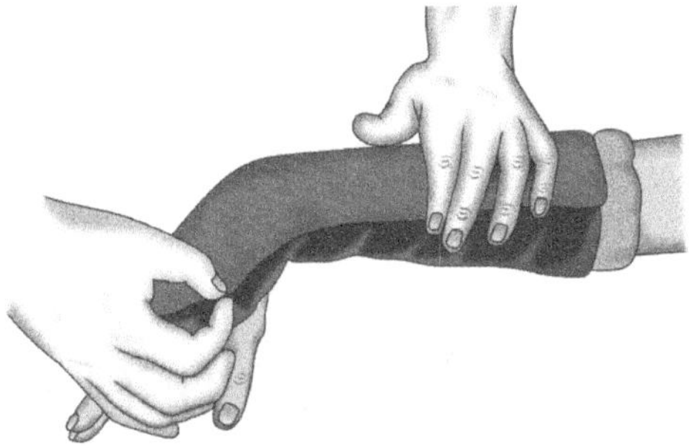

Fig. 22.23: Application of splint

CARRYING FOR A CAST AND SPLINT

- Keep the cast or splint dry at all times
- Encourage patients to try not to scratch their skin under the cast or splint with a sharp or blunt object
- Allow the cast to dry for 24 hours before putting weight on it or resting it on a hard surface
- For acute injuries, elevate the injured part for 24–48 hours and have the patient wiggle their fingers or toes frequently.

Return to the health clinic immediately if...

- Your cast or splint gets wet or becomes soft or broken
- You have increasing pain
- You experience numbness or tingling, or have difficulty moving your fingers or toes
- You see a change in skin color of the extremity
- Your cast or splint has a foul odor.

CHAPTER 23

Professional Ethics of the Physiotherapy

According to Indian Association of Physiotherapists, Ethical Rules and Guidelines are as follows: source: www.physiotherapyindia .orgs

GENERAL RESPONSIBILITIES

- Physiotherapists shall provide honest quality care, competent and accountable professional consultancy, therapeutic and otherwise, as 1st contact practitioner to any person who may seek or may be in need of the same.
- The physiotherapists shall administer only such treatment that is in the interest of the patient with the responsibility for the exercise of sound judgment with diligence.
- The physiotherapists shall respect the dignity and basic rights of the patients and professional colleagues.
- The physiotherapists shall refer the patient to the appropriate specialists whenever the problems/symptoms of the diseases of the patient so demand.
- The physiotherapists shall maintain secrecy of the patient's disease and shall not divulge the same to any other individual except to professional colleagues during scientific case discussions/ meetings.

- The physiotherapists shall provide accurate information to the patient or to the next relative if required about the problem and specific physiotherapy management of that individual's problems if required.
- The physiotherapy management shall have the prior consent of the patient/relative if the procedure adopted involves risk of any damage to the tissue, organ system or any side effects/complications after explaining the same accurately.
- The physiotherapists shall comply with the laws governing the patient's rights and cause.
- The physiotherapists shall not solicit patients through fee splitting. It shall be based upon their individual competence and ability in accordance with the accepted scientific standards.
- The physiotherapists shall constantly strive to keep himself/herself abreast of the recent and latest scientific developments related to physiotherapy and add to the knowledge fund.
- The physiotherapists shall not indulge in or associate with any activity that goes against the dignity, honour and development of the profession.
- The physiotherapists shall contribute to the planning and development of professional services which address the health needs of the community.
- Maintain high standards of professional conduct.
- Follow ethical practices outlined in the Code of Ethics. Strive to follow the ethical practices outlined in the Principles for Physiotherapy Education and practice norms.
- Balance the wants, needs, and requirements of program patients, institutional policies, laws, and sponsors. Members' ultimate concern must be the long-term well-being of physiotherapy education and practice norms.
- Resist pressures (personal, social, organizational, financial, and political) to use their influence inappropriately and refuse to allow self-aggrandizement or personal gain to influence their professional judgments.
- Seek appropriate guidance and direction when faced with ethical dilemmas.
- Make every effort to ensure that their services are offered only to individuals and organizations with a legitimate claim on these services.

IN THEIR PROFESSIONAL PREPARATION AND DEVELOPMENT, MEMBERS SHALL

- Accurately represent their areas of competence, education, training, and experience.
- Recognize the limits of their expertise and confine themselves to performing duties for which they are properly educated, trained, and qualified, making referrals when situations are outside their area of competence.
- Be informed of current developments in their fields, and ensure their continuing development and competence.
- Stay abreast of laws and regulations that affect their clients.
- Stay knowledgeable about world events that impact physiotherapy education and practice program patients.
- Stay knowledgeable about differences in cultural and value orientations.
- Actively uphold IAP's Ethical Rules andGuidelines when practices that contravene it become evident.

IN RELATIONSHIP WITH STUDENTS, SCHOLARS, AND OTHER MEMBERS SHALL

- Understand and protect the civil and human rights of all individuals.
- Not discriminate with regard to race, color, national origin, ethnicity, sex, religion, sexual orientation, marital status, age, political opinion, immigration status, or disability.
- Recognize their own cultural and value orientations and be aware of how those orientations affect their interactions with people from other cultures.
- Demonstrate awareness of, sensitivity to, and respect for other education and practice systems, values, beliefs, and cultures.
- Not exploit, threaten, coerce, or sexually harass others.
- Not use one's position to proselytize.
- Refrain from invoking governmental or institutional regulations in order to intimidate patients in matters not related to their status.
- Maintain the confidentiality, integrity, and security of patients' records and of all communications with treatment program, Members shall secure permission of the individuals before sharing information with others inside or outside the organization,

unless disclosure is authorized by law or institutional policy or is mandated by previous arrangement.

- Inform patients of their rights and responsibilities in the context of the institution and the community.
- Respond to inquiries fairly, equitably, and professionally.
- Provide accurate, complete, current, and unbiased information.
- Refrain from becoming involved in personal relationships with patients when such relationships might result in either the appearance or the fact of undue influence being exercised on the making of professional judgments.
- Accept only gifts that are of nominal value and that do not seem intended to influence professional decisions, while remaining sensitive to the varying significance and implications of gifts in different cultures.
- Identify and provide appropriate referrals for patients who experience unusual levels of emotional difficulty.
- Provide information, orientation, and support services needed to facilitate patient's adaptation to a new education and practice and cultural environment.

IN PROFESSIONAL RELATIONSHIPS, MEMBERS SHALL

- Show respect for the diversity of viewpoints among colleagues, just as they show respect for the diversity of viewpoints among their clients.
- Refrain from unjustified or unseemly criticism of fellow members, other programs and other organizations.
- Use their office, title, and professional associations only for the conduct of official business.
- Uphold agreements when participating in joint activities and give due credit to collaborators for their contributions.
- Carry out, in a timely and professional manner, any IAP responsibilities they agree to accept.

IN ADMINISTERING PROGRAMS, MEMBERS SHALL

- Clearly and accurately represent the identity of the organization and the goals, capabilities, and costs of programs
- Recruit individuals, paid and unpaid, who are qualified to offer the instruction or services promised, train and supervise them responsibly, and ensure by means of regular evaluation that they

are performing acceptably and that the overall program is meeting its professed goals.
- Encourage and support participation in professional development activities.
- Strive to establish standards, activities, instruction, and fee structures that are appropriate and responsive to patient's needs.
- Provide appropriate orientation, materials, and on-going guidance for patients.
- Provide appropriate opportunities for students to observe and to join in mutual inquiry into cultural differences.
- Take appropriate steps to enhance the safety and security of patients.
- Strive to ensure that the practices of those with whom one contracts do conform to IAP's Code of Ethics and the Principles for Physiotherapy Education and practice.

IN MAKING PUBLIC STATEMENTS, MEMBERS SHALL

- Clearly distinguish, in both written and oral public statements, between their personal opinions and those opinions representing IAP, their own institutions, or other organizations.
- Provide accurate, complete, current, and unbiased information.

GUIDELINES OF THE WORLD CONFEDERATION FOR PHYSICAL THERAPY

The World Confederation for Physical Therapy (WCPT) expects its member organizations to:
- Have a code of ethics or code of conduct
- Publish, promote and circulate their Code of Ethics or Code of Conduct for the benefit of their members, the general public, employers, governments and government agencies
- Have procedures for monitoring the practice of their members, disciplinary procedures and sanctions for members whose practice falls outside their Code of Ethics or Code of Conduct

WCPT offers advice and support to its member organizations wishing to develop codes of ethics or conduct.

The following statements expand on WCPT's ethical principles. They are intended to help member organizations and individuals interpret WCPT's ethical principles, with a particular view to supporting those physical therapy organizations wishing to develop Codes of Ethics that are consistent with WCPT's own ethical principles.

Ethical Principle-1

Physical therapists respect the rights and dignity of all individuals.

Everyone who seeks the services of a physical therapist has the right to service regardless of age, gender, race, nationality, religion, ethnic origin, creed, color, sexual orientation, disability, health status or politics.

Physical therapists should assure that patients/clients have the right to:

- The highest quality physical therapy services
- Information about the physical therapy services
- Make an informed consent
- Confidentiality
- Have access to their physical therapy data
- Health education and health promotion services
- Choose who should be informed on his/her behalf.

Ethical Principle-2

Physical therapists comply with the laws and regulations governing the practice of physical therapy in the country in which they practise.

Physical therapists will have a full understanding of the laws and regulations governing the practice of physical therapy. They have the right to refuse to treat or otherwise intervene when, in their opinion, the service is not in the best interests of the patient/client.

Physical therapists have the right to advocate for patient/client access to physical therapist services when, in their opinion, there is restricted access to those who have the capacity to benefit.

Ethical Principle-3

Physical therapists accept responsibility for the exercise of sound judgement.

Physical therapists are professionally independent and autonomous practitioners. They make independent judgments in the provision of services for which they have knowledge and skills.

With each patient/client, physical therapists undertake appropriate examination/assessment to allow the development of a diagnosis. In light of the diagnosis and other relevant information about the patient/client and their goals, physical therapists determine the prognosis/plan of care and implement the interventions/ treatment. When the goals have been achieved or further benefits can no longer be obtained, the physical therapist shall inform and discharge the patient/client. When the diagnosis is not clear or the required intervention/treatment is not within the realm of physical therapist practice, the physical therapist shall inform the patient/client and facilitate a referral to other professionals.

- Physical therapists shall not delegate to another health professional or support worker any activity that requires the unique skill, knowledge and judgment of the physical therapist.

If the patient/client has been referred to the physical therapist by a medical practitioner and the treatment program prescribed is not appropriate in the judgment of the physical therapist, then the physical therapist should consult with the referring medical practitioner.

Physical therapists have the right to expect cooperation from their colleagues.

Ethical Principle-4

Physical therapists provide honest, competent and accountable professional services.

Physical therapists shall:

- Ensure that their behavior and conduct is professional at all times
- Deliver timely, patient/client-specific physical therapy intervention/treatment in line with the individual's goals
- Ensure that patients/clients understand the nature of the service being provided, especially the anticipated costs (both time and financial)
- Undertake a continuous, planned, personal development program designed to maintain and enhance professional knowledge and skills
- Maintain appropriate patient/client records to allow effective evaluation of the patient's/client's care and evaluation of the physical therapist's practice
- Not disclose any information about a patient/client to a third party without the patient's/client's permission or prior knowledge, unless such disclosure is required by law
- Participate in peer review and other forms of practice evaluation, the results of which shall not be disclosed to another party without the permission of the physical therapist
- Maintain data to facilitate service performance measurement and make that data available to other agents as required by mutual agreement

- Not allow their services to be misused
- The ethical principles governing the practice of physical therapy shall take precedence over any business or employment practice. Where such conflict arises, the physical therapist shall make all efforts to rectify the matter, seeking the assistance of the national physical therapy association if required.

Ethical Principle-5

Physical therapists are committed to providing quality services.
Physical therapists shall:

- Be aware of the currently accepted standards of practice and undertake activities which measure their conformity
- Participate in continuing professional development to enhance their basic knowledge and to provide new knowledge
- Support research that contributes to improved patient/client interventions and service delivery
- Keep up to date with the best evidence available and implement it in their practice
- Support quality education in academic and clinical settings

Physical therapists engaged in research shall ensure that they:

- Abide by all current rules and policies applying to the conduct of research on human subjects
- Have obtained subjects' consent
- Protect subjects' confidentiality
- Protect subjects' safety and well-being
- Do not engage in fraud or plagiarism
- Fully disclose any research support and appropriately acknowledge any assistance
- Report any breaches of the rules to appropriate authorities
- Freely share the results of their research, especially in journals and conference presentations

Physical therapists in the role of employer shall:

- Ensure all employees are properly and duly qualified, ensuring compliance with statutory requirements
- Apply current management principles and practices to the conduct of the service, with particular attention to appropriate standards of personnel management
- Ensure policies and procedures are properly developed, implemented and monitored

- Ensure that clinical practice is appropriately evaluated and audited
- Provide adequate opportunities for staff education and personal development based on effective performance appraisal.

Ethical Principle-6

Physical therapists are entitled to a just and fair level of remuneration for their services.

Physical therapists shall:

- Ensure that their fee schedules are based on prevailing market conditions
- Ensure that fees charged offer value for money
- Ensure as much as possible that reimbursement from third-party funders are reflective of and consistent with good practice (third-party funders should not seek to exert control in any way that restricts the scope of practice of physical therapists or inhibits their right to fair remuneration)
- Ensure that influence is not used for personal gain
- Ensure that sound business principles are applied when dealing with suppliers, manufacturers and other agents.

Ethical Principle-7

Physical therapists provide accurate information to patients/clients, other agencies and the community about physical therapy and about the services physical therapists provide.

Physical Therapists:

- Shall participate in public education programs, providing information about the profession
- Shall inform the public and referring professionals truthfully about the nature of their service so that individuals are more able to make a decision about the use of the service
- May advertise their services
- Shall not use false, fraudulent, misleading, deceptive, unfair or sensational statements or claims
- Shall claim only those titles which correctly describe their professional status.

Ethical Principle-8

Physical therapists contribute to the planning and development of services that address the health needs of the community.

Physical therapists have a duty and obligation to participate in planning services designed to provide optimum community health.

Physical therapists are obliged to work toward achieving justice in the provision of health services for all people.

GLOSSARY

Codes of practice/conduct: Are ethical rules and principles that form an obligatory part of professional practice. They may be established by the physical therapy profession or incorporated into national rules and laws.

Ethics: The rules of conduct recognized in certain departments of human life.

Informed consent: It is a decision to participate in assessment, treatment or research, taken by a competent individual who has received the necessary information; who has adequately understood the information; and who, after considering the information, has arrived at a decision without having been subjected to coercion, undue influence or inducement, or intimidation. Informed consent is based on the principle that competent individuals are entitled to choose freely whether to participate in assessment, treatment or research. Informed consent protects the individual's freedom of choice and respects the individual's autonomy. In order to obtain the valid consent of patients for assessment, treatment or participation in research, they must be informed of all potential and significant risks, benefits and likely outcomes of treatment, taking into account their age, emotional state and cognitive ability, to allow valid/informed consent to be given.

Regulation of the profession: Cluster of laws, regulations, directives or rules set by the authority to legislate the physical therapy profession. The regulation can also be in form of self-regulation set by the physical therapy profession (WCPT Member Organization).

CHAPTER

24

Functional Assessment Scale and Measures

INTRODUCTION

Measurements of functional abilities and supports are commonly used across the country as a basis for differentiating among levels of care giving. Functional abilities and supports are the degrees of independence with which a consumer performs activities of daily living (ADLs) and instrumental activities of daily living (IADLs).

Points to Remember when Assessing Functional Abilities and Supports

There are three important points to remember when assessing functional abilities and supports:

- Functional abilities and supports are measures of the consumer's impairment level and need for personal assistance. In many cases, impairment level and need for personal assistance are described by the help received, but this could lead to an inaccurate assessment. For example, a disabled consumer needs help to perform an activity in a safe manner, but he/she lives alone, has no formal supports, and "receives no help." Coding the consumer's performance as "independent" because no help is received is very misleading in terms of the actual impairment level. In order to avoid this type of distortion, interpret the ADLs in terms of what is usually needed to safely perform the entire activity.

- Second, an assessment of functional abilities and supports are based on what the consumer is able to do, not what he/she prefers to do. In other words, assess the consumer's ability to do particular activities, even if he/she does not usually do the activity. Lack of capacity should be distinguished from lack of motivation, opportunity, or choice. This is particularly relevant for the IADLs mentioned above. For example, when asking someone if he/she can prepare light meals, the response may be "no", he/she does not prepare meals, even though the consumer may be able to do so. The consumer should be coded as not needing help. If a consumer refuses to perform an activity, thus putting himself/herself at risk, it is important to probe for the reason why the consumer refuses, in order to code the activity correctly. The emphasis in this section is on assessing whether ability is impaired. Physical health, mental health, cognitive, or functional disability problems may manifest themselves as the inability to perform ADL and IADL activities. If a consumer is mentally and physically free of impairment, there is not a safety risk to the consumer, and the consumer chooses not to complete an activity due to personal preference or choice, indicate that the consumer does not need help.
- The emphasis of the measurement of each of the functional activities should be how the consumer usually performed the activity over the past two weeks. For example, if a consumer usually bathes with no help or reminding/cuing, but on the date of the interview requires some assistance with bathing, code the consumer as not requiring help unless the consumer's ability to function on the date of the assessment accurately reflects ongoing need.

There are several components to each functional activity, and the coded response is based on the consumer's ability to perform all the components. For example, when assessing the consumer's ability to bathe, it is necessary to consider all of the bathing activities such as getting in and out of the tub, preparing the bath, washing, and towel drying.

Base the selection of the amount of assistance required (None, Minimal, Moderate, Extensive, and Total) on the consumer's ability to perform each activity on the day of the review. Base the selection according to how the consumer would perform each item if the consumer lived on his/her own. If the consumer has a temporary problem on the day of the review which interferes with how the activity is usually performed, base the selection on the consumer's most typical performance. If the consumer often has wide variations in performance of the activity, base the selection on the most dependent performance. When completing this functional assessment, utilize all available information. Your contacts and interviews with the consumer are important, and feedback from the family and documentation can also be helpful.

Examples of how to rate the categories on the functional assessment scale (FAS) follow.

DESCRIPTIONS/EXAMPLES OF FUNCTIONAL NEEDS

(*Note:* There is an example for each category on the measure. The scale is N = None, MI = Minimum, MO = Moderate, E = Extensive, and T = Total)

Preparing Meals

- Capable of preparing nutritious meals. (N)
- Capable of eating main meal at meal site or restaurant or receiving home-delivered meals and can fix other meals as required. (MI)
- Needs assistance to prepare main meal and can fix most other simple meals required. (MO)
- Needs assistance to prepare all meals. (E)
- Cannot prepare any meals. (T)

Eating Meals

- Can feed self, chew, and swallow solid foods without difficulty or can feed self by gastrostomy tube or catheter. (N)
- Can feed self, chew, and swallow foods but needs reminding/cuing to maintain adequate intake, or may need food cut up. (MI)
- Can feed self only if food is brought to them. (MO)
- Can feed self but needs standby assistance or cuing. May have occasional gagging, choking, or swallowing difficulty, or require assistance with feeding appliances. (E)
- Must be fed by another person by mouth, or gastrostomy tube. (T)

Toileting

- Can toilet self without physical assistance or supervision. May need grab bars/raised toilet seat or can manage own closed drainage system if has a catheter or sheath or uses protective aids. (N)
- Needs standby assistance or cuing for safety or task completion. May need some physical assistance with parts of the task such as clothing adjustment, washing hands, etc. (MI)
- Needs physical assistance with parts of the task such as wiping, cleansing, clothing adjustment. May need a protective garment. (MO)

Ambulation

- Can get around inside and outside without assistance. (N)
- Can get around inside without assistance but needs assistance outside. (MI)
- Needs occasional assistance inside and usually needs assistance outside. (MO)
- Can only get around with regular assistance both inside and outside. (E)
- Cannot move around even with regular assistance. (T)

Transferring

- Can transfer independently and can manage own position changes. (N)
- Transfers and changes position most of the time but needs assistance on occasion. (MI)
- Can assist with own transfers and position changes but needs assistance most of the time. (MO)
- Can assist with own transfers and position changes but needs assistance all of the time. (E)
- Transfers/position changes must be done by one person all of the time. (T)

Personal Hygiene

- Can manage personal hygiene without reminders, assistance, or supervision. (N)
- Can manage personal hygiene but must be reminded/cued at least some of the time. (MI)

- Performs personal hygiene but requires physical assistance to complete. (MO)
- Caregiver performs most personal hygiene but consumer assists. (E)
- Dependent on others to provide all personal hygiene. (T)

Dressing

- Can dress/undress and select clothing without assistance or supervision. (N)
- Can dress/undress and select clothing but may need to be reminded/supervised. (MI)
- Can dress/undress and select clothing with assistance. (MO)
- Caregiver dresses/undresses and selects clothing but consumer assists. (E)
- Dependent upon others to do all dressing/undressing. (T)

Bathing

- Can bathe without reminders and without assistance or supervision. (N)
- Can bathe without physical assistance but may need reminding or standby assistance. (MI)
- Requires assistance or cuing with parts of bathing, (i.e. washing back, feet, rinsing hair, etc.). Includes people who cannot get into/out of tub and may require some other assistance. (MO)
- Caregiver bathes the consumer with consumer's assistance. (E)
- Dependent on others to provide complete bath, including shampoo. (T)

Access to Transportation

- Can drive safely or is capable of using alternate transportation without assistance. (N)
- Can use available transportation but needs instruction or physical assistance to get to or from transportation vehicle. (MI)
- Can use available transportation if physical assistance or cuing is provided to both get into and out of vehicle, but assistance is not needed during trip. (MO)
- Is dependent upon being accompanied to access the community. (E)
- Medical condition is such that an ambulance is required. (T)

Finances

- Handles financial business matters. (N)
- Needs occasional assistance with financial business matters. (MI)
- Needs help with some financial business. (MO)
- Needs extensive helping managing financial business matters. (E)
- Unable to handle financial business matters. (T)

Shopping

- Can shop without assistance. (N)
- Shops without physical assistance but may need to be reminded/supervised. (MI)
- Can shop with physical assistance or cuing from caregiver. (MO)
- Caregiver shops but consumer assists. (E)
- Totally dependent upon others for shopping. (T)

Laundry

- Is capable of doing laundry. (N)
- Does laundry without assistance but may need to be reminded/supervised. (MI)
- Can do laundry but needs physical assistance or reminding/cuing from caregiver. (MO)
- Caregiver does the laundry but consumer assists. (E)
- Totally dependent upon others to do laundry within/outside the home. (T)

Housework

- Performs house-cleaning with no assistance. (N)
- Physically capable of performing all house cleaning but needs to be reminded/supervised. (MI)
- Performs light house cleaning without supervision or cuing and caregiver handles physically difficult house cleaning. (MO)
- Performs light house cleaning with supervision or cuing and caregiver handles physically difficult house cleaning. (E)
- Totally dependent upon others for all house cleaning. (T)

Night Needs

- Needs no assistance from another person during the night. (N)
- Occasionally requires assistance from caregiver at night. (MI)

- Requires care at night, but caregiver can get at least five hours of sleep during an eight-hour period. (MO)
- Requires care at night, and caregiver cannot get at least five hours of sleep during an eight-hour period. (E)
- Requires licensed staff to be up and awake all night. (T)

Emergency Response

- Needs no assistance to get outside of present dwelling or get emergency help. Is able to use the phone in emergency situations. (N)
- Needs supervision and/or verbal cuing to get outside of present dwelling or get emergency help. (MI)
- Caregiver must assist to get outside of present dwelling, but consumer can assist. (MO)
- Requires some physical assistance to get outside of present dwelling. (E)
- Requires total physical assistance to get outside of present dwelling. (T)

Medication

- Can self-administer medication without assistance. (N)
- Requires minimal physical assistance (i.e. open containers only); understands medication routine. (MI)
- Requires occasional supervision/cuing to follow medication routine. (MO)
- Requires supervision/cuing; must be reminded to take medications; does not know medication routine; may not remember if took medications. (E)
- Requires professional to administer medication. (T)

Supervision

- No supervision required beyond that included in the previous answers. (N)
- Requires occasional voice cues and prompts. (MI)
- Requires frequent voice cues and prompts. (MO)
- Requires both physical and voice prompts most of the time. (E)
- Consumer requires a behavior management program. Supervision must be available all the time, and behavior is controlled by the program with only occasional outbursts. (T)

	None (1)	*Minimal (2)*	*Moderate (3)*	*Extensive (4)*	*Total (5)*
1. PREPARING MEALS: Identify the consumer's ability to prepare own food. Consider safety issues such as whether burners are left on.					
2. EATING MEALS: Identify the level of assistance needed to perform the activity of feeding and eating with special equipment if regularly used or special tray set-up.					
3. TOILETING: Identify the consumer's ability to get to and from the toilet (including commode, bedpan, and urinal), to cleanse after eliminating, and to adjust clothing.					
4. AMBULATION: Identify the consumer's physical ability to get around, both inside and outside, using mechanical aids if needed.					
5. TRANSFERRING: Identify the consumer's ability to transfer when in bed or wheelchair.					
6. PERSONAL HYGIENE: Identify the consumer's ability to shave, care for mouth, and comb hair.					

	None (1)	*Minimal (2)*	*Moderate (3)*	*Extensive (4)*	*Total (5)*
7. DRESSING: Identify the consumer's ability to dress and undress, including selection of clean clothing or appropriate seasonal clothing.					
8. BATHING: Identify the consumer's ability to bathe and wash hair.					
9. Access to transportation-identify the consumer's ability to get to and from stores, medical facilities, and other community activities, considering the ability both to access and use transportation.					
10. FINANCES: Identify the consumer's ability to handle paying bills, managing checking/ savings accounts, and overseeing other items which are part of a household budget.					
11. SHOPPING: Identify the consumer's ability to shop for food and personal items.					
12. LAUNDRY: Identify the consumer's ability to do own laundry either at home or at Laundromat.					

	None (1)	*Minimal (2)*	*Moderate (3)*	*Extensive (4)*	*Total (5)*
13. HOUSEWORK: Identify the consumer's ability to clean surfaces and furnishings in his/her living quarters, including dishes, floors, and bathroom fixtures, and disposing of household garbage.					
14. NIGHT NEEDS: Identify the consumer's need for assistance during the night.					
15. EMERGENCY RESPONSE: Identify the consumer's ability to recognize the need for and to seek emergency help.					
16. MEDICATION: Identify the consumer's ability/willingness to administer his/her own medication.					
17. SUPERVISION: Identify the consumer's ability to manage his/her life, including needs and activities.					

Source: Developed by the Idaho Department of Health and Welfare

Directions: Check the most appropriate box to indicate the amount of assistance required for the specific daily living skill: None, minimal, moderate, extensive, and total.

Detail medical history, emphasizing on the onset, type of stroke, cause, territory of the brain affected. Following which examination of patient to confirm the extent of involvement and examine the voluntary control in limbs. Thorough assessment of sensorimotor control is also mandatory. Few assessment scales are used as standard tools.

- Stream scoring.

- The brathel index.
- Functional independence measure (FIM)
- National Institute of Health Stroke Scale (NIHSS) worksheet.

FUNCTIONAL INDEPENDENT MEASURES

The functional independence measure scale assesses physical and cognitive disability. This scale focuses on the burden of care—that is, the level of disability indicating the burden of caring for them.

Scoring

Items are scored on the level of assistance required for an individual to perform activities of daily living. The scale includes 18 items, of which 13 items are physical domains based on the Barthel Index and 5 items are cognition items.

Each item is scored from 1 to 7 based on level of independence, where 1 represents total dependence and 7 indicates complete independence. The scale can be administered by a physician, nurse, therapist or layperson. Possible scores range from 18–126, with higher scores indicating more independence. Alternatively, 13 physical items could be scored separately from 5 cognitive items.

Time

It takes 1 hour to train a rater to use the FIM scale, and 30 minutes to score the scale for each patient.

Clinical Application

The FIM scale is used to measure the patient's progress and assess rehabilitation outcomes. This scale is useful in clinical settings of rehabilitation. The FIM was carefully designed and developed with the consensus of the US National Advisory Committee, with close attention to definitions, administration and reliability. Manuals, training and videos are provided (further information can be found at www.udsmr.org). The FIM has been used in a number of countries, including the USA, Canada, Australia, France, Japan, Sweden and Germany. Studies of large samples have been published, including a study of 93,829 subjects. The FIM has been used extensively in rehabilitation, including that for stroke and multiple sclerosis. Scores are responsive to change and also reflect the patient's discharge destination.

FIM AND FAM

The functional assessment measure (FAM) includes FIM items but also adds 12 new items, mainly covering cognition, such as community integration, emotional status, orientation, attention, reading and writing skills, and employability. The FIM scale on its own had ceiling effects, so the FAM was proposed, which extends the coverage of the FIM. This scale was originally intended for patients with brain injury, but is in fact useful in all rehabilitation settings. FIM + FAM is completed by a healthcare professional for the patient.

UK FIM + FAM

This scale was developed in the UK, and was last modified by the UK FIM + FAM Group in 1999. Some of the items used in the original FAM from the US Developmental Group in California were considered to be too vague. For this reason the UK version was developed after modification of the original FAM. The UK FIM + FAM Group was coordinated by the Regional Rehabilitation Unit at Northwick Park Hospital, Middlesex, UK. This group has improved the consistency of scoring. The original 30 items and 7 levels remain the same as in the original version.

UK FIM + FAM SCALE

Self-care

1. Eating
2. Grooming
3. Bathing/showering
4. Dressing upper body
5. Dressing lower body
6. Toileting
7. Swallowing.*

Sphincters

1. Bladder management
2. Bowel management

Mobility

1. Transfers: Bed/chair/wheelchair
2. Transfers: Toilet
3. Transfers: Bathtub/shower
4. Transfers: Car*
5. Locomotion: Walking/wheelchair
6. Locomotion: Stairs
7. Community mobility.*

Communication

1. Expression
2. Comprehension
3. Reading*
4. Writing*
5. Speech intelligibility.*

Psychosocial

1. Social interaction
2. Emotional status*
3. Adjustment to limitations*
4. Use of leisure time (replaces employability in original version).*

Cognition

1. Problem-solving
2. Memory
3. Orientation*
4. Concentration (replaces attention in original version)*
5. Safety awareness (replaces safety judgment in original version)*

*FAM items

Seven Levels for Each Item

Level	*Description*
7 Complete independence	Fully independent
6 Modified independence	Requiring the use of a device but no physical help
5 Supervision	Requiring only standby assistance or verbal prompting or help with set-up

Contd...

Contd...

Level	*Description*
4 Minimal assistance	Requiring incidental hands-on help only (subject performs >75% of the task)
3 Moderate assistance	Subject still performs 50–75% of the task
2 Maximal assistance	Subject provides less than half of the effort (25–49%)
1 Total assistance	Subject contributes <25% of the effort or is unable to do the task.

Scoring Principles

- Function is assessed on the basis of direct observation
- Admission scoring is done within 10 days of admission
- Discharge scoring is done during the last week before discharge
- Scoring is done by a multidisciplinary team member
- The subject is scored on what they actually do on a day-to-day basis, not on what they could do
- Do not leave any score blank
- Score 1 if the subject does not perform the activity at all, or if no information is available
- If function is variable, use the lower score.

FALLS RISK ASSESSMENT TOOLS

Falls in the elderly represent a complex phenomenon and are rarely due to a single cause. A variety of factors are associated with risk of falling among older adults, including the following:

- Physical factors such as history of previous falls, poor gait or balance, muscle, weakness, functional limitation, poor vision, arthritis, postural hypotension, sensory deterioration and neurological disorders
- Pharmaceutical factors—use of medications
- Psychiatric factors—cognitive impairment
- Environmental factors.

Assessment of falls risk may include the following:

- Use of multifactorial assessment tools that cover a range of falls risk factors.
- This could enable screening of high-risk populations and targeting of interventions

- Functional mobility assessments that focus on postural stability, including strength, balance, gait and reaction times.

Effective assessment of fall risk requires a holistic approach, and includes review of many complex and interconnected factors. Falls could be the result of one or more complex and interrelated physiological systems impairments as well as environmental factors. The falls risk increases rapidly with advancing age above 65 years. It is difficult to determine what factors affect balance and contributes to fall, and which factors could be addressed to reduce falls.

Choice of Tool

This is difficult. A variety of tools have been assessed and evaluated for their use in predicting falls risk. Different tools have been used in a variety of settings – for example, in the community, at home, and in long-term or acute care. Some of them have focused on balance and gait assessments, while others have focused on risk factors. Target populations within a given setting have varied in studies – for example, those with cognitive impairment, and studies limited to small samples or recurrent fallers. Few tools have been tested more than once in more than one setting. Therefore, no single falls risk assessment tool can be recommended for implementation in all settings.

The choice of tool in a particular clinical context should reflect the purpose for which that tool needs to be applied. For example, the screening of a high-risk population requires a tool that is quick and easy to use, with good sensitivity and specificity. If the aim is to reduce risk, the tool should be reliably able to Identify remedial risk factors which would allow for tailoring of interventions. Comprehensive medical assessment of fallers is the focus of the prevention of falls.

A systematic review of risk assessment tools for falls in hospitalized patients was published in 2004. The authors concluded that few well-validated tools have been described, and that even the best-validated tool could fail to predict a significant number of falls, as fallers are a heterogeneous group. However, a small number of readily detectable risk factors has been repeatedly identified in studies. Perhaps the key is to look for reversible falls risk factors in all patients. Currently, the use of falls risk assessment as part of a multifactorial approach to the prevention of falls is supported by evidence of a strong association between multiple risk factors and falls, and a significant reduction in falls can be achieved where assessment is combined with tailored interventions. Some of the tools for assessing risk of falling are described below.

GROSS MOTOR FUNCTION

Gross motor skills are the abilities usually acquired during infancy and early childhood as part of a child's motor development. By the time they reach two years of age, almost all children are able to stand up, walk and run, walk up stairs, etc. These skills are built upon, improved and better controlled throughout early childhood, and continue in refinement throughout most of the individual's years of development into adulthood. These gross movements come from large muscle groups and whole body movement. These skills develop in a head-to-toe order. The children will typically learn head control, trunk stability, and then standing up and walking (Humphrey).

Types of Motor Skills

Motor skills are movements and actions of the muscles. Typically, they are categorized into two groups: *gross motor skills* and *fine motor skills*. Gross motor skills are involved in movement and coordination of the arms, legs, and other large body parts and movements. They participate in actions such as running, crawling, swimming, etc. Fine motor skills are involved in smaller movements that occur in the wrists, hands, fingers, and the feet and toes. They participate in smaller actions such as picking up objects between the thumb and finger, writing carefully, and even blinking. These two motor skills work together to provide coordination.

Development of Posture

Gross motor skills, as well as many other activities, require postural control. Infants need to control the heads to stabilize their gaze and to track moving objects. They also must have strength and balance in their legs to walk. Newborn infants cannot voluntarily control their posture. Within a few weeks, though, they can hold their heads erect, and soon they can lift their heads while prone. By 2 months of age, babies can sit while supported on a lap or an infant seat, but sitting independently is not accomplished until 6 or 7 months of age.

Standing also develops gradually across the first year of life. By about 8 months of age, infants usually learn to pull themselves up and hold on to a chair, and they often can stand alone by about 10–12 months of age. There is a new device called a "Standing Dani" developed to help special needs children with their posture.

Walking upright requires being able to stand up and balance position from one foot to the other. Although infants usually learn to walk around the time of their first birthday, the neural pathways that control the leg alternation component of walking are in place from a very early age, possibly even at birth or before. This is shown because 1- to 2-month-olds are given support with their feet in contact with a motorized treadmill, they show well-coordinated, alternating steps. If it were not for the problem of switching balance from one foot to the other, babies could walk earlier. Tests were performed on crawling and walking babies where slopes were placed in front of the path and the babies had to decide whether or not it was safe. The tests proved that babies who just learned how to walk did not know what they were capable of and often went down slopes that were not safe, whereas experienced walkers knew what they could do. Practice has a big part to do with teaching a child how to walk. Vision does not have an effect on muscle growth but it could slow down the child's process of learning to walk. According to the nonprofit Blind Children Center, "Without special training, fully capable infants who are visually impaired may not learn to crawl or walk at an appropriate age and gross and fine motor skills will not properly develop." When the child is not able to see an object then there is no motivation for the child to try to reach for it. Therefore, they do not want to learn independently. Learning to walk is usually done by modeling others and watching them. The babies will imitate others, picking up the skills a lot faster than creating their own errors. Visually impaired children may need physical therapy to help them learn these gross motor skills faster. One hour of therapy each week is not enough so parents have to make sure they are involved in this process. The parent can help by telling the baby the direction of where the object is and encourage them to get it. You must have patience because every child has their own developmental schedule and it is even truer for the children with special needs. Focusing on the progress of your child is better than focusing on comparing your child to other children (Humphrey).

Infancy Development

It has been observed by scientists that motor skills generally develop from the center to the body outward and head to tail. Babies need to practice their skills; therefore they will grow and strengthen better. They need space and time to explore in their environment and use their muscles. "Tummy-time" is a good example of this. At first they are only able to lay their belly on the floor but by around two months they start to gain muscle to raise their head and chest off the ground. Some are also able to go on their elbows. They will also start to kick and bend their legs while lying there, this helps to prepare for crawling. By four months they are able to start to control their head and hold it steady while sitting up. Rolling from belly to back movements is started. At about five months the baby will start to wiggle their limbs to strengthen crawling muscles. Infants can start to sit up by themselves and put some weight on their legs as they hold onto something for support by six months. As they enter their first year caregivers needs to be more active. The babies will want to get into everything so the house needs to become 'baby proofed'. Babies are able to start to reach and play with their toys too. It is said that the use of baby walkers or devices that help to hold the baby upright are said to delay the process of walking. Research has been found that it delays developing the core torso strength, which can lead to different issues down in their future. Around 10 months they should be able to stand on their own. Throughout their years of life different motor skills are formed (Oswalt).

Development in the Second Year

Development in the second year of life, toddlers become more motorically skilled and mobile. They are no longer content with being in a playpen and want to move all over the place. Child development experts believe that motor activity during the second year is vital to the child's competent development and that few restrictions, except for safety, should be placed on their motoric adventures. By 13–18 months, toddlers can move up and down steps and carry toys. Once they reach the top of the stairs though, they are not able to get back down. They also begin to move from one position to another more smoothly. (Oswalt) By 18–24 months, can move quicker or run for a short distance along with other motor skills. They also start to walk backwards and in circles and begin to run. They can also not only walk up the stairs with their hands and feet but are now able to hold onto the handrail and walk up. Near the end of their second year, complex gross motor skills begin to develop including throwing and kicking. Their skills become more natural. Peddling a tricycle and jumping in place is acquired. At the end they are very mobile and can go from place to place. It is normal for them to get themselves into small situations that could be dangerous such as walking into the street because their brain can't send the information fast enough to their feet. Parents need to keep an eye on their children at all times (Oswalt).

Development of Children with Special Needs

Children with special needs who are as young as seven months can learn to drive a power wheelchair. This chair may decrease the rate of development of the child's gross motor skills, but there are ways to compensate for this. These children usually work with a physical therapist to help with their leg movements. Walkers and other devices are used to help aide this process and avoid obstacles. The negative side to this is that they are limited in their mobility. There is research out to find a device to encourage children to explore their environment while gaining their gross motor skills. This will also hopefully help them with their exercise.

Childhood

As a preschooler, the child does not need any help standing alone or moving quickly. At 3 years of age, children enjoy simple movements, such as hopping, jumping, and running back and forth, just for the sheer delight of performing these activities. A study was done to assess motor skill development and the overall rate and level of growth development. This study shows that at the preschool age children develop more goal-directed behaviors. This plays a big role, because their learning focuses around play and physical activity. While assessing the gross motor skills in children can be challenging, it is essential to do so in order to ensure that children are prepared to interact with the environment they live in. Different tests are given to these children to measure their skill level. At age 4, children continue to do the same actions as they did at age 3, but further their moving. They are beginning to be able to go down the stairs with one foot on each step. At 5 years of age, they become even more adventurous. During middle and late childhood, children's motor development becomes much smoother and more coordinated than it was in early childhood. As they age, children become able to have control over their bodies and have an increased attention span . Having a child in a sport can help them with their coordination , as well as some social aspects. Teachers will suggest that their students may need occupational therapists in different situations. Students could get frustrated doing writing exercises if they are having difficulties with their writing skills. It also may affect the teacher because it is illegible. Some children also may have reports of their "hands getting tired". There are many occupational therapists out there today to give students the help they need. These therapists were once used when something was seriously wrong with your child but now they are used to help children be the best they can be.

Adolescence and Adulthood

Between the ages of 7 and 12 there is an increase in running speed and are able to skip. Jumping is also acquired better and there is an increase in throwing and kicking. They are able to bat and dribble a ball. (Age) Gross motor skills usually continue improving during adolescence. The peak of physical performance is before 30, between 18 and 26. Even though athletes keep getting better than their predecessors—running faster, jumping higher, and lifting more weight—the age at which they reach their peak performance has remained virtually the same. After age 30, most functions begin to decline. Older adults move slower than younger adults. This can be moving from one place to another or continually moving. Exercising regularly and maintaining a healthy lifestyle can slow this process. Aging individuals who are active and biologically healthy perform motor skills at a higher level than their less active, less healthy aging counterparts.

PEDIATRIC EVALUATION OF DISABILITY INVENTORY (PEDI)

The original pediatric evaluation of disability inventory (PEDI) is a descriptive measure of a child's current functional performance and can track changes over time. The PEDI measures both capability and performance of functional activities in three content domains:

- Self-care
- Mobility
- Social function.

It can be used as a comprehensive clinical assessment of key functional capabilities and performance in children between the ages of six months and seven years. The PEDI™ can be used to evaluate older children with functional abilities that are less than those expected of a 7-year-old child without disabilities.

The Pediatric Evaluation of Disability Inventory (PEDI) is an instrument with which functional status can be measured in children aged between 6 months and 90 months (7.5 years). Functional status is the extent to which a child is independent of his parents in performing daily activities. The authors, Haley, Coster, Ludlow, Haltiwanger and Andrellos, stress the importance of using functional outcome measures because functional measures are consistent with treatment goals and functional measures emphasize independence, not normality. The PEDI is based on an adaptation of the conceptual hierarchy of outcomes defined by the ICIDH, in 1990 the leading classification system of disability and health, provided by the World Health Organization (WHO). In the adapted model the concept of 'functional limitations' is added to bridge the gap between impairments and disability. Functional limitations refer to limitations that affect the ability to perform normal daily activities, whereas disability refers to problems in the performance of those daily activities. The model has been made suitable for use in pediatric rehabilitation by adding a developmental and a contextual framework. In the actual International Classification of Functioning, Disability and Health (ICF), these constructs are also incorporated, in the 'activities' component of this classification. Performance depends on the capabilities of the child: when a child does not have sufficient skills no independent performance is possible and the child needs assistance of their parents. Furthermore, performance depends on the physical and social environment the child lives in. This environment provides opportunities for the acquirement of the skills needed for an independent performance, but also has to give the child the chance of performing independently when he masters the necessary skills. The PEDI contains items to measure functional capability, and also items to measure the performance in three content domains: Self Care (SC), Mobility (M) and Social Function (SF). Capability is measured by the assessment of the functional skills of which the child has shown mastery. These skills are rated in the Functional Skills Scales (FSS) and provide sufficient detail to identify clinical patterns of deficiencies in functional skill attainment. Actual performance is measured in the Caregiver Assistance Scales (CAS) by the extent of help a parent gives in daily functioning. Therefore, the CAS is an indirect measure of capability, whereas the FSS is a direct measure. The CAS provides additional information to the results of the FSS: when children have mastered certain skills, this does not mean that they use those skills in actual performance. The Modifications Scale (MS) is a frequency count of the type and extent of environmental modifications that support functional performance. Table 24.1 gives an overview of the content of the PEDI.

The PEDI was designed to use as an instrument:

- To detect a functional deficit or delay, and if that exists, the extent and content
- Area of the delay or deficit
- To evaluate individual or group progress in pediatric rehabilitation
- To evaluate programs in pediatric rehabilitation.
- Administration of the PEDI can be done by professional judgment of a therapist or by structured interview and parent report. The PEDI can be used for children with various types of congenital and acquired disorders, and the authors believe that the PEDI is most appropriate for measuring functional status in children with moderate or severe physical or combined physical and cognitive disabilities.

Measurement Scales and Summary Scores

The items in the FSS are discrete and are accompanied by scoring criteria and sometimes examples of behavior to help clarify scoring decisions. The items can be scored 0 or 1.

0 = unable or limited in capability to perform item in most situations

1 = capable of performing item in most situations, or item has been previously mastered and functional skills have progressed beyond this level.

TABLE 24.1: Contents of PEDI

Domains	*Functional skills scale*		*Caregiver assistance scale Modifications scale*
	Subscales	*Number of items*	
Self-care	• Types of food textures • Use of utensils • Use of drinking containers • Tooth brushing • Hair brushing • Nose care • Hand washing • Washing body and face • Pullover/front-opening garments • Fasteners • Pants • Shoes/socks • Toileting task • Management of bladder • Management of bowel	4 5 5 5 4 5 5 5 5 5 5 5 5	Eating Grooming Bathing Dressing upper body Dressing lower body Toileting Bladder management Bowel management
Mobility	• Toilet transfers • • Chair/Wheelchair transfers • Car transfers • Bed mobility/transfers • • Tub transfers • Indoor locomotion methods • Indoor locomotion—distance/speed • Indoor locomotion—pulls/carries objects • Outdoor locomotion methods • Outdoor locomotion—distance/speed • Outdoor surfaces • Upstairs • Downstairs	5 5 5 4 5 3 5 5 2 5 5 5 5	Chair and toilet transfer Car transfers Bed mobility/transfers Tub transfers Indoor locomotion Outdoor locomotion Stairs

Contd...

Contd...

Domains	*Functional skills scale*		*Caregiver assistance scale Modifications scale*
	Subscales	*Number of items*	
Social function	• Comprehension of word meanings • Comprehension of sentence • Complexity • Functional use of communication • Complexity of expressive communication • Problem-resolution • Social interactive play (adults) • Peer interactions (child of similar age) • Play with objects • Self-information • Time orientation • Self-protection • Community function	5 5 5 5 5 5 5 5 5 5 5 5	Functional comprehension Functional expression Joint problem-solving Peer play Safety

The CAS assesses the amount of help the child receives to complete a complex functional activity using a six-point ordinal scale.

0 = total assistance: child totally depends on the caregiver.

1 = maximal assistance: caregiver does more than half the effort needed for performance, but the child does provide some meaningful assistance.

2 = moderate assistance: child does more than half the effort, but the caregiver provides substantial assistance.

3 = minimal assistance: child does more than half the effort, the caregiver provides some assistance.

4 = supervision: caregiver does not provide physical assistance, but supervises the performance.

5 = independent: child performs the activity independent of the caregiver.

The MS is not a measurement scale but a frequency count of types of Modification required in performing the activity under ordinary circumstances:

N = no modifications.

C = child-oriented modifications, commonly used, nonspecialized equipment.

R = rehabilitation equipment, equipment normally not needed by non-disabled children.

E = extensive modifications such as a wheelchair or major architectural alterations.

The manual of the American PEDI describes two kinds of summary scores:

Normative Standard Scores and Scaled Scores. The Normative Standard Scores are transformed scores that depend on the age of the child: with these scores discrimination between children with and without disabilities is possible. For each age group, the scores have a mean of 50 and a standard deviation of 10, therefore a normative standard score can be directly interpreted in terms of deviation from the mean score in that age group. Scaled Scores give an indication of functional performance independent of age. The Scaled Scores vary from 0–100: 0 means that a child is not capable of performing even the easiest item, 100 means that the child has mastered all the items. Finally, with the aid of a computer program, goodness-of-fit tests can be computed in the original PEDI, to see whether the development of a child is consistent with the development of non-disabled children with the same raw score. There is an absence of fit when a child is capable of performing relatively difficult items but not capable of performing relatively easy items, a score pattern typically seen in children with particular disabilities.

CHAPTER

25

Home Exercise Program for Various Physiotherapy Conditions

HOME EXERCISE PROGRAM FOR CARDIAC REHABILITATION

A home exercise walking program has been planned for you to help you safely increase your strength during your recovery period.

- Begin your walking program the day after your discharge from the hospital
- Make sure you are well-rested; plan to walk at least 1 hour after a meal
- Walk at a comfortable pace; you should be able to carry on a conversation without feeling short of breath; the walk should feel easy to somewhat hard at the most
- Walk for a specific amount of time; start with three to five minutes, four times per day; increase the amount of time walked as tolerated
- Continue your walking program until you start phase II cardiac rehabilitation.

General Instructions for Exercise

- Wear loose, comfortable clothing
- Wait one hour after eating to exercise
- Do not exercise if you are experiencing symptoms of a cold, fever, flu or an increase in your heart-related symptoms; your body needs energy to overcome an illness.

- Breathe in a slow, deep and rhythmic manner while exercising; never hold your breath
- Shoes should fit properly, offer good support and be comfortable; rubber-soled shoes are recommended
- Be certain to take all your medications as prescribed
- Get in the habit of practicing relaxation techniques; these are helpful in reducing blood pressure and heart rate
- There is no best time to exercise
  - Review your daily routine and decide what time will be best for you
  - Do not pick a time that will be difficult for you to exercise
- Avoid exercise when the weather is extreme
  - High heat and humidity can interfere with your body's ability to cool off
  - An excessive rise in your body temperature can increase your heart rate, blood pressure and oxygen usage; the same principle applies to excessively cold and windy days.

Exercise Precautions

1. Walk indoors during the first few days at home; when walking outdoors, pay attention to the temperature, humidity and wind-chill factors
   - <20° Fahrenheit—exercise indoors
   - 30–70° Fahrenheit—ideal
   - 70–80° Fahrenheit with <60% humidity—exercise with caution; drink plenty of water
   - 80° Fahrenheit with >60% humidity—exercise in air conditioned area.
2. Avoid home exercise equipment
3. Avoid hills and rugged terrain
4. Consider walking with a partner in the first few weeks or carry a cell phone for safety purposes
5. Stop and rest if you experience:
   - Shortness of breath
   - Unusual pain or discomfort
   - Angina or chest pain
   - Nausea or vomiting
   - Light-headedness or dizziness
   - Palpitations or fast heartbeat
   - Extreme fatigue
   - Call your cardiologist if these symptoms persist.

HOME EXERCISE PROGRAM FOR MANAGEMENT OF CERVICAL SPONDYLOSIS

Spondylosis is a disorder that is caused by the degeneration of the discs which are soft cushions, present between the vertebrae. This results in the vertebrae rubbing together and exerting pressure on the nerves. As the condition progresses, the bones may move out of their natural positions, causing pain and disability.

1. Sleeping posture: Use firm mattress and keep your head at level. Use pillows which do not bend the back more than 15 degrees. Do not sleep on your stomach. It extends the neck. Sleep on your back or on your side.
2. Motion exercises:
   - Motion exercises slowly turn your head to the right until it hurts, hold, and return it to the center. Do the same to the left.
   - Drop your chin down slowly towards your chest, hold, and relax. Bring your head backup.
   - Tilt your head straight over towards your left ear, hold, and return it to the center. Do the same on the right side. Tilt your head backwards so you can see the ceiling, hold, then bring your head back down.
3. Isometric exercises:
   - Do not hold your breath as you do these. For each exercise, press for 5–6 counts, then relax. Press your forehead into your palms. Resist any motion.
   - Press your hand against the side of your head. Try to bring your ear to the shoulder, but resist any motion.
   - Press both hands against the back of your head. Try to pull your head up, but resist any motion.
   - Press your hand against your temple. Try to turn your chin to your shoulder, but resist any motion. You can do all these exercises 5 times each twice a day.
4. Cervical collar: When exercises don't help and pain worsens, the doctor may ask the patient to use cervical collar to restrict neck movements and reduce pain.
5. Neck traction: In some cases, neck traction may also be suggested in addition to the cervical collar.
6. Surgical decompression: Surgical decompression of the spinal cord in the neck may be required in severe cases if there is loss of movement, sensation or function.

7. Heat or ice: Applying heat or ice to your neck can ease sore neck muscles.
8. Soft neck brace: The brace allows your neck muscles to rest. However, a neck brace should be worn for only short periods of time because it can eventually weaken neck muscles.

HOME EXERCISE PROGRAM FOR ROTATOR CUFF INJURY

This program is broken up into three parts:

Range of motion: You should do this every day to help get your motion back.

Flexibility: You should do this every day to help stretch tight tissues.

Strengthening: You should do this 3 or 4 days each week to help get your strength back.

For most of the exercises you will do a certain number of repetitions (or reps) and a certain number of sets. Example: 3 sets/10 reps

Set 1: Do the exercise 10 times and then rest for a few seconds

Set 2: Do the exercise 10 times and then rest for a few seconds

Set 3: Do the exercise 10 times and then rest for a few seconds. Then move onto the next exercise.

Range of Motion Exercises

Do these every day.

Pendulum Exercises

Move your body and let the movement of your body move your shoulder. Example: Rest your good hand on a table and bend over a little at your waist. Make circles with your hips/body which will cause your injured arm to make circles. Repeat this by moving your hips/body in different directions. Do not use your shoulder muscles. Do each motion 20 times.

Let the injured arm hang over the side of the table. Make 20 small circles in one direction and then 20 small circles in the other direction. Make forward and backward motions 20 times and then side to side motions 20 times.

Posture Exercises

These exercises should be done within the pain free range. In other words you should not have any pain while doing these exercises. Do this exercise 20 times—put your hands on your hips, lean back and hold for 20 seconds.

Active Assisted Range of Motion

Use a cane/broomstick/pulley system so the good arm moves the injured arm.

Do 3 sets/10 reps for each exercise.

Lying on your back, hold the cane with both hands. Raise your arms using the good arm to help guide the injured arm. Next use the good arm to move the injured arm to the side. Lastly, use the good arm to move the injured arm up to the side and up. You may start to use your injured arm more as it starts to feel more comfortable. Again as you start to feel more comfortable you can also do these standing up.

Active Training of the Scapula Muscles

Two exercises are shoulder shrugs and pinching your shoulder blades.

Do 3 sets/10 reps for each exercise—Shoulder shrugs: Pull shoulders up and back and hold. Pinch the back of the shoulder blades together using good posture.

Chair Press

Do 3 sets/10 reps. While seated put your hands on the seat or on the arm rests. Then press down with your arms, lifting your body off chair. Try to keep your back straight.

Shrugs

Like the shoulder shrugs. Except this time you use weights. Do 3 sets/10 reps—stand with weights in hands. Roll shoulders back and hold.

Press Up

Do 3 sets/10 reps—lie on back, elbow locked straight, arms stretched up towards the ceiling with weights in hands. Move/push arms up towards the ceiling as far as possible.

Pushup Plus

Do 3 sets/10 reps—do a pushup (either on your hands or forearms) and then really push to bring your spine to the ceiling. Kneeling on the floor, place your hands or forearms on the floor. Start by doing a pushup, then round your back. Really push to try to touch your spine to the ceiling.

Posterior Deltoid

Do 3 sets/10 reps—lying on your stomach hang your arm over the side of the bed or couch. While holding a weight, bring the arm out to the side and hold for 20 seconds.

Flexibility

Do these every day.

Hold each stretch for 30 seconds and rest for about 10 seconds in between. Repeat five times per day.

Door Stretch

Place your hands or forearms at shoulder level on each side of a door frame or in a corner of a room. Lean forward into door or corner and hold. Next place your hands or forearms over your head on each side of the door, lean forward and hold.

Sleeper Stretch

On a flat surface lie on your side with your injured shoulder down. Raise your arm to shoulder height and then bend your elbow. Use your good arm to push your forearm (of the injured shoulder) down towards the floor or bed.

Golfer Stretch

Bring the injured arm across in front of body. Hold elbow with other arm. Gently pull your forearm (of your good arm) towards your chest/ face which will pull the injured arm across chest until a stretch is felt in the back of shoulder.

Towel Stretch

Place the hand of your good arm behind your neck and the hand of the injured shoulder by your back pocket. Grab a towel with both hands.

Use the good arm to pull upward, bringing the injured arm up the back. Hold your good arm over shoulder with towel as shown. Grasp the towel with your injured arm. Slowly pull upward with your good arm until a gentle stretch is felt.

Strengthening

Do these 3 to 4 times per week

- Repetitions and/or resistance can be increased as tolerated
- Be sure to use good form
- If you have moderate or severe discomfort reduce the level of resistance or decrease the range of the exercise until it is comfortable.

Rotator Cuff Strengthening

Isometrics against a wall

Do 3 sets/10 reps—press the outside of your forearm against a wall for 20 seconds (Relax).

Next press the inside of your forearm against a wall for 20 seconds. Relax.

Internal/External Rotation against Resistance

Stand up when using elastic bands or lie on side to use hand weights. If you are using elastic bands please tie them to a doorknob in order to secure them. Keep the arm against the body. Internally rotate against resistance for internal rotation. Externally rotate against resistance for external rotation. Do 3 sets/10 reps.

Secure elastic at waist level. Hold elbow at 90° with arm at side. Pull hand away from the body. Secure elastic at waist level. Hold elbow at 90° arm at side. Pull hand across body. Or Lie on injured side, elbow bent at 90°, arm at side. With or without weight, pull hand towards your belly. Lie on side, injured side up. Arm at side, elbow bent, with or without weight, move hand away from your belly.

Jackins' Exercises

If you have a hard time raising your arm, you should try these Jackins' exercises. Do 3 sets/10 reps. for each exercise—begin by lying flat on your back. While lying on your back lift your injured arm over your head, using your good arm to help. Once this gets easier, try raising the injured arm by itself. Once this gets easier, try raising the injured arm with a small weight in your hand. Once this gets easier raise your back by resting on pillows or sitting in a recliner and start the whole process over. Keep raising your back and starting the process over again until you are standing straight up.

Low Trapezius Exercise

Do 3 sets/10 reps—stand straight up. Grab the elastic bands with both hands. Keep elbows straight and pull your arms backwards, trying to reach behind you.

HOME EXERCISE PROGRAM FOR OSTEOARTHRITIS

Exercise Program Components

The exercise intervention has designed to include multiple components that would address the individual features of dysfunction associated with knee osteoarthritis and collectively improve the functional capacity and pain of the patients. The main areas of dysfunction addressed were muscle weakness, muscle fatigue, reduced locomotor function and reduced balance. The exercise program was designed to address recommended goals of treatment:

- Reduction of impairment and improvement of function
- Protection of the joint by reducing stress on the joint, attenuating joint forces and improving biomechanics
- Prevention of disability and poor health secondary to inactivity by increasing daily physical activity.

Muscle weakness was addressed by including muscle strengthening exercises.

- Sitting to standing: this exercise involved the patient rising from sitting to standing and then lowering themselves gently back to the chair seat. This exercise was repeated to a number of repetitions. The number of repetitions was determined at initial assessment.
- While standing, the patient contracted the quadriceps femoris muscle group maximally and held the contraction for a period determined at initial assessment.
- While sitting, the patient extended the knee from 90° of flexion to the maximum degree of extension they could obtain and held the

leg in this position for 10 seconds. The knee was then slowly flexed to 90°. The number of repetitions was determined at assessment.

Muscle fatigue was addressed by the performance of a muscular endurance exercise. This involved the patient rising from a seated position to a position of approximately 45° of knee flexion. The patients then held that position by maintaining isometric tension in the lower limb extensors for a period determined at initial assessment.

Range of movement increase was addressed by the performance of three stretches.

- An anterior thigh and hip stretch was obtained by gentle translation of the pelvis anteriorly, while standing. This maneuver stretches the anterior thigh, rectus femoris muscle and hip of the posteriorly placed leg, while also stretching the calves and ankles.
- A posterior calf stretch was obtained by gently flexing the knees while standing, ensuring that the heels remained in contact with the floor.
- A posterior stretch of the knee was obtained by contracting the quadriceps femoris group while standing, thus generating an extension moment to place tension on the posterior knee musculature, joint capsule and ligaments.

Standing balance was addressed by patient standing on one leg (close to a supporting surface), thereby placing themselves in a situation requiring increased conscious balance control and integration. The number of times that balance was lost was recorded by patients while they performed the exercise for 2 minutes.

HOME EXERCISES FOR TREATING FROZEN SHOULDER SYNDROME

Shoulder exercises are generally recommended to regain mobility and range of motion. Physical therapy maneuvers and exercises are especially effective in stiffness stage and recovery stage. Some of the best exercises for frozen shoulder syndrome suggested by healthcare providers are discuss below:

Shoulder Abduction

- Physical therapist suggests active-passive exercises to restore joint range of motion. A variety of pulley exercises are devised by Dr Phil for such patients like shoulder abduction.
- Attach a pulley to a door (as high and as secure as possible)

- Use a chair or stool with your back facing the door and grasp the two ends of the pulley with your both hands
- Now extend your injured arm using pulley handle as fulcrum to the side of your body while using the non-injured arm as your overhead support
- Now pull down the non-injured arm to the side of your body while extending and lifting the injured arm overhead
- Repeat the exercise for 10 minutes twice a day

This exercise is helpful in restoring full range of motion with minimal pain and discomfort.

Shoulder External Rotation

The basic principle of all shoulder exercises in adhesive capsulitis or frozen shoulder syndrome is to improve the range of motion by allowing passive movements with minimal discomfort. Moreover, since the weight of upper body is supported by the pulleys, the movements are less stressful for the body that helps in directing all the force towards the joint components.

- For this exercise, secure the pulley around the door knob and extend your elbows while keeping your forearms parallel to the ground level
- With gentle traction on injured arm, stretch your non-injured arm and rotate the pulley strings between two arms alternately.

The benefit of this exercise is loosening of ligaments that control rotatory motion of shoulder joint.

Shoulder Flexion

It is very important to perform all the shoulder stretching exercises with your elbows fully extended. This exercise involves securing a pulley on top of a door or with a hook on wall.

- Once pulley is secure, stand straight with your back supported by the wall
- Now using pulley handle, lift your normal arm in the air in full-extended motion, while your injured arm is stretched by the side of your body (shoulder joint is flexed in this position)
- Hold the position for a few seconds and extend your injured arm overhead while your normal arm is stretched by the side of your body

- Repeat the exercise for a few minutes every day at periodic intervals.

This exercise helps in decreasing stiffness by promoting joint activity in vertical motion.

Arm Circles

Arm circle is a common fitness exercise that is often advised to athletes to improve their overall range of motion. Instructions are simple and benefits are immense and almost immediate.

- Lie down on a flat horizontal surface-like a table on your right side
- Place your left hand on your left shoulder and try to make small circles in the air
- Start off by making small circles and gradually increase the size and circumference of the circle by using elbow joint as the center point of focus
- After making at least 20 clockwise circles, make 20 counter-clockwise circles
- Repeat the activity with right side

The most wonderful benefit of this exercise is increased flow of blood across the joint capsule and tissues that increase the pace of healing.

Back Clasp

Black clasp is another exercise that primarily aims at improving the flexibility of shoulder muscles and joint ligaments. It ensures pain-free movements and to restore full range of motion.

- Stand straight with your legs wide apart
- Next step is to use your hands and clasp on your back
- Stabilize your arm and slowly raise the arms over your head
- Stop the arm movement at the point of maximum resistance and hold your position for 30 seconds

Start from the base-level again and you will see that slowly your range of motion has increased by the time you are done with the exercise (at least for 5–8 minutes thrice a day).

Wall Climbing

Wall climbing is an exercise or recreational activity that allows your shoulders to work in synchronous motion with the rest of your upper limb components. Since, it is also a recreational activity, you may be able to work up your joint apparatus for a longer period of time without conscious perception.

- Stand straight with your legs wide apart
- Now use your fingers to crawl or climb the wall and as you move up, stop and hold the position at every 6 inch to feel the grip
- Discontinue when you begin to feel pain.

THE ROLE OF PHYSICAL THERAPY FOR HERNIATED DISK

Physical therapy with a trained professional may be useful if pain has not improved after 3–4 weeks. It is important for any person who has chronic low back pain to have an exercise program. Professionals who understand the limitations and special needs of back pain, and can address individual health conditions, should guide this program. One study indicated that patients who planned their own exercise program did worse than those in physical therapy or doctor-directed programs.

Physical therapy typically includes the following:

- Education and training the patient in correct movement
- Exercises to help the patient keep the spine in neutral positions during all daily activities
- Incorrect movements or long-term high-impact exercise is often a cause of back pain in the first place. People vulnerable to back pain should avoid activities that put undue stress on the lower back or require sudden twisting movements, such as football, golf, ballet, and weight lifting
- Exercises performed after a simple discectomy do not seem to provide much added benefit over time
- Specific and regular exercise under the guidance of a trained professional is important for reducing pain and improving function, although patients often find it difficult to maintain therapy.

Exercise and Acute or Sub-acute Back Pain

- Exercise does not help acute back pain. In fact, overexertion may cause further harm. Beginning after 4–8 weeks of pain, however, a rehabilitation program may benefit the patient.
- An incremental aerobic exercise program (such as walking, stationary biking, and swimming) may begin within 2 weeks of

symptoms. Jogging is usually not recommended, at least not until the pain is gone and muscles are stronger.

- Patients should avoid exercises that put the lower back under pressure until the back muscles are well-toned. Such exercises include leg lifts done in a facedown position, straight leg sit-ups, and leg curls using exercise equipment.
- In all cases, patients should never force themselves to exercise if, by doing so, the pain increases.

Exercise and Chronic Back Pain

- Exercise plays a very beneficial role in chronic back pain. Repetition is the key to increasing flexibility, building endurance, and strengthening the specific muscles needed to support and neutralize the spine. Exercise should be considered as part of a broader program to return to normal home, work, and social activities. In this way, the positive benefits of exercise not only affect strength and flexibility but also alter and improve patients' attitudes toward their disability and pain. Exercise may also be effective when combined with a psychological and motivational program, such as cognitive-behavioral therapy.
- There are different types of back pain exercises. Stretching exercises work best for reducing pain, while strengthening exercises are best for improving function.

Exercises for Back Pain Include

- Low impact aerobic exercises: Such as swimming, bicycling, and walking can strengthen muscles in the abdomen and back without over-straining the back. Programs that use strengthening exercises while swimming may be a particularly beneficial approach for many patients with back pain. Medical research has shown that pregnant women who engaged in a water gymnastics program have less back pain and are able to continue working longer.
- Spine stabilization and strength training: Exercises called lumbar extension strength training are proving to be effective. Generally, these exercises attempt to strengthen the abdomen, improve lower back mobility, strength, and endurance, and enhance flexibility in the hip, the hamstring muscles, and the tendons at the back of the thigh.

- Yoga, Tai Chi, Chi Kung: Practices originating in Asia that combine low-impact physical movements and meditation may be very helpful. They are designed to achieve a physical and mental balance and can be very helpful in preventing recurrences of low back pain.
- Flexibility exercises: It may help to reduce pain. A stretching program may work best when combined with strengthening exercises.

Specific Exercises for Low Back Strength

Perform the following exercises at least three times a week:

- Partial Sit-ups: Partial sit-ups or crunches strengthen the abdominal muscles
- Keep the knees bent and the lower back flat on the floor while raising the shoulders up 3–6 inches
- Exhale on the way up, and inhale on the way down
- Perform this exercise slowly 8–10 times with the arms across the chest
- Pelvic tilt: The pelvic tilt alleviates tight or fatigued lower back muscles
- Lie on the back with the knees bent and feet flat on the floor
- Tighten the buttocks and abdomen so that they tip up slightly
- Press the lower back to the floor, hold for 1 second, and then relax
- Be sure to breathe evenly
- Over time increase this exercise until it is held for 5 seconds. Then, extend the legs a little more so that the feet are further away from the body and try it again
- Stretching lower-back muscles. The following are three exercises for stretching the lower back:
  - Lie on the back with knees bent and legs together. Keeping arms at the sides, slowly roll the knees over to one side until totally relaxed. Hold this position for about 20 seconds (while breathing evenly) and then repeat on the other side.
  - Lying on the back, hold one knee and pull it gently toward the chest. Hold for 20 seconds. Repeat with the other knee.
  - While supported on hands and knees, lift and straighten right hand and left leg at the same time. Hold for 3 seconds while tightening the abdominal muscles. The back should be straight. Alternate with the other arm and leg and repeat on each side 8–20 times.

Note: No one with low back pain should perform exercises that require bending over right after getting up in the morning. At that time, the disks are more fluid-filled and more vulnerable to pressure from this movement.

EXERCISE PROGRAM FOR RHEUMATID ARTHRITIS

Physically active individuals are healthier, happier and live longer than those who are inactive and unfit. This is especially true for people with arthritis. Yet, arthritis is one of the most common reasons people give for limiting physical activity and recreational pursuits. Inactivity, in addition to arthritis-related problems, can result in a variety of health risks, including Type II diabetes, cardiovascular disease and osteoporosis.

In addition, decreased pain tolerance, weak muscles, stiff joints and poor balance common to many forms of arthritis can be made worse by inactivity. For many older people with arthritis, joint and muscle changes due to aging can make matters worse. Therefore, for the person with arthritis, the right kind of exercise is very important.

Fast Facts

Physical activity is made up of daily tasks, both occupational and leisure activities that are usually affected by arthritis. Exercise or planned physical activity then becomes that much more important.

People with arthritis who exercise regularly have less pain, more energy, improved sleep and better day-to-day function.

Starting off slowly with a few, low-intensity exercises will help to ensure a safe and successful exercise program.

What Exercises are Helpful and Safe?

Aquatic exercise is a safe form of aerobic exercise.

The three main levels of exercise are:

1. Therapeutic/rehabilitative
2. Recreational/leisure and
3. Competitive/elite. Finding the right balance is key.

Therapeutic/Rehabilitative

Therapeutic exercises, prescribed by health professionals, address specific joints or body parts affected by the arthritis or arthritis-related surgery. A therapeutic exercise program is often a necessary first step for individuals who have been inactive, have restricted joint motion or muscle strength, are experiencing joint paint or are recovering from surgery such as a joint replacement.

Recreational/Leisure

Recreational or leisure activities can range from walking and swimming to cross country skiing and running. Appropriate forms are those that can be done in a controlled and safe manner, have little risk of injury, and place little stress and loads on affected joints. In most cases, participating in recreational exercise does not do away with the need for therapeutic exercises.

Competitive/Elite

Competitive or elite level activities are performed at higher intensities, for longer durations and require greater skill and training. There are limited reports of people with arthritis continuing or returning to a competitive level of sport participation. However, as a general rule, exercising at this level is not recommended for individuals with inflammatory arthritis or with joint problems that may be adversely affected by the sporting activity (e.g. marathon running with hip or knee arthritis). If you have mild or early arthritis and wish to continue exercising at this level, first talk to your rheumatologist or a physical therapist who has experience in arthritis and knowledge of the specific sport.

Who should Exercise?

Everyone! Research shows that people with many forms of arthritis can participate safely in appropriate, regular exercise. Long-term studies have shown that even people with inflammatory arthritis such as rheumatoid arthritis (RA) can benefit from moderate intensity, weight-bearing activity. Other benefits include less bone loss and small-joint damage associated with RA and no increase in pain or disease activity. For individuals with osteoarthritis (OA) in the knee or elsewhere, research suggests programs that combine strengthening and aerobic exercise, reduce symptoms, improve joint motion and function, enhance coordination and balance, and control body weight. Regular moderate exercise even has been found to improve cartilage health in individuals at risk for developing knee OA. Having weak thigh muscles (quadriceps) is a risk factor for both developing OA in the knee and having greater disability.

What Exercises are Best?

There are four major types of exercise that make up all exercise programs, regardless of the level of participation. Each can have a positive effect on reducing arthritis-related pain and disability.

Flexibility Exercises

Both range-of-motion (ROM) and stretching exercises help to maintain or improve the flexibility in affected joints and surrounding muscles. This contributes to better posture, reduced risk of injuries and improved function.

ROM exercises usually are performed 5–10 times on a daily basis. People with RA may find doing ROM exercises in the evening helps reduce joint stiffness the next morning. It is recommended that stretching exercises be done at least 3 days a week with each stretch being held for about 30 seconds.

While ROM exercises are more common in therapeutic programs, stretching activities are important in all levels of exercise. Recreational activities such as yoga incorporate both ROM and stretching movements into their routines.

Strengthening exercises: These more vigorous exercises are designed to work muscles a bit harder. As the muscle becomes stronger, it provides greater joint support and helps reduce loading and stress through the painful joint. Strong muscles, which also contribute to better function, help reduce bone loss related to inactivity, some forms of inflammatory arthritis and the use of certain medications (corticosteroids).

One set of 8–10 exercises for the major muscle groups of the body 2-3 times a week is recommended. Most persons should complete 8–12 repetitions of each exercise. Older individuals may find that 10–15 repetitions with less resistance are more appropriate. The resistance or weight needs to be of sufficient intensity to challenge the muscles without increasing joint pain. Resistance can take the form of lifting a limb against gravity, using hand-held weights or elastic bands, or pushing/pulling against resistance using a weight machine. Even movement against water can provide resistance when done at faster speeds. Gradually increase the amount or form of resistance for ongoing improvements in strength.

Aerobic exercises: Also referred to as cardiorespiratory conditioning, these exercises include activities that use the large muscles of the body in a repetitive and rhythmic manner. Aerobic exercise improves heart, lung and muscle function. For people with arthritis, this type of exercise has benefits for weight control, mood, sleep and general health.

Safe forms of aerobic exercise include walking, aerobic dance, aquatic exercise, bicycling or exercising on equipment such as stationary bikes, treadmills or elliptical trainers. Daily tasks and leisure activities such as mowing the lawn, raking leaves, playing golf or walking the dog also are aerobic if carried out at a moderate intensity level.

Current recommendations for aerobic activity are, to do 150 minutes of moderate intensity exercise a week, preferably spread out over several days. You can accumulate this amount of exercise in several 10-minute bouts over the course of the day or week for similar health benefits as sustained exercise sessions. This provides greater options in scheduling aerobic exercise sessions, and allows those individuals with greater pain and fatigue to do shorter sessions within their personal tolerance level. Moderate intensity is the safest and most effective exertion level for aerobic exercise. This means the exerciser can speak normally (Talk Test), doesn't get short of breath or over-heated, and can carry on the activity for a sustained period of time in comfort.

Body awareness exercises: A fourth—and less recognized, though very important—group of exercises is referred to together as body awareness exercises. These include activities to improve posture, balance, joint position sense (proprioception), coordination and relaxation. While some of these improvements can be achieved through the first 3 types of exercise, problems in these areas often require different exercises. Tai chi and yoga are examples of recreational exercises that incorporate elements of body awareness.

When a joint and its surrounding muscles are affected by arthritis, or if a joint has been replaced, the result is often impaired coordination, position awareness, balance and an increased risk of falling. A health professional experienced in arthritis exercise prescription can determine which of these exercises will help improve your overall functioning and reduce the risk of injury.

Tai chi and yoga are examples of a recreational exercise that incorporates elements of body awareness.

When to Exercise?

Finding the right time of day to exercise will help you establish a routine and obtain the greatest benefits. For those with a lot of morning stiffness, gentle ROM exercises may be helpful, but getting to a fitness class may be too difficult. If fatigue is a problem, breaking up the exercise program into several short bouts during the day may be more manageable. Trouble sleeping at night? Avoid doing aerobic exercises within 2 hours of bedtime; however, stretching and relaxation exercises may help with sleep.

It is important to be aware of any changes in your arthritis symptoms such as periods of more joint pain and stiffness. You may need more rest and less exercise during these times.

Where to Exercise?

The best place to exercise is a personal choice. Some people prefer to exercise in the comfort, convenience and privacy of their own home with an exercise DVD or video such as the Arthritis Foundation's Take Control with Exercise. Others enjoy the social aspect of getting out of the house and attending a class or gym in the community. A community-based program offers greater options than exercising at home and, for some people, the support and guidance offered by an instructor or fitness trainer provides the needed motivation to stick with a program.

Aquatic or pool-based exercise is another good option for people with arthritis. The buoyancy effects of water result in less stress on the weight-bearing joints and marked pain relief for many people with arthritis. The Arthritis Foundation's Aquatic Program is a good starting point to learn appropriate exercises in the pool. [Check with your local Arthritis Foundation chapter for arthritis exercise programs in your community.]

How to Get Started?

Starting a regular exercise program can be very challenging. Understanding the benefits of exercise for people with arthritis and having the support and guidance from your rheumatologist will help. Physical and occupational therapists can suggest exercises that are safe and customized to your specific needs, teach you how to monitor your body's response to exercise, and modify your exercise routine as needed. Make an exercise plan or contract including when, how often and for how long you will exercise. Other tips to help you stay motivated are:

- Set realistic short-and long-term goals, and reward yourself when you have achieved them.
- Exercise with a friend or family member
- Keep an exercise log or chart your progress on a calendar
- Identify problems or obstacles that are likely to get in the way of your exercise program and plan ahead how you will deal with them
- Choose activities that are convenient, relatively inexpensive and fun!

Discuss your exercise program and any concerns you have with your rheumatologist and/or other arthritis health professionals on a regular basis. With their support and guidance, you will be able to build regular physical activity and exercise into your daily routine and reap the benefits of an active and healthy lifestyle.

HOME-BASED ARM LOADING EXERCISES FOR OSTEOPOROSIS

The following exercises increase bone mineral density in the wrist and load the forearm in various directions. They should be done three times a week and repeated 10–15 times on each occasion. Keep breathing easily and try not to hold your breath while doing these exercises.

Arm Press

Stand facing a wall, about 50 cm away from it, with your feet slightly apart, arms bent at the elbows and hands at shoulder height.

- Lean your body forwards towards the wall by bending your elbows in a controlled movement.
- Push your body back to the starting position.

Wrist Curl

This is an easy exercise that will work your forearm muscles. You can do it with a light weight or water bottle, and progress further by increasing the weight—(the safe limit is 5 kg (11 lbs) in each hand.

- Sit towards the front of a chair with your feet hip-width apart and your knees over your ankles. Sit with your forearms resting on your thighs, holding a dumbbell in an underhand grip with your palms facing up.
- Position your wrists so that they are just beyond your knees.
- Start with your wrists flat, dumbbells resting on your fingers.
- In one movement, curl your fingers up, followed by your wrists.
- Hold for two seconds then slowly lower back down.
- Repeat 10 times.

Turn your forearm over and exercise more effective. Repeat using an overhand grip.

Tip: Keep your elbows in contact with your thighs, parallel to your wrists. This will make the exercise more effective.

All Fours

Support yourself on your hands and knees on the floor, on a firm mat or carpet. Your fingers should point forwards, and you should have right angles at the wrists, shoulders, hips and knees. While doing this, keep your shoulders level, tighten your abdominal muscles and squeeze your buttocks. Making small, controlled movements, walk your hands forwards as far as you can without over-arching your back or moving your knees or feet. Hold, then walk your hands back to the start position. Rest, then repeat.

PHYSIOTHERAPY MANAGEMENT DURING REHABILITATION OF SPINAL CORD INJURY

The most essential need of spinal cord injury (SCI) patient is some amount of mobility in the bed. The very first thing that he attempts is going on to the side by using upper trunk movements and scapular movements. The therapist can assist him initially by just doing passive rotation and asking him to assist as much as possible. Next he is asked to do this by himself and the therapist helping only as much as he wants. When the patient can do by himself, more and more resistance has to be applied. He may use momentum and facilitate movements it also strengthen the muscle.

These activities give awareness that with swift movement of the upper trunk he can initiate lower trunk movements.

Rolling can be made easy if he flexes his one hip and knee or both hip are flexed.

BED MOBILITY FOR PARAPLEGICS

Outcome: Patient should do all bed motilities independently and without any specific equipment.

How to Achieve

- Rolling to the left and right.
- Rolling from prone to supine and back.
- Sitting with extended legs from supine as well as with flexed knees.
- Moving to either side of bed.
- Moving to head and foot of the bed.
- Doing pushups in bed to relieve pressure.
- Coming to quadruped (all fours) position.
- Crawling
- Kneel.

Consideration

- Upper extremity strength and ROM
- Spasticity
- Pressure sore
- Age
- Obesity.

Process

- Evaluate and improve motor skill routinely
- Appropriate bed mobility techniques
- Make a routine exercise programme to improve corresponding muscles.

Pressure Relief

Due to lack of sensation, they don't perceive the discomfort of pressure on certain vulnerable points because of squeezing of local blood supply and resulting in to ischemia over certain area and that will lead in to pressure sore. They also do not have the ability to move the part to relieve the pressure. Therefore, they have to develop new methods consciously. Patient who have very pointed bony prominences are prone to develop pressure sores than others (e.g. some have anatomically pointed ischial tuberosities) therefore therapist have to make a protocol for each patient and see as to how often they have to do the pressure relieving measures. After the patient become active in wheelchair activities, the chances of getting pressure sore are much less. Therefore, careful clinical observations can help a patient to develop a treatment protocol which he can follow by himself.

Pressure relieving maneuvers:

- Pushups with hands on arm rest of wheelchair lifting buttocks off the Seat. (Strong triceps and shoulder extensors essentials.)
- Forward leaning: trunk muscle, pectoral muscles, triceps are essential. However, I passively leaning forward can also relieve pressure to some extent.
- Side lean by hooking on the rim of the wheelchair on the opposite side and leaning to one side and then the other. For doing this he needs strong biceps.
- Electrically operated reclining wheelchair can also relieve the pressure.

Cushions

It is proven that no perfect cushion exists which is suitable for all the patients. We have to look in to the lifestyle needs. Some of the cushions are too expensive. Some are easily punctured. Foam cushions need to be replaced every 6–18 months. Arteriolar pressure in skin capillaries is appropriately 32 mm Hg but none of the cushions available in the market can maintain pressure below 32 mm. Perhaps, it is the postural control that matters most foam cushion has the benefit of being more porous with less moisture formation.

However, it is essential that the covering should be of light cotton material and not plastic. Another disadvantage of foam cushion is that if the atmospheric pressure is high the skin temperature also tends to increase. Older patients tend to have lower skin capillary pressures (even as low as 20 mm). Thin patient has less fat to cover bony prominence so also flaccid patients. For these patients, cushion with lower contact pressure relief are recommended.

Those who have sensation intact, find contoured foam cushions uncomfortable. Those who have bladder bowel incontinence, less porous cover have to be given. With contoured cushions, transferring is more difficult. These entire factors should be taken into consideration. No cushion can substitute for frequent pressure releasing maneuvers, like weight shifting and pushups. Other factor like protein deficiency, anemia and infection also should be controlled in order to prevent pressure sores.

Mechanical Methods

Electrically operated reclining wheelchair is probably the best pressure relieving method especially for higher level paraplegic and tetraplegics.

Relieve pressure on ischium, sacrum, and greater trochanter. Factors to be considered are ROM (especially hip and elbow), tone obesity, cushions, adjustable arm rests, ability to do pushups and other pressure relief skills like forward leaning, side leaning, etc.

TRANSFERS

Moving from one surface to other is a major task for almost all SCI cases and need special training and effort. They need the support of their strong hands to do that. They have to take extra care that they do not fall on the ground while transferring and also see that they do not hurt themselves.

As an initial step they are taught to maneuver to move themselves on the bed itself. Firmer beds are essential for the initial training. One has to learn step by step and may take several days in achieving each step. For example,

- Lifting and moving the legs to the left and right with the own hands.
- Managing to lift their body up by pushing on the bed.
- Shifting the body to the left and right on the bed, maintaining their balance. Some of their require improving their sitting balance specially the higher level paraplegic some may require strengthening their triceps. Some may require improving their ROM like rotation of trunk, elbow movement. How the various components to be continued will depends on his skill. He should be encouraged to try different methods and should see that he never gives up trying. It would be ideal to show other patients

who have achieved the task by trying different methods and have managed. Many times the therapists have to try different methods before the patient find a better method for him, i.e. much experimentation to be made.

- After achieving the ability to move from one end of the cot to the other he has to learn to transfer from the cot to the wheelchair. It would be easy for him if the wheelchair is at a lower height he can easily go from the cot to wheelchair but would find it difficult to transfer back. One needs very strong upper extremities. A transfer board would facilitate the movements especially for higher level SCI cases who cannot maintain balance while transferring. However with repeated attempts they learn to manage well even to a higher level. Keeping the transfer board under the mid thigh is the most difficult thing.
- The next transfer the paraplegics to learn to transfer to the floor and back, though this is not a very easy maneuver for obese and higher level paraplegics. Before attempting this it would be ideal for them to try it step by step. As a first step they can try corner-shifting in one attempt, then they can try holding on the two cots they can go up to the floor and back. Next, they could go on to the floor with one hand on the floor and then going up with both hands on the cot and twisting their body. This is possible for patients with lower level of paraplegia and with satisfactory abdominal muscles. Prior to learning, these transfer activities, it is necessary for the patient to develop good abdominals. He should attempt to go on all four position and do cat and camel exercises. Next, he should attempt to do side-sitting on either side. Next he could attempt kneel standing with a hyper lordotic lumbar spine and balance. If he has a strong quadratus lumborum and lattissimus dorsi he can be taught kneel walking in parallel bars. All these exercises are preparatory exercises for walking with orthosis.
- Next, he can learn a stand pivot transfer. This he can perform only if he has strong abdominals and trunk balance.

DEPENDENT TRANSFERS

1. One man pivot transfer
   - Anterior arm around shoulder.
   - Sideways arm around the waist.
2. Two-men lifts.

3. Three-men lifts.
4. Mechanical lifts.
   - Swivel bar transfer: Useful in cases of limited hip ROM due to spasticity or ectopic bone formation around hip joints.
   - Bathroom transfers: Before beginning these transfers, it is important to assess the patient's own bathroom, i.e. size of the bathroom, width of the entrance door, age, safety, amount of assistance required to transfer and time consumption. If the wheelchair would fit, lateral transfer is very practical. Raised toilet seats, grab bars are necessary. There is no one way to approach bath transfers selection of specific techniques will depends on each individual patients.

TRANSFER TO CAR AND BACK TO WHEELCHAIR

Difficulties is because of limited space for movement and bringing the wheelchair closer to the car seat. Therefore, longer sliding boards are required. One man pivot transfer is also difficult because of the limited space. Finding the right method is a matter of experimentation usually while getting in legs should go in last and while getting out legs should come out first.

TRANSFER FROM WHEELCHAIR TO FLOOR

This is frightening maneuver for a patient who does not have strong abdominals and triceps. However, repeated attempts would give them confidence. First they have to scoot to the edge of the wheelchair and then come down straight on one hand and then the other with both knees following and coming on all fours position. The other alternative is going on the sides with straight legs sliding forward while landing on one hand, talking full weight with extended elbow and gradually, bringing down the buttocks.

FLOOR TO WHEELCHAIR

1. One of the easiest method is to have an intermediate step and then lifting the body to the wheelchair.
2. Another method in which patient has to get in to kneeling position and then pull himself in to the wheel chair. However getting into kneeling position is not that easy. Patient needs a lot of strength and balance. Removing the foot pedals is important.

3. Yet another method is using the extensor tone which would assist in the pushing back to wheelchair. Here again the upper limb/ lower limb strength and extensor tone are very important.

The factors determine the process of transferring independently are the following:

- Age
- Obesity
- Pressure sore
- Spasticity
- Range of motion.

The actual process includes:

- Positioning of the wheelchair and management of its part viz. brakes, detachable arm rests, foot rests
- Positioning of transfer board (if necessary)
- Ability to maintain sitting balance. Ability to lift bodyweight with elbows extended
- Ability to slide from one surface to the rest (lateral transfer), including the management of both lower extremities.

WHEELCHAIR MOBILITY

As a first step, the paraplegic has to accept concept of using wheelchair for mobility. This is not an easy thing for a person who was walking and running or driving a vehicle a few days of month back. For him to accept this slow moving mode of mobility is very difficult. Not only that, the stigma attached to the wheelchair is too much.

However, when he realizes that he is bedridden and that without moving from the bed, life becomes monotonous and a desire could come to him to get in to a wheelchair. If he observes another wheel chair bound patient moving around comfortably, he too would consider getting in to a wheelchair and attempt moving at least within house. When he observes people even get out of the house in a wheel chair and face other people in the society, slowly he gets a desire to accept a wheelchair for mobility rather than remain in a bedridden condition. This acceptance is the first step towards rehabilitation.

SCI above 1st lumbar spine should almost always consider wheel chair as a mode of mobility where as cauda equina lesion with good abdominal muscles along with quadratus lumborum, should think of appliances in the form of orthosis like knee ankle foot orthosis (KAFO) and a pair of crutches either elbow crutches or auxiliary crutches. Between wheelchair and orthosis the energy consumption is a much more with orthosis. However, everyone has a desire in him for walking than being on a wheelchair. But when he realizes that wearing a caliper and crutches take time he would think in terms of getting into wheelchair and moving fast. However, wheelchair needs more space to maneuver. Some of the bathrooms may not have enough space for movement. Achieving good wheelchair mobility is essential for all high level paraplegics. For developing wheelchair skills, it is essential to have a good posture of the trunk and strong upper extremity. The muscle to be developed are shoulder flexors and extensors, elbow flexors and extensors, so also good hand grip. Maintaining a good posture is essential for various reasons mainly for conservation of energy, proper chest expansion, endurance, prevention of pressure sore (as awkward sitting can cause unequal pressure leading to pressure sore).

Bad alignment cause postural pain in the back. Wheelchair with higher back may help patient in maintaining a good posture. However, wheelchairs with higher back support are not good for fast movement. With lower back support, the movements of arm are swifter.

A good pelvic support is essential. If there is any pelvic obliquity it needs to be corrected. Sling seat causes adduction of lower extremities and causes the base of support becoming smaller and this would cause instability. Sometimes legs steps are necessary to keep the lower extremities in abduction.

Gel cushion also may cause instability. Some prefer higher foot rests in order to get pelvic stability, preventing forward movement of the pelvis. Slight inclined back support with lumbar roll is a good option the lumbar roll will maintain in a good position; prevent kyphosis, scoliosis and pelvic obliquities. It also helps in maintain the pressure anterior to the ischial tuberosities and thighs. Adjustment of the height of the arm rest is also important as they are essential for adjusting and maintaining the trunk in a good posture. Wheelchair movements are better with strong upper extremities. However, more than the strength, good timing and coordination would help in skillful movement. For forward movement, the muscle essential are: shoulder flexors, adductors and external rotators whereas for back ward movements: Shoulder extensors and adductors and internal rotators.

Propelling of wheelchair

- Trunk flexors and extensors would facilitate forward push
- Avoid holding the tyre as it can get caught in the brake and cause injury. Grip should be always on the rim.

Wheelies

Wheelies one of the advanced skills, a paraplegics can learn, i.e. to lift the front wheels up and maintain the balance on the back wheels only. This position would help a patient to negotiate curbs up. Without achieving a "full wheelies" a patient can negotiate curbs up to 2 inches. When he approaches the curbs, he stop and raise the front wheel then lean forward push the back wheel up. For negotiating higher curbs, i.e more than 2 inches, one has to gain momentum by going fast for 5–10 feet and go in to wheelie and drop front casters on the curb and then lean forward then push the rear wheels. One needs good rhythm and timing which every one cannot achieve. For a patient to become independent in mobility both indoors and outdoors, he has to do step by step training like:

- Trunk mobility in sitting
- Balance and equilibrium reach outs in sitting
- Use of reach out
- Use of upper extremity in sitting
- Wheelies
- Improve endurance
- Forward, backward and turns
- Management of brakes and removing and putting back arm rests, foot rests, etc.
- Movement on surfaces-like tiles, carpets, etc.
- Movement through narrow passages, elevators, ramps
- Movement curbs bumps, cracks inside walk, etc.
- Crossing the street safely.

GAIT TRAINING

A gait with orthosis like KAFO and crutches requires very high energy consumption because the patient has to maintain the balance in *a paraplegic stance* both in the dynamic movement and while resting, i.e. keeping the spine in a hyperextended position and taking the weight on the crutches. Therefore, the patient gets exhausted after walking a few steps. It is essential that the energy consumption should be bare minimum. Depending on the patients muscle power, *"four point gait" or swing to gait"* are the easiest to learn. If he can master these gaits, he can easily negotiate narrow spaces. Wheelchair may not pass through very narrow passages. Swing through gait needs more strength, coordination and are difficult to learn but once mastered the energy consumption is less. Gait training should be started in the parallel bars first. Initially, patient is taught to be in the paraplegic's stance, i.e. hip in extension and spine in hyperlordotic posture. The therapists stand on the side and push the shoulders backwards and pelvis forward. Optimum position of the ankle is also important as with hyperdorsiflexion and planter flexion, one tends to loose balance. High boots with posterior steel shank can maintain ankle mobility in neutral position with minimal ankle mobility required for ambulation. After this, patient is able to balance in standing. He is taught four point gait pattern which is easiest to learn. It is easier for patients who have some power in hip flexors. If he has no hip flexors, he may use adductors by externally rotating at the hips and dragging his feet alternatively. The third option is by hiking the pelvis by quadratus lumborum. The other option is by *swing to or swings through gait.*

Once he is able to move comfortably in the parallel bars he is brought out first in the walker and later with crutches. Initially, he could be given axillary crutches and later on elbow crutches. Older patients prefer walker as it gives much more balance than any of the crutches. Once he gains confidence in moving indoor, he can be brought out door. Initially he is taught to walk long distances so as to gain confidence and endurance. The next step could be climb stairs. Initially, he is taught to hold on to one side on the railings and the other side on the crutch and lift his body up and climb one step and bring the crutch to the standing level and then lift once again holding the crutch and railing climb another step.

Another method is facing the railing and holding it with both hands, swing one limb in one pendulum cycle and then hike the hip and place the foot on the higher step; then bring the other foot up. This is possible only if has strong hip flexors or quadratus lumborum. There is yet another way of climbing up, i.e. jack kniving. Here the patient has to lift himself up higher than the height of a step with back facing the stair case and swinging both legs backwards so as to reach the higher step. The person has to use one crutch in one hand and holding the railing with the other hand or using crutches in both hands. This is possible only for patients who have very good control of the trunk as well as very strong triceps and shoulder muscles.

Home-based Exercise Program for People with Spinal Cord Injury

The following exercise program is designed for people with spinal cord injury (SCI) who are long-term wheelchair users. The aim is to provide patients with a resource that they can use in their own homes with limited equipment. Arms ergometers have been shown to be particularly useful for increasing cardiovascular fitness in people with SCI. However, this equipment is expensive. It was therefore decided to modify a 2nd-hand Exercycle in the hope of providing a cost-effective alternative.

The exercises have been selected based on a review of the current literature on cardiovascular and strength training in the SCI population. Because shoulder pain is a common problem among people following SCI, exercises have been designed to specifically prevent shoulder injuries.

Circuit Training

It has been shown that circuit training increases both cardiovascular, and strength Parameters and can also have psychological benefits.

A circuit consists of alternating strength exercises with cardiovascular exercises. Each exercise is known as a 'station' and participants progress from one station to the next. It is important to set up the circuit in advance to minimize stopping between stations. Ideally rest periods should be between 15–30 seconds. This enables the heart rate to remain elevated so that cardiovascular and metabolic benefits are received. The circuit will be divided into sections. 2 resistance stations will be performed after each other, followed immediately by 5 minutes of arm cranking. This will be followed by a rest period of 15–30 seconds, and then the 'section' will be repeated for exercises 3 + 4, and 5 + 6. This comprises one 'circuit,' which will be performed twice in one session.

Exercise 1	
Exercise 2	
Arm cranking	
Exercise 3	
Exercise 4	
Arm cranking	To be performed twice
Rest	
Exercise 5	
Exercise 6	
Arm cranking	
Rest	

How Much How Often?

- The circuit should be performed 3–5 times per week. Results may not appear until approximately eight weeks. The key is to persevere and to make exercise a part of patient daily routine. Patient should feel muscle soreness rather than pain.

Resistance Exercises

When performing resistance exercises, do 15 repetitions (on each arm) in a row, for each exercise. You will be using either theraband or hand weights, which are both readily available.

Hand Weights

To do most of the following strength exercises, patient need to lift or push weights, and patient need to keep gradually increasing the amount of weight use. He/she can use the hand weights sold in sporting-goods stores, or can use things like emptied milk jugs filled with sand or water, or socks filled with beans and tied shut at the ends. Use a minimum of weight initially, then gradually build up the weight. Starting out with weights that are too heavy can cause injuries. At the same time, remember that patient have to gradually add a challenging amount of weight in order to benefit from strength exercises. If they do not challenge your muscles, they would not benefit from strength exercises.

Take three seconds to lift or push a weight into place; hold the position for one second, and take another three seconds to lower the weight. Do not let the weight drop; lowering it slowly is very important.

Theraband

- Remember to have the theraband firmly attached. Pull the band in the desired direction for 2–3 seconds holds at maximal stretch for 1 second, and then slowly release. Try to maintain some stretch on the band even at its most slack position (i.e. do not return to a starting position where the band is slack).

Safety

- Do not hold your breath during strength exercises. Breathe normally. Holding your breath while straining can cause changes in blood pressure. Avoid jerking or thrusting movements, instead use smooth, steady movements. Breathe out as you move the Theraband or weight, and breathe in as you relax.
- When exercising with the weight or Theraband in one hand, you may need to hold the chair with the other hand to maintain balance. A security strap may also be necessary to add stability.
- Muscle soreness lasting up to a few days and slight fatigue are normal after muscle-building exercises, but exhaustion, sore joints, and unpleasant muscle pulling aren't. The latter symptoms mean you are overdoing it. None of the exercises you do should cause pain.

Arm Cranking

You will perform five minutes of arm cranking per section. This will be divided into four minutes at a moderate level (base) and one minute at a higher intensity (peak). The arm crank should be secured to a table at shoulder height, with the hand straps attached.

How Hard should You Exercise?

The key is to listen to your body. Researchers have found that the level of effort you feel you are putting into an activity is likely to agree with what actual physical measurements would show. In other words, if your body tells you that the exercise you are doing is moderate, measurements of things like how hard your heart is working would probably show that it is working at a moderate level.

One way you can estimate how hard to work is by using something called the Borg scale. The 15-point Borg scale is illustrated below. As an example a 6 would be the equivalent of sitting down doing nothing, 13 a steady exercising pace and 19/20 the hardest exercise you have ever done. Your aim is to work at a 12–13 throughout the circuit (moderate—moderately hard).

6
7 — Very, very light
8
9 — Very light
10
11 — Fairly light
12
13 — Moderately hard
14
15 — Hard
16
17 — Very hard
18
19 — Very, very hard
20 — Exhaustion

Arm Cranking

- During the four minute (base) period, continue to work at 12–13 on the Borg scale. However for the one minute peak increase your intensity to 13–14 (moderately hard+)

Resistance Exercises (Theraband and Hand Weights)

Select a weight that you can lift or push 15 times in a row. If you can't manage 15 times in a row, it is too heavy for you. Reduce the amount of weight. If you can lift a weight more than 20 times in a row, it is too light for you. Increase the amount of weight.

CIRCUIT

Warm Up

Begin with 5 minute of gentle arm cranking (10–11 on the Borg scale).

Stretch

Stretches are to be performed with the wheelchair in a door way so that the arm to be stretched will just fit behind the frame without having to lean forward or backward in the wheelchair.

You should feel some tension in the muscle, but not a sharp pain. Hold each stretch for 20–30 seconds, and repeat for 2 repetitions. Stretching should never cause pain, especially joint pain. If it does, you are stretching too far, and you need to reduce the stretch so that it doesn't hurt. Mild discomfort or a mild pulling sensation is normal.

Never "bounce" into a stretch; make slow, steady movements instead. Avoid "locking" your joints into place when you straighten them during stretches. You should always have a very small amount of bending in your joints while stretching.

Below is a list of stretches, perform those which you are able.

Circuit

Below are 10 resistance exercises. Trial the exercises, and select from the list those that you can manage. You aim is to have at least 6 different exercises. If you can complete more than six exercise, either add the others to the circuit (depending on how long it takes you) or select six on one day and vary the exercise so that you perform a different selection of the following exercise day. Most exercises have a second exercise following that can be used as a progression.

Perform your first exercise, followed immediately by the second. After completing the second exercise, begin the arm cranking station (four minutes, at 12–13 on Borg Scale, followed by 1 minute at a 13–14). Rest for 15–30 seconds, then repeat the same procedure for your third and fourth exercise, followed by your fifth and sixth. Now complete the whole regime through once more!!

Cooldown: 2 minutes of gentle arm cranking (7-8 on the Borg Scale).

Progressing

Every 6 weeks your exercise program should be reassessed. If the circuit is becoming easy you can progress it in a number of ways:

- Increase the base of the arm cranking by 1 minute
- Increase the peak of the arm cranking by 30 seconds

- Increase the number of repetitions on the resistance exercises by five
- Gradually increasing the amount of weight you use.

CIRCUIT

Cranking	
Rest	
Warm up	
Exercise 1	
Exercise 2	
Arm Exercise 3	
Exercise 4	
Arm cranking	
Rest	
Exercise 5	
Exercise 6	
Arm cranking	To be performed twice
Rest	
Cool down	

All stretches are to be held for 20–30 seconds, and performed twice on each side.

Stretch 1:

- With elbow at shoulder height and elbow bent to 90°, place forearm on door frame making contact from elbow to wrist
- Lean slightly forward until a firm stretch is felt in the chest region keeping elbow and wrist in contact with the frame at all times
- Repeat with other arm.

Stretch 2:

- Place outstretched arm at 45° from your body, elbow straight and thumb up
- Place lower forearm against the door frame
- Rotate wheelchair AWAY from arm until you feel a stretch in the front of your arm
- Repeat on other arm.

Stretch 3:

- Lean forward. Cross your arms and grasp your thighs near your knees
- Pull you trunk up and back (still holding your thighs)
- You should feel the stretch between you shoulder blades.

Stretch 4:

- Place one arm straight out in front of you, palm facing in
- Move your arm to cross your body, keeping your shoulder down
- With opposite hand pull the arm into your body, while keeping the elbow straight.

Stretch 5:

- Sit tall in your chair
- Tilt your head so that your ear moves toward your shoulder on the same side (keep the opposite shoulder down)
- Repeat on the other side.

Stretch 6:

- Place one arm in the air above your head
- Bend at the elbow and reach as far as you can down your back
- With the other arm add resistance by pulling the elbow across
- Repeat on the other side.

Stretch 7:

- Sit tall in your chair
- Rotate you body to the left
- Use your arms to help pull you around
- Repeat on the other side.

RESISTANCE EXERCISES

Remember to hold onto your chair for balance, when exercise one arm. A security strap may be used to add stability.

External Rotation

- Position yourself parallel to a closed door
- Attach the band to your wrist or hold in your hand that is furthest from the door and to the door handle
- Place yourself far enough away so that the band's tension allows your hand to rest on your abdomen, with your elbow bent to 90° and at your side

- Without moving your elbow, pull your wrist away from the door as far as you can
- Your elbow should stay at your side and bent throughout the motion
- Return slowly to the starting position
- Complete 15 repetitions. Repeat with other arm.

To Progress from the above Exercise Use Hand Weights

External Rotation

- Holding a weight or with wrist cuff attached, begin with your shoulder out to the side at 90°, elbow bent to 90°, and palm facing down
- While keeping the shoulder and elbow in this position, move your forearm toward the roof as far as it will go
- Return slowly to the starting position
- Complete 15 repetitions. Repeat with the other arm.

Internal Rotation

- Position yourself parallel to a closed door
- Attach the band to your wrist or hold in your hand that is closes to the door
- Place yourself far enough away so that the band is taut when your elbow is bent to 90° and at your side
- Keeping your elbow at your side and bent, pull your forearm away from the door and bring your wrist to sit on your abdomen
- Your elbow should stay at your side and bent throughout the motion
- Return slowly to the starting position
- Complete 15 repetitions. Repeat with other arm.

To Progress from the above Exercise Use Hand Weights

Internal Rotation

- Holding a weight or with wrist cuff attached, begin with your shoulder out to the side at 90°, elbow bent to 90°, and palm facing down
- While keeping the shoulder and elbow in this position, lower your forearm, until your fist faces the floor

- Return slowly to the starting position
- Complete 15 repetitions. Repeat with the other arm.

Scapular Retraction

- Attach the band to your wrists or hold in each hand
- Face the door so that the band is in front of you with your arms straight
- With the arms at chest level, pull back in a rowing motion
- Return slowly to the starting position
- Complete 15 repetitions.

To Progress from the above Exercise Use Hand Weights

Scapular Retraction

- Holding a weight in each hand or using wrist cuffs, begin with arms straight out in front of you
- Pull your elbows out and back in a rowing motion
- Return slowly to the starting position
- Complete 15 repetitions.

Shoulder Adduction

- Turn wheelchair so that you are at a 90° angle to the door
- The band should be attached to the door knob and to your wrist or held in your hand that is closest to the door
- Pull you wrist down toward your side while keeping your elbow straight and thumb pointing forward
- Return slowly to the starting position
- Complete 15 repetitions. Repeat on the other arm exercise.

Shoulder Abduction

- Sit in your chair with your arm hanging down over your wheel with your elbow straight
- Attach the band to your chair at floor level and to your wrist on the same side
- Pull you arm out and up towards shoulder level while keeping your elbow straight and thumb pointing forward or slightly up
- Return slowly to the starting position
- Complete 15 repetitions. Repeat on the other arm.

To Progress from the above Exercise Use Hand Weights

Shoulder Abduction

- Sit in your chair with your arm hanging down over your wheel. Hold a weight or attach wrist cuffs
- Extend your arm out to the side (keeping your elbow straight) until shoulder height
- Return slowly to the starting position
- Complete 15 repetitions. Repeat on the other arm
- *Note:* If this is too difficult bend the elbow to 90º, and keep in this position throughout the movement.

Bicep Curl

- Attach the band to your wrist (or hold in your hand) and to your chair, near the floor, on the same side
- Begin with arm straight, palm facing forward
- Bend at the elbow, until hand is in front of your shoulder
- Slowly lower your wrist to the starting position
- Complete 15 repetitions. Repeat with the other arm.

To Progress from the above Exercise Use Hand Weights

Bicep Curl

- Hold a weight in your hand or attach wrist cuffs
- Start with your arm hanging straight down beside your chair
- Keeping the shoulder still, bend at the elbow, bringing hand toward your shoulder
- Slowly lower your wrist to the starting position
- Complete 15 repetitions. Repeat with the other arm.

Triceps Extension

- Attach the band to your wrist, and to the wheel of your chair
- Begin with your elbow bent and close to you body
- Straighten your elbow until inline with the back of your chair (elbow remains at your side)
- Return slowly to the starting position
- Complete 15 repetitions. Repeat with the other arm.

To Progress from the above Exercise Use Hand Weights

Triceps Extension

- Holding a weight or with wrist cuff attached, begin with your arm straight above you
- Keeping your shoulder in this position, bend at the elbow, so that your hand moves behind your head
- Return slowly to the starting position
- Complete 15 repetitions. Repeat with the other arm.

Anterior Deltoid

- Attach the band to your wrist, (or hold in your hand) and to the chair near the floor
- Begin with your elbow as straight as possible and down beside your chair
- Raise your arm, with your elbow remaining straight, until inline with your shoulder
- Return slowly to the starting position
- Complete 15 repetitions. Repeat with the other arm.

To Progress from the above Exercise Use Hand Weights

Anterior Deltoid

- Holding a weight or with wrist cuffs attached, begin with your arm beside your chair
- With your elbow straight and your palm facing down, straightened your arm in front of you, until shoulder height
- Return slowly to the starting position
- Complete 15 repetitions. Repeat with the other arm.

Shoulder Girdle Depression

- Sitting in your chair, lean slightly forward, keeping your back and shoulders straight. Grasp the seat of the chair.
- Slowly lift yourself up, by straightening your arms.
- Slowly lower yourself back down
- Repeat 15 times.

Chest, Pectorals

- Attach two bands to a door knob behind you
- Drape the Theraband over each shoulder and attach to you wrist (or hold in your hands)
- Start with your hands near each shoulder, and move your arm in a circle out and forward, until they meet in front of you (as if hugging a barrel)
- Return slowly to the starting position. Complete 15 repetitions.

To Progress from the above Exercise Use Hand Weight

Chest, Pectorals

- Holding weights or with wrist cuffs attached, begin with both hands by your shoulders
- Start with your hands near each shoulder, and move your arm in a circle out and forward, until they meet in front of you (as if hugging a barrel)
- Return slowly to the starting position
- Complete 15 repetitions.

CHAPTER

26

International Health Organizations

International Health Organizations are usually divided into three groups: Multilateral Organizations, Bilateral Organizations, and Non-governmental Organizations (NGOs). The term multilateral means that funding comes from multiple governments (as well as from non-governmental sources) and is distributed to many different countries. The major multilateral organizations are all part of the United Nations.

WORLD HEALTH ORGANIZATION

World Health Organization (WHO) is the premier International Health Organization. Technically, it is an "intergovernmental agency related to the United Nations." WHO and other such intergovernmental agencies are "separate, autonomous organizations which, by special agreements, work with the UN and each other through the coordinating machinery of the Economic and Social Council." According to its constitution (1948) its principal goal is "the attainment by all peoples of the highest possible level of health."

WHO has three main divisions. The governing body, the World Health Assembly, meets once a year to approve the budget and decide on major matters of health policy. All the 190 or so member nations send delegations. The World Health Assembly elects 31 member nations to designate health experts for the Executive Board, which meets twice a year and serves as the liaison between the Assembly and the Secretariat, which carries on the day-to-day work of the WHO. The Secretariat has a staff of about 4,500, with 30% of the employees at headquarters in Geneva, 30% in six regional field offices, and 40% in individual countries, either as country-wide WHO representatives or as representatives of special WHO programs. The principal work of WHO is directing and coordinating international health activities and supplying technical assistance to countries. It develops norms and standards, disseminates health information, promotes research, provides training in international health, collects and analyzes epidemiologic data, and develops systems for monitoring and evaluating health programs.

PAN AMERICAN HEALTH ORGANIZATION

The Pan American Health Organization (PAHO) serves as the regional field office for WHO in the Americas and, since it predates WHO, carries on some additional autonomous activities.

WHO has a biannual budget. Assessed contributions from the member nations constitute the regular budget. In recent years voluntary ("extrabudgetary") contributions—from governments and private philanthropies—have exceeded the regular budget. Donors may earmark voluntary contributions for special programs; WHO allocates assessed contributions.

UNITED NATIONAL CHILDREN'S FUND

Three subsidiary agencies of the UN Economic and Social Council are heavily committed to International Health programs. The United Nation Children's Fund (UNICEF) spends the majority of its program (nonadministrative) budget on health care. UNICEF makes the world's most vulnerable children its top priority, so it devotes most of its resources to the poorest countries and to children younger than 5. In 1994 UNICEF, received about $1 billion in contributions, all voluntary—70% from governments and 30% from private sources. (The US government is the largest single donor to UNICEF, but the per capita contribution from the US, including private sources, is much less than that from Canada, Switzerland, the Netherlands, and the Scandinavian countries.) In 1994, UNICEF spent $202 million on child health, $81 million on water supply and sanitation, $30 million on child nutrition, and $216 million on emergency relief. UNICEF runs many of the child health programs in cooperation with WHO. The United Nations Population Fund (UNFPA) spent about $130 million of its $260 million budget for 1994 on family planning programs, with 59 priority countries receiving 70% of this money. (Priority is based on rate of population growth and poverty.)

UNITED NATIONS DEVELOPMENT PROGRAM

The United Nations Development Program (UNDP) allocated $141 million, out of a total budget for field expenditures of $1 billion, to "health, education, employment". Its major health concerns are acquired immune deficiency syndrome (AIDS)maternal and child nutrition, and excessive maternal mortality. In conjunction with WHO and the World Bank it sponsors the Special Program for Research and Training in Tropical Diseases (TDR).

BILATERAL AGENCIES

United States Agency for International Development

Bilateral agencies are governmental agencies in a single country which provide aid to developing countries. The largest of these is the United States Agency for International Development (USAID). Most of the industrialized nations have a similar governmental agency. Political and historical reasons often determine which countries receive donations from bilateral agencies and how much they receive. For example, France concentrates on its former colonies, and Japan gives mostly to developing countries in Asia. In 1994, USAID, through its Center for Population, Health, and Nutrition, donated $1,050 million for long-term health care in developing countries. USAID channels most of this aid through "cooperating agencies" - private international health agencies which contract with USAID.

Nongovernmental Organizations

Nongovernmental organizations (NGOs), also known as private voluntary organizations (PVOs), provide approximately 20% of all external health aid to developing countries. Most of these organizations are quite small; many are church-affiliated. In the very poorest countries, hospitals and clinics run by missionary societies are especially important. Data from Uganda indicates that church mission hospitals are much more efficient than government health facilities, with mission doctors treating five times as many patients as their counterparts in government facilities and mission nurses attending twice the number of patients that government nurses do. The largest NGO devoted to international health in the United States is *Project Hope,* with an annual budget exceeding $100 million. Worldwide, the most important NGO in long-term international health is probably *Oxfam,* International. Founded in the United Kingdom in 1943, it now has affiliates in 10 other countries, including the United States.

Refugee and Disaster Relief Organizations

In most natural disasters, e.g. earthquakes, floods, volcanic eruptions, the majority of deaths occur in the first few hours or days, and likewise most of the lives that are saved are saved early and saved by local efforts at disaster relief. A major disaster, however, can overwhelm the resources of a poor country and, by destruction of an already somewhat tenuous economic and social infrastructure, set the stage for famine and epidemics. The aid provided by international relief organizations in the days immediately following the disaster can play a major role in averting health crises and re-establishing a functioning society.

In contrast to natural disasters, famines and refugee crises tend to develop slowly, often preceded by warning signs of the impending emergency, so that international agencies can coordinate relief efforts with national agencies in a timely fashion. The United Nations agencies are probably the most important of the international relief organizations, but there are several very large NGOs active in refugee and disaster relief. Two of these, *the International Committee of the Red Cross (ICRC)* and Medicines Sans Frontieres, perform special functions that will be discussed below.

United Nations Organizations

Six major UN organizations are involved in refugee and disaster relief. The Department of Humanitarian Affairs, established in 1992, coordinates UN activities in this area. The Department operates on a 24-hour basis the UN Disaster Assessment and Coordination Team, which can be deployed immediately to an affected country. Three of the six major agencies are mentioned above in the section on long-term health care. UNICEF allocated $216 million to emergency relief in 1994. The WHO budget does not contain a line item for disaster relief, but WHO is active in this area through its Division of Emergency and Humanitarian Action, which coordinates the response of the international relief community and supplies technical assistance and emergency drugs and equipment. UNDP allocated $59 million to disaster relief in 1994; its special function is organizing efforts at rehabilitation in the disaster-struck area.

World Food Program

The World Food Program (WFP) supplies food relief in disasters and coordinates the activities of NGOs involved in food relief, as well as assisting them with transportation and logistics. In 1994, it spent $874 million on relief. The WFP also supports agricultural and rural development ($181 million), and education ($131 million).

UN High Commissioner for Refugees

The Office of the UN High Commissioner for Refugees (UNHCR) provides international protection to refugees and also attempts to find long-lasting solutions to their problems. UNHCR is the major international organization for the world's 20 million refugees. It aids refugees directly and coordinates the work of NGOs involved in refugee relief. Although, it has no formal authority over displaced persons), upon request of the UN General Assembly and the Secretary General, UNHCR has provided assistance to displaced persons in such countries as Bosnia and Herzegovina, Somalia, and Rwanda in recent years. In 1994, UNHCR spent almost $1.2 billion on its programs.

Food and Agriculture Organization

The sixth of the UN organizations involved in relief work is the Food and Agriculture Organization (FAO). Like the World Bank and WHO it is technically an "intergovernmental agency related to the UN". It helps developing countries prepare for famine through its Global Information and Early Warning System and its Food Security Assistance Scheme, which helps developing countries set-up national food reserves. In disasters its principal role is to assist in the re-establishment of agricultural production.

United Nations Educational Scientific and Cultural Organization

United Nations Educational Scientific and Cultural Organization (UNESCO) was formed during 1945 and currently has 188 members. The main objective is to get peace and security in the world by promoting collaboration among nations through education. Science, culture and communication. It publishes world education report annually.

International Labour Organization

The International Labour Organization (ILO) was founded in 1919, in the wake of a destructive war, to pursue a vision based on the premise that universal, lasting peace can be established only if it is based on social justice. The ILO became the first specialized agency of the UN in 1946. Only tripartite UN agency, since 1919 the ILO brings together governments, employers and workers representatives of 187 member States, to set labor standards, develop policies and devise programs promoting decent work for all women and men.

The main aims of the ILO are to:

- Promote rights at work
- Encourage decent employment opportunities
- Enhance social protection
- Strengthen dialogue on work-related issues.

The unique tripartite structure of the ILO gives an equal voice to workers, employers and governments to ensure that the views of the social partners are closely reflected in labor standards and in shaping policies and programs.

United States Agency for International Development

The United States Agency for International Development (USAID) is the United States Government agency which is primarily responsible for administering civilian foreign aid.

President John F Kennedy created USAID from its predecessor agencies in 1961 by Executive Order. USAID's programs are authorized by the Congress in the Foreign Assistance Act, which the Congress supplements through directions in annual funding appropriation acts and other legislation. Although, it is technically an independent agency, USAID operates subject to the foreign policy guidance of the President, Secretary of State, and the National Security Council. USAID operates in Africa, Asia, Latin America, the Middle East, and Eastern Europe.

Goals

Responding to President Barack Obama's pledge in his 2013 State of the Union Address to "join with our allies to eradicate extreme poverty in the next two decades," USAID has adopted as its mission statement "to partner to end extreme poverty and to promote resilient, democratic societies while advancing the security and prosperity of the United States".

USAID's decentralized network of resident field missions is drawn on to manage US Government (USG) programs in low-income countries for a range of purposes.

- Disaster relief
- Poverty relief
- Technical cooperation on global issues, including the environment
- US bilateral interests
- Socioeconomic development.

Swedish International Development Cooperation Agency

The Swedish International Development Cooperation Agency (SIDA) is a government agency of the Swedish Ministry for Foreign Affairs. SIDA is responsible for organization of the bulk of Sweden's official development assistance to developing countries.

Danish International Development Agency

Danish International Development Agency (DANIDA) was established by the government of Denmark. It is providing assistance in 3 major health programs in India DANLEP, DANTB and DANPCB, i.e. respectively leprosy, tuberculosis and blindness' The Danish International Development Agency is the section of the Danish Ministry of Foreign Affairs dedicated to providing aid and financing pro-development activities in developing countries worldwide.

The new strategy for Denmark's development cooperation "The Right to a Better Life" creates the foundation for an effective Danish development cooperation, which aims to combat poverty and promote human rights. Economic growth is central to the strategy, but growth should be green and promote social progress in order for it to contribute to improving the lives of poor people and their ability to create a better life for themselves.

Denmark has been granting development assistance since the end of the Second World War. It is one of the five countries in the world that meets the United Nations' target of granting 0.7% of gross national income (GNI) in development assistance.

Cooperative for Assistance and Relief Everywhere

Cooperative for Assistance and Relief Everywhere (CARE) is a major international humanitarian agency delivering emergency relief and long-term international development projects. It was founded in 1945, CARE is nonsectarian, impartial, and nongovernmental. It is one of the largest and oldest humanitarian aid organizations focused on fighting global poverty. In 2014, CARE reported working in 90 countries, supporting 880 poverty-fighting projects and humanitarian aid projects, and reaching over 72 million people.

CARE's programs in the developing world address a broad range of topics including emergency response, food security, water and sanitation, economic development, climate change, agriculture, education, and health. CARE also advocates at the local, national, and international levels for policy change and the rights of poor people. Within each of these areas, CARE focuses particularly on empowering and meeting the needs of women and girls and promoting gender equality.

CARE International is a confederation of fourteen CARE National Members, each of which is registered as an autonomous nonprofit nongovernmental organization in the country. The fourteen CARE National Members are CARE Australia, CARE Canada, CARE Denmark, CARE Deutschland-Luxembourg, CARE France, CARE India, CARE International Japan, CARE Netherland, CARE Norge, CARE Österreich, Raks Thai Foundation (CARE Thailand), CARE International UK, CARE USA, and CARE Peru. Programs in developing countries are usually managed by a country office, but CARE also supports projects and may respond to emergencies in some countries where they do not maintain a full country office.

Care began its operation in India in1950 by funding through the following services:

- Mid day School Meal program
- Integrated Child Development Scheme (ICDS)
- Educational and vocational training
- Distribution of garden tools, pump sets seeds for raising vegetable garden in schools
- Improvement of medical care by supplying medical equipment, mobile vans, X-ray machines, diagnostic sets, eye glasses, glass frames, drugs, books, and medicine to Indian hospitals
- It is helping in the project such as nutrition and health project, anemia control project, adolescent girl's project child survival project, reproductive and family health project.

ROCKEFELLER FOUNDATION

This philanthropic organization was established in USA in 1913 by Mr John Rockefeller with the objective of promoting the well-being of mankind all over world. In the early days it confined to medical education and public health. Later, it expanded its fields to social sciences. It started its functioning in India from 1920, with a scheme for the control of hookworm diseases in the Madras presidency. Since, the ford foundation has been associated with several medical and public health programs in India.

Activities

It has helped in the establishment of All India Institute of Hygiene and Public Health (Kolkata); All India Institute of Medical Science (New Delhi); King George Medical College (Lucknow); Christian Medical College (Vellore); Christian Medical College (Ludhiana); SGS Medical College (Mumbai); Field Demonstration Project (Ballabhgarh); National Institute of Virology (Pune), etc.

- It sponsors educational training for advanced training of health professionals of India to other countries through fellowship and travel grant.
- It sponsors the visit of specialist from USA.
- It provide grant in aid to the selected institutions for carrying out researchers. Libraries and medical education.
- Currently, it is giving active support for the improvement of agriculture, family planning and rural development.

RED CROSS SOCIETY

Red Cross Society was founded by John Henry Dunant, a Swiss businessman. World Red Cross day is celebrated on 8th May of every year. Red Cross Society is an independent, nongovernment organization concern with humanitarian assistance in war time and piece time disastrous situations. Thus, red cross offers relief and rehabilitation services not only to the wounded and disabled individuals afflicted by war, but also later, it was extended to the people affected in famine, earthquake, floods and other natural or manmade calamities.

Red Cross Society in India was established in 1920 by an Act of Indian legislature with the three objective of improvement of health, prevention of disease and mitigation of suffering.

Its activities are:

- Provision of amenities to soldiers in time of war.
- Organizing disaster relief services, in the form of milk, medicine, food, vitamin, clothes, blankets, etc.
- Maintaining blood banks and promoting blood donation for the benefit of those wounded in war of disasters.
- Development of maternity and child welfare services.
- In peace time, it provides to the patient of military hospitals with such amenities as newspapers, periodicals, musical instruments and other comfort goods.
- It maintains Red Cross Home at Bengaluru for permanently disabled ex-service man, which is one of the pioneer institutions of its kind in Asia. It provide nursing and rehabilitative care of disabled and paralytic ex-service man.
- It contributes health care by providing equipment drugs and supplies to the hospitals. It conduct health education campaigns.
- It provides first aid services to the deserving cases and also training in first aid through St. John Ambulance Association of India.

The Junior Red Cross is one of the most active sections of the society. It gives an opportunity to lakhs of boys and girls all over India, to be associated with the activities, such as upliftment of villages, provision of first aid, control of outbreaks of diseases, building up of an international fraternity of youth, thus, the promoting international friendliness, understanding and cooperation.

CHAPTER

27

Industrial Health and Ergonomics

Occupational health refers to the identification and control of the risks arising from physical, chemical, and other workplace hazards in order to establish and maintain a safe and healthy working environment. These hazards may include chemical agents and solvents, heavy metals such as lead and mercury, physical agents such as loud noise or vibration, and physical hazards such as electricity or dangerous machinery. Since 1986, the National Institute of Environmental Health Science (NIEHS) has supported training and education program designed to protect workers and their communities from exposure to toxic materials encountered during hazardous waste operations and chemical emergency response. This includes safety and health training for workers who are involved in hazardous waste removal and comprehensive training and environmental restoration for residents living near heavily polluted industrial waste sites.

Industrial health is differ from occupational health industrial health deals with workers in the industries and mines. Where as occupational health is concerned with man in any occupation. Industrial health is older concept of occupational health. Industrial health used to be concerned with the hazards at the place of work.

ERGONOMICS

Ergonomics means fitting the job to the worker after making a scientific study of the relationship between man and his working environment. It is derived from a Greek words, 'Ergon' meaning work and 'Nomos' meaning law. The discipline of ergonomics includes designing of machines, tools, etc. layout of working places and methods of work for improvement of human and machines efficiency.

OCCUPATIONAL HAZARDS

The five main types of occupational hazards and diseases are as follows: 1. Physical hazards, 2. Chemical hazards, 3. Biological hazards, 4. Environmental hazards, 5. Psychological hazards.

Physical Hazards

These are the hazard occurring due to following physical agents:

Heat

The effect are the heat syncope (fainting attack due to pooling of blood in the lower limb), heat cramps (painful and spasmodic contractions of muscles due to loss of sodium and chloride), heat exhaustion (loss of salt leading on to circulatory failure), heat stroke, heat hyperpyrexia (failure in heart regulating mechanism, resulting in high temperature is about 106°F), prickly heat, burns, etc.

Cold

Frostbite, Reynaud disease, erythromelalgia, erythrocyanosis, chilblains, trench foot, gangrene, etc. all because of cutaneous vasoconstriction.

Light

Its effect occur either due to inadequate light or excessive light.
Inadequte light: Headache, eye strain, eye fatigue, (visual fatigue) chronic effect is miner's mystagmus.
Excessive light: Bright light results in glaring, visual fatigue, bluring of vision discomfort and accidents.

Radiation

Ionizing radiation: X-ray, radioactive isotopes like cobalt-60, phosphorus-32.

- Acute effects: acute radiation syndrome.
- Chronic effect; somatic effect; leukemia, aplastic anemia, cancer, tumor induction, pancytopenia.
- Genetic effect; stillbirths, congenital defects, neonatal death, sex chromosome, anuploidy, sterility.

Non ionizing radiation

- *Ultravoilet radiation:*
  - On the skin; darkening of the skin, thickening of the skin, erythma, cancer of the skin.
  - On the eye; (e.g. welding) photophobia, conjuctivitis, keratitis, corneal ulcer, blindness (weldors flash), snow blindness.
- *Infrared radiation:* Cataract
- *Microwaves:* Microwave sickness
- *Laser radiation:* Thermal burns, cataract, retinal burns.

Atmospheric Pressure

- *High atmospheric pressure (as in mines):* Caissons disease (compressed air illness), syncope and pain in joints, air embolism, cardiorespiratory distress, paralysis.
- *Low atmospheric pressure* (as in high attitude): Deafness (due to blocking eustachian tube) pain in ears, rupture of eardrums, expansion of gases in the sinuses and body cavities, headache, pulmonary edema, dyspnea, etc.

Electricity

Electric shock, burns, venttricular flutter.

Noise

- *Auditory effects:* Deafness (temporary or permanent), tinnitus (buzzing in the ears) degeneration of cochlea and eight nerve.
- *Nonauditory effect:* Fatigue, irritability, nervousness, interference with speech and communication, increased intracranial tension, hypertension, peptic ulcer, higher environmental stress.

Vibration

Working with pneumatic tools like drills and hammers: Numbness, white fingers, injuries.

Chemical Hazards

The common chemical substances, such as carbon monoxide, carbon dioxide, nitrogen dioxide, sulfur dioxide, hydrocarbons, sulfuric acid, tannic acid, acetic acid, fumeric acid, ozone, limes and alkalies cause injury to the employee when they are absorbed through skin and inhaling or ingesting. Workers may suffer from respiratory diseases, skin diseases, allergy, heart disease, cancer and neurological disorders.

These diseases may be temporary or chronic in nature. Often a disease may be difficult to diagnose because either its symptoms may appear after a long dormant period or may not be apparent at all. These diseases often shorten employee's life expectancy.

Biological Hazards

These hazards are manifested by diseases caused by bacteria, fungi, viruses, insects, dietary deficiencies, excessive drinking, allergies, brain fever, imbalances, tetanus, stresses and strains. All these tell upon employee's health. Biological hazards are from animals and soil. These are common in agriculture industries.

- *From the animals:* They are called "zoonotic diseases", e.g. anthrax, bovine tuberculosis, salmonellosis, Japanese encephalitis, rabies, plague, etc.
- *From the soil:* Tetanus, ankylostomiasis, gas gangrene, malignant edema, anthrax, aspergillosis, coccidioidomycosis, mycetoma.

Environmental Hazards

Environmental hazards may include noise pollution, vibration and shocks, illumination, radiation, heat, ventilation, air and water pollution. These hazards cause redness of eyes, genetic disorders, cancer, sterility, hearing loss, nerve injury, etc. to workers.

Psychological Hazards

Industrial/job stress caused by various stressors such as task and role demands, organizational leadership, lack of group cohesion, inter-group and interpersonal conflicts, life and career changes, etc. lead to emotional disturbances which, in turn, lead to fatigue and exhaustion. All these affect health of employees. Apart from occupational hazards, there are some occupational diseases also that impair health of employees in industries. Psychological hazards are of two types:

- *Psychological (behavioral) changes:* Such as hostility, aggressiveness, anxiety, depression, frustration, tardiness, alcoholism, drug addiction, sickness absenteeism, etc.
- *Psychosomatic ill health:* Such as neurosis, fatigue, propensity to peptic ulcer, hypertension, asthma, heart disease and rapid aging.

PREVENTIVE MEASURES

- Education regarding hazards and steps for prevention of the same
- Personal hygiene including washing hands thoroughly after handling toxic chemicals
- Use of personal protective devices like gloves, etc.
- Preventive maintenance of machinery used
- Boiling of milk, regular health check-up of cattle that is in use
- Regular intervals of rest in shady places
- Health promotional measures like maintenance of nutritional status.

Stress Management and Physiotherapy

Stress and its management in the community is a growing issue for many health practitioners.

Physiotherapists offer a number of stress management techniques and treatments which can help improve a patient's health and well-being, whether it be specially designed stress management programs, exercise programs, massage, muscle relaxation or general fitness advice.

Role of Physiotherapy

Physiotherapists use an initial assessment to clarify the nature of the problem and develop strategies and treatment which are acceptable to the individual.

Treatment can take the form of individual consultation, group relaxation classes, relaxation audio tapes or information sessions for the general public. As part of the treatment program, physiotherapists offer close professional follow-up with the patient to ensure a positive treatment outcome.

Physiotherapists with a special interest in stress management can offer many different types of relaxation therapy including guided imagery, progressive muscle relaxation, breathing techniques, thought stopping, stretching, massage and general fitness advice.

Benefits of Physiotherapy

Research continues to indicate a positive correlation between a person's ability to cope with stressors and the likelihood of disease during their lifetime.

Physiotherapy can assist by:

- Reducing muscle tension
- Increasing vitality and decreasing reported tiredness
- Improving concentration span
- Improving feeling of general well-being
- Decreasing blood pressure
- Reducing risk of cardiovascular disease
- Improving attitude to work and leisure activity
- Reducing pain states such as headache, chronic pain syndrome and work-related anxiety
- Possibly decreasing dosage of psychoactive medication.

CHAPTER

28

Common Pediatric Diseases and Disorders

There are many diseases and disorders seen in a pediatric practice. The following table lists some of the more common ones along with their sign and symptoms.

Disease	*Description*	*Signs and symptoms*
Asthma	Lung disease in which the airways become inflamed and obstructed as a response to various stimuli, including allergens	• Airway obstruction, wheezing, coughing, inability to speak, fatigue and cyanosis, which may result in severe distress
Diaper dermatitis	A rash anywhere in the groin region or gluteal folds of the buttocks which may become infected with bacteria or yeast	• Patches of reddened skin that may contain fluid and pustules
Eczema	Skin inflammation resulting from allergies and irritants	• Vesicles, redness, oozing, crusting, scaling and itching
Gastroenteritis	A syndrome of vomiting and diarrhea that may cause dehydration and electrolyte imbalance	• Diarrhea, vomiting, dehydration, lethargy, anorexia, weight loss, fever and decreased urination

Contd...

Contd...

Disease	*Description*	*Signs and symptoms*
Impetigo	Superficial skin infection characterized by vesicles and pustules	• Lesions on the skin, exudate, crusting, and itching
Otitis media	Bacterial or viral infection of the middle ear	• Severe earache, fever, nausea and vomiting, and diarrhea
Pinworms *(Enterobius vermicularis)*	Small worms that infest the large intestine	• Irritation of the anal region, allergic skin reaction, intense itching, and secondary infection
Scabies	Contagious skin infestation caused by the itch mite	• Severe itchy rash characterized by fine wavy dark lines. • Lesions may occur between the fingers, at the wrist or elbow, in the axilla, and on the trunk or extremities
Strep throat	Severe throat infection caused by the *Streptococcus* genus of bacteria	• Red, sore throat, pustules, and high fever
Urinary tract infection	An infection of the kidneys, ureters, or bladder caused by microorganisms	• Painful and frequent urination, foul-smelling urine, and hematuria

Other Pediatric Conditions

In today's society, we hear a lot about issues that can have a profound effect on the pediatric patient's learning abilities and social interactions. Conditions such as attention deficit hyperactivity disorder (ADHD), autism, Down syndrome, cerebral palsy and childhood obesity are more prevalent now and need to be dealt with in a professional but helpful manner.

Attention Deficit Hyperactivity Disorder

Although first described in 1845, this condition appears to be on the increase in current years. It may first be apparent in preschool, while others cases are diagnosed in late adolescence and even adulthood. The most classic symptoms of ADHD are:

- Being overly impulsive
- Unable to maintain attention during important tasks
- Hyperactivity

Usually, the child is viewed as one who is disruptive and highly active. Another child with ADHD might be a day dreamer. Poor concentration is a term often used to describe the patient. This condition is difficult to diagnose as these symptoms may also be an indication of other physical or emotional problems. If diagnosed, the patient can be treated with medication and support by the health care team.

Autism

Autism is a brain disorder that hinders a person's ability to communicate or relate to others. It is thought to be a genetic disorder, as it often runs in families. This disorder can also affect how a child understands and processes information that is sensory in nature.

Autism is usually diagnosed by the time a child reaches the age of three; however, some cases are not diagnosed until later. Typically parents are the first to notice the signs and seek the advice of their pediatrician. There are diagnostic guidelines that have been established by the American Academy of Child and Adolescent Psychiatry (AACAP) which the clinician will use to determine if the child has the core symptoms of autism. Signs and symptoms may include:

- Toddlers who do not begin to talk or do not interact like other children do
- Little or no eye contact with others
- Plays alone
- Delayed language development
- Repetitive patterns of behavior such as rocking, keeping to a certain routine or ritual, and resistance to any change.

There is no "mold" that all persons with autism fit into. Some need help with the simplest aspects of daily living, while others are able to function at a level high enough that permits them to attend school in a regular class and participate in sports and other activities.

Treatment methods include: Behavioral, speech, and occupational therapy, parent education, and sometimes medications. Since, each child with autism is different, treatment methods are usually individualized. Collectively, most children with autism need to be in a structured and specialized educational program in order to achieve their highest potential.

Down Syndrome

Down syndrome is a common birth defect that occurs in approximately one in every 800 to 1,000 newborns. This syndrome includes mild to moderate mental retardation and other health problems such as cardiac valvular disease, along with specific physical characteristics which include a sloping forehead, low-set ears, and short, broad hands.

The most common form of Down syndrome, trisomy 21, is caused by the presence of an extra 21st chromosome. The cause of the occurrence of this extra chromosome is unknown but appears to be related to the age of the mother and usually occurs in women over the age of 40.

Cerebral Palsy

Cerebral palsy is a term that is used to describe a range of disorders that impairs control of movement due to damage to the brain during its developmental stage. It is one of the most common causes of disability in children. While CP is not a progressive disease, symptoms may get better for a time only to worsen later on. The exact cause of CP is unknown but is thought to be related to the oxygen levels in the brain before, during, and after birth, infections, and injuries occurring during the birth process. Children with CP not only have physical disabilities, but may also have some level of retardation, learning disabilities, and vision, speech, hearing, and language problems.

Pediatric Disorders Related to Abnormal Vital Signs and Measurements

The following table identifies some possible medical conditions related to abnormal measurements. The medical assistant should be familiar with pathology related to pediatric patients. Familiarity with common diseases and disorders helps to increase communication opportunities with patients and family members, thus enabling better patient education and patient compliance.

Abnormal vital sign	*Possible pediatric pathology*
Low weight (less than 5th percentile)	GI disease, neurological disorder, environmental influences, failure to thrive
Low height, short stature	Endocrine disorder, growth hormone deficiency, Inflammatory bowel disease, renal disease, celiac disease (disorder of the immune system that damages lining of the small intestine if foods are consumed that contain gluten)
Small head circumference	Premature suture closure, chromosomal abnormalities, infection, maternal metabolic disorder
Large head circumference	Hydrocephalus, subdural hematoma, brain tumor, benign brain growth
Elevated blood pressure	Renal artery disease, coarctation (stricture) of the aorta, primary hypertension, drugs
High pulse rate (Tachycardia)	Supraventricular tachycardia
Low pulse rate (Bradycardia)	Hypoxia, intracranial disorders, heart block, drug ingestion, anorexia
Rapid, shallow respirations	Cardiac disease, metabolic acidosis, bronchiolitis, pneumonia
Fever	Infections, anxiety, dressing the infant too warmly

MENTAL RETARDATION

Mental retardation (MR) is a condition diagnosed before age 18, usually in infancy or prior to birth, that includes below-average general intellectual function, and a lack of the skills necessary for daily living. When onset occurs at age 18 or after, it is called dementia, which can coexist with an MR diagnosis.

Intellectual disability (ID), also called mental retardation (MR) is a generalized neurodevelopmental disorder characterized by significantly impaired intellectual and adaptive functioning. It is defined by an IQ score under 70 in addition to deficits in two or more adaptive behaviors that affect everyday, general living. Once focused almost entirely on cognition, the definition now includes both a component relating to mental functioning and one relating to individuals' functional skills in their environments. As a result of this focus on the person's abilities in practice, a person with an unusually low IQ may not be considered intellectually disabled. Intellectual disability is subdivided into syndromic intellectual disability, in which intellectual deficits associated with other medical and behavioral signs and symptoms are present, and non-syndromic intellectual disability, in which intellectual deficits appear without other abnormalities. Down syndrome and fragile X syndrome are examples of syndromic intellectual disabilities.

Intellectual disability affects about 2–3% of the general population. 75–90% of the affected people have mild intellectual disability. Non-syndromic or idiopathic cases account for 30–50% of cases. About a quarter of cases are caused by a genetic disorder. Cases of unknown cause affect about 95 million people as of 2013.

The terms mental retardation and mentally retarded were invented in the middle of the 20th century to replace the previous set of terms, which were deemed to have become offensive. By the end of the 20th century, these terms themselves have come to be widely seen as disparaging, politically incorrect, and in need of replacement. The term intellectual disability is now preferred by most advocates and researchers in most English-speaking countries. As of 2015, the term "mental retardation" is still used by the World Health Organization in the ICD-10 codes, which have a section titled "Mental Retardation" (codes F70–F79). In the next revision, the ICD-11 is expected to replace the term mental retardation with either intellectual disability or intellectual developmental disorder, which the DSM-5 already uses. Because of its specificity and lack of confusion with other conditions, the term "mental retardation" is still sometimes used in professional medical settings around the world, such as formal scientific research and health insurance paperwork.

Signs and Symptoms

The signs and symptoms of intellectual disability are all behavioral. Most people with intellectual disability do not look like they are afflicted with such, especially if the disability is caused by environmental factors such as malnutrition or lead poisoning. The so-called typical appearance ascribed to people with intellectual disability is only present in a minority of cases, all of which are syndromic.

Children with intellectual disability may learn to sit up, to crawl, or to walk later than other children, or they may learn to talk later. Both adults and children with intellectual disability may also exhibit some or all of the following characteristics:

- Delays in oral language development
- Deficits in memory skills
- Difficulty learning social rules
- Difficulty with problem-solving skills
- Delays in the development of adaptive behaviors such as self-help or self-care skills
- Lack of social inhibitors.

Children with intellectual disability learn more slowly than a typical child. Children may take longer to learn language, develop social skills, and take care of their personal needs, such as dressing or eating. Learning will take them longer, require more repetition, and skills may need to be adapted to their learning levels. Nevertheless, virtually every child is able to learn, develop and become a participating member of the community.

In early childhood, mild intellectual disability (IQ 50–69) may not be obvious, and may not be identified until children begin school. Even when poor academic performance is recognized, it may take expert assessment to distinguish mild intellectual disability from learning disability or emotional/behavioral disorders. People with mild intellectual disability are capable of learning reading and mathematics skills to approximately the level of a typical child aged nine to twelve. They can learn self-care and practical skills, such as cooking or using the local mass transit system. As individuals with intellectual disability reach adulthood, many learn to live independently and maintain gainful employment.

Moderate intellectual disability (IQ 35–49) is nearly always apparent within the first years of life. Speech delays are particularly common signs of moderate ID. People with moderate intellectual disability need considerable supports in school, at home, and in the community in order to participate fully. While their academic potential is limited, they can learn simple health and safety skills and to participate in simple activities. As adults, they may live with their parents, in a supportive group home, or even semi-independently with significant supportive services to help them, for example, manage their finances. As adults, they may work in a sheltered workshop.

People with severe or profound intellectual disability need more intensive support and supervision their entire lives. They may learn some activities of daily living. Some require full-time care by an attendant.

Cause

Down syndrome is one of the common genetic causes of intellectual disability.

Among children, the cause is unknown for one-third to one-half of cases. Down syndrome, velocardiofacial syndrome, and fetal alcohol spectrum disorders are the three most common inborn causes. However, doctors have found many other causes. The most common are:

- *Genetic conditions.* Sometimes disability is caused by abnormal genes inherited from parents, errors when genes combine, or other reasons. The most prevalent genetic conditions include Down syndrome, Klinefelter's syndrome, Fragile X syndrome (common among boys), neurofibromatosis, congenital hypothyroidism, Williams syndrome, phenylketonuria(PKU), and Prader-Willi syndrome. Other genetic conditions include Phelan-Mc Dermid syndrome (22q13del), Mowat-Wilson syndrome, genetic ciliopathy, and Siderius typeX-linked intellectual disability (OMIM 300263) as caused by mutations in the *PHF8* gene (OMIM 300560). In the rarest of cases, abnormalities with the X or Y chromosome may also cause disability. 48, XXXX and 49, XXXXX syndrome affect a small number of girls worldwide, while boys may be affected by 47, XYY, 49, XXXXY, or 49, XYYYY.
- *Problems during pregnancy.* Intellectual disability can result when the fetus does not develop properly. For example, there may be a problem with the way the fetus' cells divide as it grows. A pregnant person who drinks alcohol (see fetal alcohol spectrum disorder) or gets an infection like rubella during pregnancy may also have a baby with intellectual disability.
- *Problems at birth.* If a baby has problems during labor and birth, such as not getting enough oxygen, he or she may have developmental disability due to brain damage.
- *Exposure to certain types of disease or toxins.* Diseases like whooping cough, measles, or meningitis can cause intellectual disability if medical care is delayed or inadequate. Exposure to poisons like lead or mercury may also affect mental ability.

- *Iodine deficiency,* affecting approximately 2 billion people worldwide, is the leading preventable cause of intellectual disability in areas of the developing world where iodine deficiency is endemic. Iodine deficiency also causes goiter, an enlargement of the thyroid gland. More common than full-fledged cretinism, as intellectual disability caused by severe iodine deficiency is called, is mild impairment of intelligence. Certain areas of the world due to natural deficiency and governmental inaction are severely affected. India is the most outstanding, with 500 million suffering from deficiency, 54 million from goiter, and 2 million from cretinism. Among other nations affected by iodine deficiency, China and Kazakhstan have instituted widespread iodization programs, whereas, as of 2006, Russia had not.
- Malnutrition is a common cause of reduced intelligence in parts of the world affected by famine, such as Ethiopia.
- Absence of the arcuate fasciculus.

Diagnosis

According to the fifth edition of the Diagnostic and Statistical Manual of Mental Disorders (DSM-IV), three criteria must be met for a diagnosis of intellectual disability: deficits in general mental abilities, significant limitations in one or more areas of adaptive behavior across multiple environments (as measured by an adaptive behavior rating scale, i.e. communication, self-help skills, interpersonal skills, and more), and evidence that the limitations became apparent in childhood or adolescence. In general, people with intellectual disability have an IQ below 70, but clinical discretion may be necessary for individuals who have a somewhat higher IQ but severe impairment in adaptive functioning.

It is formally diagnosed by an assessment of IQ and adaptive behavior. A third condition requiring onset in childhood is used to distinguish intellectual disability from dementia such as Alzheimer's disease or due to traumatic brain injuries.

Bibliography

1. A review regarding "Human Dignity, Respect and Consideration for Mentally Disabled Adults" was published as "Official. Recommendations from the National Swedish Board of Health and Welfare" in Stockholm, Sweden, 1987. See also: Human Dignity, Respect and Consideration for Mentally Disabled Adults. Official Recommendations from the National Swedish Board of Health and Welfare, Stockholm, Sweden, 1987.
2. Barbotte E, Guellimin F, Chan N, Lorhandicap Group. Prevalence of impairments, disabilities, handicaps and quality of life in the general population: a review of recent literature. Bull World Health Organ. 2001;79:1047-55.
3. Brundtland GH. The Importance of Snow World Health Organization. Geneva, Switzerland Talk, Washington, D.C., 28 October 1998.
4. Buck C, Llopis A, Nájera E, Terris M. The challenge of Epidemiology: Issues and selected readings. Scientific Publication No. 505. Pan American Health Organization. Washington, DC; 1998 .p3.
5. Census of India 2001. Data on disability. Office of the Registrar General and Census Commissioner, India. Available from: Http://www.censusindia.net/disabilioty/disability_mapgallery.html. [Last accessed on 9 Aug 2004].
6. Changing Concepts: Background to Epidemiology". Duncan & Associates. Retrieved. 2008-02-03.
7. Community medicines. S Suryakant 2009-97893807-04319
8. Council of International Organizations of Medical Science. Ethical Guidelines for Biomedical Research Involving Human Subjects. London, UK: CIOMS; 2008. (Access date 23rd March 2010).
9. Cumaiyi C, Glynn R. Community based rehabilitation: relevance for indigenous Australians in remote areas, an investigation. The Winston Churchill Memorial Trust of Australia; 1999.
10. Curry R. Allied Health Therapy Services in Aged and Disability Care in Remote Aboriginal Communities of the Northern Territory: a Framework for quality service provision. Top End Division of General Practice. Darwin; 1999.
11. Doctor John Snow Blames Water Pollution for Cholera Epidemic, by David Vachon UCLA Department of Epidemlology, School of Public Health May & June; 2005.

12. Ethical issues have during the past 20 years or so become major preoccupation in the industrialized countries. See B. Duncan and D. Woods (Ed.): Ethical Issues in Disability and Rehabilitation, New York, USA, published by the World; 1989.
13. European Region of World Confederation for Physical Therapy. European Core Standards of Physiotherapy Practice. Brussels, Belgium: ER-WCPT; 2008. (Access date 22nd March 2010).
14. European Region World Confederation for Physical Therapy. European Region World Confederation for Physical Therapy Glossary of Terms. Brussels, Belgium: ER-WCPT; 2010.
15. European Region World Confederation for Physical Therapy. European Region World Confederation for Physical Therapy Glossary of Terms. Brussels, Belgium: ER-WCPT; 2010.
16. Ganesh KS, Das A, Shashi JS. Epidemiology of disability in a rural community of Karnataka. Indian J Public Health. 2008;52:125-9.
17. Glynn R, Mattiazzo V, Lowell A, Baker L, Lynch A, Wanatjura E. Developing partnerships between community based workers and visiting workers for the delivery of aged and disability services in remote indigenous communities. Territory Health Service. Darwin; 1999.
18. Greenspan SI. Building Healthy Minds, Perseus Books; Prizant BM, Wetherby AM, Roberts JE (2000). Communication Disorders in Infants and Toddlers, In: Zeanah C (Ed.) Handbook of Infant Mental Health, Second Edition, New York: Guilford Press; and Wetherby AM. 1999 Babies Learn to Talk at an Amazing Rate, FIRST WORDS Project, Florida State University; 1999.
19. Hall KM, Mann N, High WM, et al. Functional measures after traumatic brain injury: ceiling effects of FIM, FIM+FAM, DRS and CIQ. J Head Trauma Rehabil. 1996;11:27-39.
20. Hamilton BB, Granger CV, Sherwin FS, et al. A uniform national data system for medical rehabilitation. In: Fuhrer MJ, (editor). Rehabilitation Outcomes: analysis and measurement. Baltimore, MD: Brookes; 1987. pp. 137-47.
21. Hippocrates. (~200BC). Airs, Waters, Places.
22. Historical Developments in Epidemiology. Chapter 2. Jones & Bartlett Learning LLC.
23. Hornby AS Oxford advanced learner's dictionary of current english, Oxford University Press, Oxford, UK; 1987.
24. Ilene Beal; Frances P. Glascoe PhD.; Rebecca Landa, PhD.; and Robert H. Wharton, MD.
25. John Snow, Father of Epidemiology NPR Talk of the Nation. 2004; September 24.
26. John Snow. John Snow, Inc. and JSI Research & Training Institute, Inc.
27. Jonathan S. Gulliver's Travels: Part IV. A Voyage to the Country of the Houyhnhnms. Retrieved 2008-02-03.

28. Joshi K, Kumar R, Avasthi A. Morbidity profile and its relationship with disability and psychological distress among elderly people in Northern India. Int J Epidemiol. 2003;32:978-87.
29. Kuipers P, Allen O. Preliminary guidelines for the implementation of Community Based Rehabilitation (CBR) approaches in rural, remote and Indigenous communities in Australia. Rural and Remote Health. 2004;4 Available at: http://www,rrb.org.au
30. Kumar SG, Das A. Are the disability data in India appropriate? Natl Med J India. 2009; 22:278.
31. McKendrick AG. Statistical methods in epidemiology. In: Karl Pearson, Ronald Ross, Major Greenwood, Austin Bradford Hill, 1900 - 1945. Trust Centre for the History of Medicine at UCL, London
32. Merrill RM. Introduction to epidemiology. Jones & Bartlett Learning. 2010 .p. 24.ISBN 0-7637-6622-4.
33. Merril RM, "An Introduction to epidemiology, Fifth Edition". Chapter 2: Historic Developments in Epidemiology. Jones and Bartlett Publishing, 2010. Web. 17 Sept. 2012.
34. Morabia A. A history of epidemiologic methods and concepts, 2004. Birkhäuser. p. 93. ISBN 3-7643-6818-7.
35. National Sample Survey Organization. A report on disabled persons. New Delhi: Department of Statistics, Government of India; 2003.
36. Nutter FW Jr.. "Understanding the interrelationships between botanical, human, and veterinary epidemiology: the Ys and Rs of it all". Ecosys Health. 1999;5(3):131-40. doi:10.1046/j.1526-0992.1999.09922.x
37. Ogino S, Fuchs CS, Giovannucci E. How many molecular subtypes? Implications of the unique tumor principle in personalized medicine. Expert Rev Mol Diagn. 2012;12:621-8.doi:10.1586/erm.12.46.
38. Ogino S, Lochhead P, Chan AT, Nishihara R, Cho E, Wolpin BM, et al. Molecular pathological epidemiology of epigenetics: Emerging integrative science to analyze environment. Mod Pathol. 2013;26(4):464-84.
39. Onions CT. The Shorter Oxford English Dictionary, (3rd Ed). Oxford, UK: Clarendon Press; 1985.
40. Origins and early development of the case-control study.
41. Plato. The Republic. The Internet Classic Archive. Retrieved. 2008-02-03.
42. Porta M. A Dictionary of Epidemiology (6th ed.). New York: Oxford University Press. ISBN 978-0-19-997673-7. Retrieved, 2014.
43. Reeves B. The natural history of frozen shoulder syndrome. Scandinavian Journal of Rehumatology. 1975;4(4):193-6.
44. Sharma RK, Bajekal RA, Bhan S/Frozen shoulder syndrome. International orthopaedics. 1992;17(5):275-8.
45. Sheridan MA, Hanna TA. fin upper extremity emphasis on frozen shoulder. Ortho clin north am. 2006;37(4):p531-9.

46. Social Workers at the Ottawa Hospital Rehabilitation Centre, Ontario, Canada.
47. S sunder text book of rehabilitation. 2004.
48. Stineman MG, Jette A, Fiedler R, et al. Impairment-specific dimensions within the functional independence measure. Arch Phys Med Rehabil. 1997;78:636-43.
49. The Chartered Society of Physiotherapy. Core standards of physiotherapy practice. London, UK: Chartered Society of Physiotherapy; 2005. (Access date 22nd March 2010).
50. The World Health Organization. Training in the community for people with disabilities. Geneva: WHO; 1989.
51. Thomas M, Thomas MJ, Henley JE and Twible R. Lidcombe NSW, Australia Information Center Japanese Society for Rehabilitation of Persons with Disabilities (JSRPD) Marina Runno.
52. Turner-Stokes L, Nyein K, Turner-Stokes T, et al. The UK FIM+FAM: development and evaluation. Clin Rehabil. 1999;13:277-87.
53. World Confederation for Physical Therapy. Ethical Principles. London, UK: WCPT; 2011. (Access date 22nd September 2011)
54. World Health Organization. International Classification of Functioning, Disability and Health 2001. Available from http://www.who.int/classifications/icf/en/. [Lastaccessed on 2011 Oct 30].
55. World Health Organization. WHO Multi-country survey study on health and responsiveness 2000-01. Available from http://www.who.int/healthinfo/survey/whspaper37.pdf. [Last accessed on 2011 Oct 30].
56. World Health Organization. World Report on Disability. Geneva; WHO; 2011.
57. Zhao T, Kwok JHF. Evaluating Community Based Rehabilitation: Guidelines for Accountable Practice.
58. Ólöf Garðarsdóttir; Loftur Guttormsson (June 2008). An isolated case of early medical intervention. The battle against neonatal tetanus in the island of Vestmannaeyjar (Iceland) during the 19th century. Instituto de Economía y Geografía. Retrieved 2011-04-19.
59. Ólöf Garðarsdóttir; Loftur Guttormsson. Public health measures against neonatal tetanus on the island of Vestmannaeyjar (Iceland) during the 19th century. The History of the Family. 2009;14(3):266 79.doi :10.1016/j.hisfam.2009.08.004. Statisticians of the centuries. By C C Heyde, Eugene Senet.
60. "A Dissertation on the Origin and Foundation of the Inequality of Mankind". Constitution Society.

Index

Page numbers followed by f refer to figure, t refer to table

A

B

C

D

E

F

G

H

M

N

O

P

R

S

V

W

X

Z